Workbook to Accompany

Introductory Medical-Surgical Nursing

TENTH EDITION

BARBARA K. TIMBY, RN, BC, BSN, MA
Professor Emeritus
Medical-Surgical Nursing
Glen Oaks Community College
Centreville, Michigan

NANCY E. SMITH, MS, RN
Professor and Chair
Health Science Division and Department of Nursing
Southern Maine Community College
South Portland, Maine

Wolters Kluwer | Lippincott Williams & Wilkins
Health

Philadelphia · Baltimore · New York · London
Buenos Aires · Hong Kong · Sydney · Tokyo

Executive Acquisitions Editor: Elizabeth Nieginski
Product Manager: Betsy Gentzler
Editorial Assistant: Laura Scott
Art Director, Design: Joan Wendt
Art Director, Illustration: Brett MacNaughton
Art Coordinator: Robert Galindo
Manufacturing Coordinator: Karin Duffield
Production Services: Cadmus Communication

10th Edition

9 8 7 6 5 4 3 2 1

Printed in China.

ISBN: 978-1-60547-064-1

Care has been taken to confirm the accuracy of the information presented and to describe generally accepted practices. However, the authors, editors, and publisher are not responsible for errors or omissions or for any consequences from application of the information in this book and make no warranty, expressed or implied, with respect to the currency, completeness, or accuracy of the contents of the publication. Application of this information in a particular situation remains the professional responsibility of the practitioner; the clinical treatments described and recommended may not be considered absolute and universal recommendations.

The authors, editors, and publisher have exerted every effort to ensure that drug selection and dosage set forth in this text are in accordance with the current recommendations and practice at the time of publication. However, in view of ongoing research, changes in government regulations, and the constant flow of information relating to drug therapy and drug reactions, the reader is urged to check the package insert for each drug for any change in indications and dosage and for added warnings and precautions. This is particularly important when the recommended agent is a new or infrequently employed drug.

Some drugs and medical devices presented in this publication have Food and Drug Administration (FDA) clearance for limited use in restricted research settings. It is the responsibility of the health care provider to ascertain the FDA status of each drug or device planned for use in his or her clinical practice.

LWW.COM

Contributors

Tina M. Berry, RN, MSN, MBA, HCM
Nursing Instructor
Columbus State Community College
Columbus, Ohio

Sarah A. Taulbee, MS, RN
Assistant Professor
Kettering College of Medical Arts
Kettering, Ohio

Preface

This Workbook was developed and updated by subject matter experts to accompany the 10th edition of *Introductory Medical-Surgical Nursing* by Barbara K. Timby and Nancy E. Smith. The Workbook is designed to help you practice and retain the knowledge you've gained from the textbook, and it is structured to integrate that knowledge and give you a basis for applying it in your nursing practice. Each chapter of the Workbook is divided into three sections: Assessing Your Understanding, Applying Your Knowledge, and Getting Ready for NCLEX.

ASSESSING YOUR UNDERSTANDING

The first section of each Workbook chapter concentrates on the basic information of the textbook chapter and helps you to remember key concepts, vocabulary, and principles. Types of exercises include

- **Fill in the Blanks**. Fill in the blank exercises test important chapter information, encouraging you to recall key points.
- **True/False**. True or false exercises test your understanding of important facts.
- **Labeling**. Labeling exercises are used where you need to remember certain visual representations of the concepts presented in the textbook.
- **Match the Following**. Matching questions test your knowledge of the definition of key terms.
- **Sequencing**. Sequencing exercises ask you to remember particular sequences or orders, for instance testing processes and prioritizing nursing actions.
- **Short Answers**. Short answer questions will cover facts, concepts, procedures, and principles of the chapter. These questions ask you to recall information as well as demonstrate your comprehension of the information.

APPLYING YOUR KNOWLEDGE

The second section of each Workbook chapter consists of exercises that ask you to begin to apply the knowledge you've gained from the textbook chapter and reinforced in the first section of the Workbook chapter. Activities include short answer questions and critical thinking exercises.

GETTING READY FOR NCLEX

The third and final section of the Study Chapters helps you practice NCLEX-style questions while further reinforcing the knowledge you have been gaining and testing for yourself through the textbook chapter and the first two sections of the Workbook chapter. In keeping with the NCLEX, the questions presented are multiple-choice and scenario-based, asking you to reflect, consider, and apply what you know and to choose the best answer out of those offered.

ANSWER KEY

The answers for all of the exercises in the Workbook are provided with the Instructor's Resources that accompany the main textbook. Your instructor may share answers with you to allow you to check your own work, or he or she may assign Workbook chapters as assignments.

We hope you will find this Workbook to be helpful and enjoyable, and we wish you every success in your studies toward becoming a nurse.

—*The Publishers*

Contents

UNIT **16**

CARING FOR CLIENTS WITH INTEGUMENTARY DISORDERS

UNIT **17**

CARING FOR CLIENTS WITH PSYCHOBIOLOGIC DISORDERS

Concepts and Trends in Healthcare

1. Explain the concepts of health, holism, wellness, illness, disease, and the health–illness continuum.
2. Describe how clients with chronic illness may still be considered healthy.
3. Differentiate health maintenance and health promotion.
4. Identify members of the healthcare team.
5. Describe three levels of care that the healthcare delivery system provides.
6. Describe problems related to access to healthcare.
7. Describe Medicare, Medicaid, and Medigap insurance.
8. Explain how a prospective payment system (PPS) works.
9. Explain how the different types of managed care organizations work.
10. Discuss the difference between capitation and fee-for-service insurance.
11. Discuss the effects of cost-driven changes on healthcare.
12. Discuss methods for monitoring quality of care.
13. Describe national and worldwide healthcare campaigns designed to improve healthcare and healthcare outcomes.
14. Identify trends that influence future healthcare policy.

SECTION I: ASSESSING YOUR UNDERSTANDING

Activity A *Fill in the blanks by choosing the correct word from the options given in parentheses.*

1. _____ is a state of being sick. *(Sickness, Illness, Disease)*

2. The _____ is an active partner in nursing care. *(HMO, PPO, Client)*

3. _____ refers to the full range of services available to people seeking prevention, identification, treatment, or rehabilitation of health problems. *(Home care delivery system, Healthcare delivery system, Fitness programs)*

4. _____is a state of complete physical, mental, and social well-being and not merely the absence of disease and infirmity. *(Holism, Wellness, Health)*

5. _____ is a federally funded, state-run program that provides medical assistance for individuals and families with limited incomes and resources. *(Medicare, Medicaid, Medigap)*

Activity B *Mark each statement as either "T" (True) or "F" (False). Correct any false statements.*

1. T F Nurses educate clients, family members, and staff to manage resources, and act as advocates for clients.

2. T F Physically disabled people are considered healthy if they are physiologically stable and also engaged in personal and social activities they find meaningful.

3. T F Clients who are ill may not take responsibility for meeting their health maintenance and may not actively participate in treatment decisions regarding health restoration.

4. T F A preferred provider organization (PPO) provides the strongest incentives for limiting expensive services and focusing healthcare on health maintenance and health promotion.

5. T F Medicare does not cover long-term care and limits coverage for health promotion and illness prevention.

Activity C *Write the correct term for each description below.*

1. A perspective of viewing a person's health as a balance of body, mind, and spirit.

   _____

2. A group of people that consists of specially trained personnel who work together to help clients meet their healthcare needs.

   _____

3. A federally run program financed primarily through employee payroll taxes. _____

4. An inpatient hospital classification system used to group services for clients with similar diagnoses. _____

5. A constant and intentional effort to stay healthy and achieve the highest potential for well-being. _____

Activity D *Match the types of care given in Column A with the descriptions given in Column B.*

Column A

_____ 1. Tertiary care

_____ 2. Home hospice care

_____ 3. Primary care

_____ 4. Skilled nursing care

_____ 5. Secondary care

Column B

a. Occurs in facilities or units that offer prolonged health maintenance or rehabilitative services such as long-term care or extended care facilities.

b. Includes referrals to facilities for additional testing, such as cardiac catheterization, consultation, and diagnosis.

c. Care is provided in hospitals where specialists and complex technology are available.

d. Resources for terminally ill clients and their families.

e. The first resource person or agency that clients contact about a health need. This initial contact is often with a family practitioner, internist, or nurse practitioner.

Activity E *Identify how these managed care systems work, cost control measures, and the use of resources.*

Managed care system	How it works	Cost control and use of resources
Health maintenance organizations (HMOs)		
Preferred provider organization (PPOs)		
Point-of-service plans (POS)		
Physician hospital organizations (PHOs)		

Activity F *Briefly answer the following questions.*

1. What is the difference between illness and disease?

   _____
   _____
   _____

2. What are the components of health maintenance and health promotion?

   _____
   _____
   _____

3. Which individuals are covered by Medicare?

_____

_____

_____

4. Identify the members of the healthcare team.

_____

_____

_____

5. Which groups of people are most likely to be underserved by the healthcare system?

_____

_____

_____

SECTION II: APPLYING YOUR KNOWLEDGE

Activity G *Give rationale for the following questions.*

1. Why do individuals with adequate resources purchase private Medigap insurance?

_____

_____

_____

2. Why must members of a health maintenance organization receive authorization for secondary care?

_____

_____

_____

3. Why do some individuals delay seeking early treatment for their health problems?

_____

_____

_____

4. Why is there much criticism of the prospective payment system?

_____

_____

_____

Activity H *Answer the following questions related to concepts and trends in healthcare.*

1. What are the various methods used to ensure the quality of care?

_____

_____

_____

2. What is managed care? What are the goals of managed care?

_____

_____

_____

3. What is an integrated delivery system? What are the services provided by a fully integrated delivery system?

_____

_____

_____

4. What is the role of the nurse in illness prevention and early detection?

_____

_____

_____

Activity I *Think over the following questions. Discuss them with your instructor or peers.*

1. What are the concerns related to cost-driven changes in healthcare? What are the benefits of cost-driven health care?

_____

_____

_____

2. What are the advantages of utilizing a clinical pathway to provide client care?

_____

_____

_____

3. Discuss issues with access to care and health disparities in your communities.

_____

_____

_____

4. Discuss the role of the nurse in national and worldwide healthcare campaigns.

_____

_____

_____

SECTION III: GETTING READY FOR NCLEX

Activity J _Answer the following questions by choosing the best answer._

1. When using a holistic approach to nursing care, the nurse must address which of the client's needs?
   a. Physical, emotional, developmental, psychological, and basic needs.
   b. Spiritual, psychological, developmental, individual, and emotional needs.
   c. Sociocultural, developmental, spiritual, physical, and psychological needs.
   d. Individual, spiritual, basic, developmental, and physical needs.

2. The nurse is on a busy Medical-Surgical unit on the 3–11 p.m. shift. The role of the nurse in caring for clients on this floor includes which of the following activities?
   a. Diagnosing illness and communicating the diagnosis to the client.
   b. Prescribing medication and communicating with the pharmacy about the dosage.
   c. Advocating for the physician and carrying out orders.
   d. Collecting data and diagnosing human responses to health problems.

3. A 50-year-old female client is instructed by the nurse to take all medications just ordered by the physician, to get screened in six months for a mammogram, and to obtain a colonoscopy. These activities by the client represent which of the following?
   a. Health promotion
   b. Health maintenance
   c. Health prevention
   d. Health detection

4. For which of the following clients should the nurse recommend Medicare?
   a. 75-year-old client with high blood pressure

   b. 35-year-old client with urinary tract infection
   c. 55-year-old client with signs of hepatic disease
   d. 15-year-old client with asthma and breathlessness

5. A client is set up for a cardiac catheterization to determine if he has a blockage in his coronary arteries. What type of care does this represent in the health care system?
   a. Tertiary care
   b. Secondary care
   c. Primary care
   d. Hospice care

6. Three clients come to the hospital for different surgeries. One has a total hip replacement, the second has a total knee replacement, and the third has a shoulder replacement. All of these inpatient hospital surgeries are classified the same way and are reimbursed at the same rate under DRG 209. This is an example of what type of financial payment system?
   a. Managed care organization (MCO)
   b. Preferred provider organization (PPO)
   c. Prospective payment system (PPS)
   d. Health maintenance organization (HMO)

7. A nurse is assigned to the Outcomes Measurement Committee for the hospital. Which of the following is the goal of this committee?
   a. To identify clients of interest to the hospital.
   b. To measure quality through the use of surveys.
   c. To determine which cases are Risk Management issues for the hospital.
   d. To use standardized indicators to measure healthcare quality.

8. A nurse is providing care to a client using a standard set of guidelines that determine aspects of care appropriate for a specific type of client. This set of guidelines is called which of the following?
   a. Case Management Trend Report
   b. Guideline for Client Safety
   c. Critical Pathway
   d. Diagnosis-Related Report

9. Nurses in Community Health use the National Health Goals, which were created in 2005 by which agency to help increase quality and years of healthy life and eliminate health disparities through the Healthy People 2010 initiative?
   a. Center for Disease Control
   b. United States Department of Health and Human Services
   c. United States Surgeon General
   d. Institute for Healthcare Improvement

10. The LPN identifies from the client's interaction that the 25-year-old African American client does not have the ability to pay for healthcare for herself and her family. This represents what kind of issue?
    a. Access to Financial Help Issue
    b. Access to Charity Care Issue
    c. Access to Quality Issue
    d. Access to Care Issue

CHAPTER 2

Settings and Models for Nursing Care

Learning Objectives

1. Define nursing.
2. Describe the different roles of the LPN/LVN and RN.
3. List three ways to classify healthcare agencies in which nurses practice.
4. Describe settings in which nurses practice and nurses' roles in each setting.
5. Compare nursing care delivery models.
6. Define case management and explain the nurse case manager's role.

SECTION I: ASSESSING YOUR UNDERSTANDING

Activity A *Fill in the blanks by choosing the correct word from the options given in parentheses.*

1. _____ have been the traditional sites for much of the nursing workforce. *(Inpatient units, Dialysis units, Same-day surgery units)*

2. _____ emerged in the 1950s to accommodate staff with varying levels of education and skill. *(Patient-focused care, Total care, Team nursing)*

3. _____ maximizes fiscal outcomes without sacrificing quality through careful oversight of a client's healthcare. *(Case management, Patient-focused care, Primary nursing)*

Activity B *Mark each statement as either "T" (True) or "F" (False). Correct any false statements.*

1. T F Case management involves aggressive management of every client.

2. T F Florence Nightingale (1859) described the role of the nurse as putting "the patient in the best condition for nature to act upon him."

3. T F The licensed practical nurse or licensed vocational nurse (LPN/LVN) provides care to clients independently.

4. T F Many models of nursing care are used today and may vary in different settings, depending on client needs and costs of service.

5. T F In patient-focused care, the nurse may be held accountable for outcomes of nursing care, such as skin breakdown.

Activity C *Write the correct term for each model of nursing care delivery description given below.*

1. The method by which one nurse provides all the services that a particular client requires.

   _____

2. The method of nursing where distinct duties are assigned to specific personnel. _____

3. The updated version of primary care and team nursing that uses an RN partnered with an

LVN/LPN, respiratory therapist, and/or unlicensed personnel. _____

Activity D *Match the facilities or settings given in Column A with the clients who would receive the type of care provide in Column B.*

Column A

____ 1. Acute care

____ 2. Long-term acute care

____ 3. Subacute care

____ 4. Skilled nursing care

____ 5. Intermediate care facilities

____ 6. Rehabilitation care

____ 7. Hospice care

____ 8. Ambulatory care

____ 9. Home care

____ 10. Community health centers

____ 11. Alternative healthcare settings

Column B

a. Nursing homes that provide custodial care for clients who cannot care for themselves because of mental or physical disabilities.

b. Clients are relatively healthy and do not need extended care, but may need some assistance with ADLs.

c. Service clients with complicated or high-risk surgeries, massive trauma, or critical illness.

d. Clients who receive outpatient surgeries or treatments such as diagnostic tests or dialysis.

e. Clients who require care that is more intense than traditional long-term care, but less intense than acute inpatient care.

f. Clients receive care in the home setting; care addresses long-term and short-term needs, and can provide comprehensive services.

g. Clients who require long-term wound care, ventilator support, or have other conditions that are potentially unstable but do not have rapid changes.

h. Provides care for clients ?diagnosed with a terminal illness

whose life expectancy is fewer than 6 months.

i. Clients who have the potential to regain function but need skilled observation and care during an acute illness.

j. Provide a range of services to clients within the districts, counties, or communities they serve.

k. Clients receive physical and occupational therapy to help them regain as much independence with ADLs as possible.

Activity E *Given below are some settings that provide alternative care for seniors and adults with physical or mental disabilities. Compare these using the criteria listed.*

	Congregate housing	Boarding homes	Assisted-living facilities
Description of the facility			
Profile of clients who need the facility			
Examples of services provided			
Disadvantages			

Activity F *Briefly answer the following questions.*

1. What is total care? What is the focus of total care? Where is this model of nursing often used?

_____
_____
_____

2. What is the goal of alternative care facilities?

_____
_____
_____

3. What is the role of the registered nurse in the home health nursing?

_____

_____

_____

4. What is an important function of the case manager? What tools are used by case managers to help them plan and coordinate care?

_____

_____

_____

SECTION II: APPLYING YOUR KNOWLEDGE

Activity G _Give rationale for the following questions._

1. Why is functional nursing confusing for the client?

_____

_____

_____

2. How did the concept of team nursing emerge?

_____

_____

_____

3. Why is the approach of primary nursing expensive? Can this model be used effectively in contemporary nursing?

_____

_____

_____

4. Why doesn't Medicare reimburse intermediate care facilities (ICFs)?

_____

_____

_____

Activity H _Answer the following questions related to settings and models for nursing care._

1. Describe the LPN/LVN's role in providing nursing care.

_____

_____

_____

2. Why did the case method become impractical? What is the contemporary model of the case method?

_____

_____

_____

3. Who are the team members involved in team nursing? What is the unique feature of team nursing?

_____

_____

_____

4. What type of care is provided by hospice? What type of special training does hospice staff receive?

_____

_____

_____

Activity I _Think over the following questions. Discuss them with your instructor or peers._

1. What is your definition of nursing? How does your definition align with the American Nurses Association (ANA) description of the six essential features of contemporary nursing practice?

_____

_____

_____

2. What type of nursing model would you prefer to practice? Why?

_____

_____

_____

SECTION III: GETTING READY FOR NCLEX

Activity J *Answer the following questions by marking the best response.*

1. Which of the following statements represents one of the six essential features of the American Nurses Association 2003 definition of nursing?

   a. Attention to the range of experiences and responses to health and illness within the physical and social environments

   b. Putting the patient in the best condition for nature to act upon him

   c. Carrying out those activities contributing to health, recovery, or a peaceful death

   d. Regaining independence through the use of knowledge and self-care

2. An LPN delivers care to a client in a nursing home and encounters a problem with the client's care that she is unable to resolve on her own. In this situation, what action by the LPN is appropriate?

   a. Call the director of the facility for instructions.

   b. Ask for assistance from the client's family member.

   c. Obtain advice from another LPN.

   d. Obtain further direction from the registered nurse who supervises her.

3. The nurse works in a subacute setting. Which of the following distinguishes the subacute setting?

   a. RNs manage this setting and LPNs do not participate in this level of care.

   b. Clients are in these facilities for 120 days or longer.

   c. Frequent assessment and periodic review of the client's progress is necessary.

   d. The client's condition changes rapidly and requires highly skilled care.

4. Which of the following describes hospices?

   a. They provide custodial care for people who cannot care for themselves.

   b. They provide physical and occupational therapy to clients and their families.

   c. They provide care for clients diagnosed with a terminal illness.

   d. They provide skilled nursing and rehabilitative care.

5. What types of clients require more intensive case management?

   a. Clients who experience complications.

   b. Clients who do not have chronic illnesses.

   c. Clients who undergo unnecessary diagnostic testing.

   d. Clients on whom expensive resources are overused.

6. How do insurance companies assess the case manager's effectiveness?

   a. By evaluating the case manager's use of tools, such as critical pathways.

   b. By assessing whether the case manager's priority is "bottom line."

   c. By determining the volume of outcome data collected by the case manager.

   d. By measuring the cost of services provided to the case manager's clients.

7. Which of the following describes the service provided by home health nurses?

   a. A 24-hour accountability for the client's care

   b. Plan of care in the primary nurse's absence

   c. Assumption of all care for small group of clients

   d. Covers both long-term and short-term health needs

8. Which of the following describes the total care model of hospital-based nursing care?

   a. One nurse provided all the services that a particular client required.

   b. Practiced in intensive care units where nurses are assigned one or two clients.

   c. Distinct duties are assigned to specific personnel.

   d. Uses an RN partnered with one or more assistive personnel to care for a group of clients.

9. Which of the following statements is the definition of nursing given by Virginia Henderson?

    a. Helping people carry out those activities contributing to health.

    b. Application of scientific knowledge to the processes of diagnosis and treatment.

    c. Promotion of a caring relationship that facilitates health and healing.

    d. Integration of objective data with knowledge gained from an understanding of the client's subjective experience.

10. Which of the following describes the case method of nursing?

    a. A nurse assumes all the care for a small group of clients.

    b. Distinct duties are assigned to specific personnel.

    c. Accommodates staff with varying levels of education.

    d. One nurse provides all the services that a particular client requires.

The Nursing Process

Learning Objectives

1. State the purpose of the nursing process.
2. Describe the five steps of the nursing process.
3. Define assessment.
4. Discuss the parts of a nursing diagnostic statement.
5. Differentiate types of nursing diagnoses.
6. Explain the five levels of human needs as identified by Maslow.
7. Explain how nurses use the hierarchy of needs to establish nursing priorities.
8. Define expected outcomes.
9. Explain the implementation phase of the nursing process and its relationship with documentation.
10. Explain the purpose of evaluation.
11. Give reasons why expected outcomes may not be accomplished.
12. Define critical thinking and its relevance to the nursing process.
13. List characteristics of critical thinkers.
14. Discuss the use of concept mapping as a means to master the nursing process and develop critical thinking skills.

SECTION I: ASSESSING YOUR UNDERSTANDING

Activity A *Fill in the blanks by choosing the correct word from the options given in parentheses.*

1. _____ serves as a comparison for future signs and symptoms and provides a reference for determining whether a client's health is improving. *(Baseline data, Client database, Ongoing assessment)*

2. _____ identifies and defines a health problem that independent or physician-prescribed nursing actions can prevent or solve. *(Assessment, Nursing diagnosis, Evaluation)*

3. The plan of care identifies _____ for achieving the outcomes. *(Interventions, Diagnoses, Assessments)*

Activity B *Mark each statement as either "T" (True) or "F" (False). Correct any false statements.*

1. T F Initial and ongoing assessment is essential to the provision of nursing care.

2. T F Respecting the client's right to participate in healthcare is an important ethical principle.

3. T F During the implementation step in the nursing process, a nurse compares the actual outcomes to the expected outcomes.

Activity C *Write the correct term for each description given below.*

1. Specific nursing directions so that all healthcare team members understand what to do for the client. _____

2. The process that provides a systematic method for nurses to plan and implement client care to achieve desired outcomes. _____

3. The step of the nursing process that carries out the written plan of care, performs the interventions, monitors the client's status, and assesses and reassesses the client before, during, and after treatments. _____

Activity D *Match the type of nursing diagnoses given in Column A with the corresponding explanation given in Column B.*

Column A

_____ **1.** Actual nursing diagnosis

_____ **2.** Health promotion nursing diagnosis

_____ **3.** Risk nursing diagnosis

_____ **4.** Wellness diagnosis

_____ **5.** Syndrome diagnosis

Column B

a. Identifies a potential problem.

b. Identifies a diagnosis associated with a cluster of other diagnoses.

c. Describes a client's transition from one level of wellness to a higher level of wellness.

d. Identifies an existing problem.

e. Reflects clinical judgment of a client's motivation to increase well-being and advance health behaviors.

Activity E *Differentiate between the role of licensed practical or vocational nurse (LPN/LVN) and the registered nurse (RN) in the nursing process based on the given criteria.*

	Role of the LPN/LVN	Role of the RN
Assessment		
Nursing diagnosis		
Planning		
Implementation		
Evaluation		

Activity F *Given below are the human needs developed by Abraham Maslow in a jumbled order. Arrange the levels of needs according to priorities in the boxes.*

1. Esteem and self-esteem needs

2. Safety and security needs

3. Physiologic needs

4. Self-actualization needs

5. Love and belonging needs

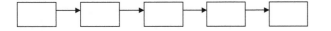

Activity G *Briefly answer the following questions.*

1. How does a collaborative problem differ from a nursing diagnosis? What is the goal of a collaborative problem?

_____

_____

_____

2. What are the parts of a diagnostic statement?

_____

_____

_____

3. A client's lack of progress may result from which deficits in the nursing care plan?

_____

_____

_____

4. How does the nursing process assist nurses to acquire critical thinking and problem-solving skills?

_____

_____

_____

SECTION II: APPLYING YOUR KNOWLEDGE

Activity H *Give rationale for the following questions.*

1. Why should the nurse actively involve the client and family in care planning?

_____

_____

_____

2. Why should expected outcomes be specific, realistic, measurable, and client-centered?

_____

_____

_____

3. Why are first-level needs given highest priority?

_____

_____

_____

Activity I *Answer the following questions related to the nursing process.*

1. What are the responsibilities of the nurse during the assessment of a client?

_____

_____

_____

2. What are the characteristics of nursing interventions and orders?

_____

_____

_____

3. What are the functions served by accurate and thorough documentation in the medical record? What information should a nurse document?

_____

_____

_____

4. What are the specific cognitive and mental activities a nurse must use when thinking critically?

_____

_____

_____

Activity J *Think over the following questions. Discuss them with your instructor or peers.*

1. You are assessing a client with post-operative right hip pain following a total hip arthroplasty. What information will you need to gather?

_____

_____

_____

2. What nursing diagnoses will you consider? What are the types of nursing diagnoses you will list?

_____

_____

_____

3. What level of priority will you give the diagnoses?

_____

_____

_____

4. How can you actively involve the client in planning and achieving positive outcomes?

_____

_____

_____

5. What would be specific, realistic, measurable, and client-centered outcomes? What would be appropriate time frames to measure the client's responses?

_____

_____

_____

6. How would you evaluate the client's responses and compare the actual outcomes to the expected outcomes?

_____

_____

_____

7. What information will be included in your documentation?

_____

_____

_____

SECTION III: GETTING READY FOR NCLEX

Activity K *Answer the following questions marking the best response.*

1. As the nurse educator teaches a group of new students she begins by discussing the

nursing process and explains that the purpose of the nursing process is to what?

a. To systematically plan and implement care to meet a client's desired outcomes.

b. To allow the nurse to follow steps to ensure consistency of care among professionals.

c. To provide a language that only nurses can understand that allows for client safety.

d. To provide a step by step process that anyone can follow regardless of education.

2. There are five steps to the nursing process. When Nurse A begins with setting priorities, defining expected outcomes, and determining interventions, which step is she using?

a. Assessment

b. Diagnosis

c. Planning

d. Implementation

3. The nurse has developed a nursing diagnosis with a client who has determined that she wants to learn more about diet and exercise. What type of nursing diagnosis reflects the motivation by a client to increase well being?

a. Actual nursing diagnoses

b. Risk for diagnoses

c. Wellness diagnoses

d. Health promotion nursing diagnoses

4. Client A has been admitted to the hospital with severe internal bleeding following a motor vehicle accident and the loss of two of his family members. According to Maslow, which of the following need (level) is the highest priority for the nurse when caring for a client?

a. Love and belonging needs.

b. Self-actualization needs.

c. Esteem and self-esteem needs.

d. Physiological needs.

5. A nurse manager has put a veteran nurse in charge due to her critical thinking skills. Critical thinking is outlined in the text as which of the following?

a. Structured, biased, and logical thinking.

b. Intentional, contemplative, and outcome-directed thinking.

c. Broad, scientific, and one-directional thinking.

d. Outcome-directed, broad, and biased thinking.

6. The nurse arrives on the unit, gets report, and enters the client's room. What is the first step in the nursing process that the nurse will utilize?

a. Planning

b. Implementation

c. Assessment

d. Evaluation

7. A nurse educator is teaching a group of students about concept mapping. The nurse educator discusses with a student the second step in the concept mapping process listed in the textbook by Schuster (2008). What is the second step in this process?

a. Identify goals, outcomes, and interventions.

b. Analyze and categorize data.

c. Develop a basic skeleton diagram.

d. Label and analyze nursing diagnosis relationships.

8. A nurse on the floor implements the nursing care plan for a client admitted to the unit but fails to document in the medical record the interventions and the response to these interventions. The five functions of documentation in the medical record (Alfaro-LeFevre, 2006) that come from accurate and thorough documentation include which of the following (**select all that apply**)?

a. Creating a legal document.

b. Communicating care.

c. Supplying validation for reimbursement

d. Substantiating the care provided by ancillary staff.

9. A nurse's expected outcome for a client who is postpartum includes a goal of minimal pain of 3 on a scale of 1–10 by the end of the 7 a.m. to 3 p.m. shift. The client has taken Motrin every 4 hours as ordered: at 8 a.m. (pain level of 6 and 30 minutes later pain level of 2) as well as at 12 noon (pain level of 5 and 30 minutes later pain level of 2). Which part of the nursing process is the nurse using when she looks at the above data?

   a. Assessment

   b. Evaluation

   c. Implementation

   d. Diagnosis

10. A nursing diagnosis is formulated for a client who has just returned from surgery. The nursing diagnosis formulated is the following: acute pain related to total knee replacement as evidenced by verbalization of pain of 8 on scale of 1–10, restlessness, and inability to concentrate. What part of the nursing diagnosis above is the name or label?

    a. Related to knee replacement

    b. As evidenced by verbalization of pain of 8 on scale of 1–10

    c. Acute pain

    d. Inability to concentrate

CHAPTER 4

Interviewing and Physical Assessment

Learning Objectives

1. Explain the purpose of the interview and physical assessment.
2. Define subjective and objective data, symptoms, and signs.
3. Summarize the three phases of the interview process.
4. Explain the components of an interview.
5. Differentiate a systems method of assessment from a head-to-toe method of assessment.
6. Identify four assessment techniques.
7. Describe general assessment measures that all nurses can perform.

SECTION I: ASSESSING YOUR UNDERSTANDING

Activity A *Fill in the blanks by choosing the correct word from the options given in parentheses.*

1. _____ are statements the client makes about what he or she feels. *(Subjective data, Objective data, Baseline data)*

2. When objective data are abnormal, they are called _____. *(Symptoms, Signs, Chief complaints)*

3. The nurse should ask _____ questions when interviewing a client. *(Exhaustive, Open-ended, Closed)*

4. The _____ method of physical assessment begins at the top of the body and progresses downward. *(Systems, Chief complaint, Head-to-toe)*

Activity B *Mark each statement as either "T" (True) or "F" (False). Correct any false statements.*

1. T F Subjective data often supports the objective data.

2. T F A feeling of discomfort described by the client is called a sign.

3. T F When performing the physical examination, the nurse should avoid showing surprise or concern at any findings to prevent increasing the client's anxiety level.

4. T F When performing auscultation, a nurse describes normal and abnormal sounds using descriptive terms such as high-pitched, low-pitched, harsh, blowing, crackling, loud, distant, and soft.

5. T F Objective data are facts obtained through observation, physical examination, and diagnostic testing.

Activity C *Write the correct term for each description below.*

1. A client's feelings of discomfort. _____

2. An assessment that determines how well a client can manage activities of daily living (ADLs). _____

3. Asking for detailed information about one body system or problem. _____

4. The approach used during the physical examination, which assesses each body system separately. _____

5. The current reason the client is seeking care. _____

Activity D *Match the assessment techniques given in Column A with the corresponding assessments given in Column B.*

Column A

____ 1. Inspection

____ 2. Palpation

____ 3. Percussion

____ 4. Auscultation

Column B

a. Detects tenderness in the body.

b. Detects changes in skin color.

c. Detects abnormal lung sounds.

d. Detects changes in skin texture.

Activity E *Compare the percussion sounds based on the given criteria.*

	Origin	Sound	Examples
Tympany			
Resonance			
Hyperresonance			
Dullness			
Flatness			

Activity F *Describe the following assessment techniques.*

1. Describe the procedure used for inspection.

2. Describe the procedure used for palpation.

3. Describe the procedure used for percussion.

4. Describe the procedure used for auscultation.

Activity G *Briefly answer the following questions.*

1. What is the importance of the initial assessment performed by a nurse?

2. What information regarding psychosocial and cultural history should a nurse collect when conducting an interview with a client?

3. What does the nurse examine and observe during the physical assessment of a client?

4. The technique of inspection should include what measures?

SECTION II: APPLYING YOUR KNOWLEDGE

Activity H *Give rationale for the following questions.*

1. Why does the nurse establish a rapport and ensure that the client is comfortable during an interview process?

2. Why does the nurse inquire about the client's use of alcohol and tobacco when collecting the health history?

_____

_____

_____

3. Why does the nurse obtain a family history when collecting the health history?

_____

_____

_____

4. When assessing a client, why should a nurse ask general questions about each body system?

_____

_____

_____

Activity I *Answer the following questions related to interviewing and physical assessment.*

1. What does the nurse identify through the systemic assessment of a client?

_____

_____

_____

2. What practices should the nurse follow during the pre-interview period?

_____

_____

_____

3. What information should the nurse obtain when discussing the client's past medical problems?

_____

_____

_____

4. What practices should the nurse follow when performing a physical examination on a client?

_____

_____

_____

Activity J *Think over the following questions. Discuss them with your instructor or peers.*

1. What necessary modifications will the nurse need to make when interviewing and performing an assessment on an older adult with Alzheimer's disease?

_____

_____

_____

SECTION III: GETTING READY FOR NCLEX

Activity K *Answer the following questions by marking the best response.*

1. A nurse performs an assessment on an older adult who is physically challenged. Which of the following assessment components is important when assessing older adults or physically challenged clients?

   a. Chief complaint

   b. Psychosocial history

   c. Functional assessment

   d. Past health history

2. A nurse is interviewing a client who cannot remember the name of the drug that has caused an allergy in the past. What should a nurse do if a client or family member is unable to remember the name of the drug causing allergy?

   a. Identify the drug from another source such as the prescribing physician or past hospital records.

   b. Ask the client or family member to describe the symptoms of allergy.

   c. Inquire about the client's use of alcohol and tobacco.

   d. Inquire about the family history.

3. Nurse A is taking care of an elderly client and needs to interview and assess the client. Which of the following nursing interventions should the nurse perform when interviewing and performing physical assessments on older adults?

   a. Keep the room cool and with draft on.

   b. Allow rest during the physical examination.

c. Observe the client performing ADLs.

d. Ensure that the client has easy access to the rest room.

e. Ensure that the client's family member is present.

4. A nurse enters the room and determines that a client is ashen gray in color. What assessment skill has the nurse utilized?

   a. Palpation

   b. Percussion

   c. Auscultation

   d. Inspection

5. A nurse enters the room of a client and begins the interview. The client responds to a question regarding his respiratory system by stating the following: "I had pneumonia in 1995 and was hospitalized for 2 weeks. It was frightening because I almost died." What kind of data has the nurse collected?

   a. Objective data

   b. Subjective data

   c. Symptomatic data

   d. Chief complaint data

6. An LPN/LVN takes the blood pressure of a client and documents the finding as 130/80. The LVN/LPN has collected which type of data?

   a. Objective data

   b. Subjective data

   c. Symptomatic data

   d. Psychological data

7. The nurse is conducting an interview and asks the client an open-ended question. Which of the following questions are considered open-ended?

   a. "Can you explain what brought you to the hospital?"

   b. "Are you feeling pain right now?"

   c. "Does your abdomen hurt in this location?"

   d. "Can you elaborate on the comment you made about feeling alone?"

8. An RN enters a client's room and detects pulsations in the client's carotid area. The actual use of the fingertips to detect pulsations is identified as what assessment technique?

   a. Palpation

   b. Percussion

   c. Inspection

   d. Auscultation

9. The RN identifies that a client is having difficulty breathing and listens with the stethoscope to identify normal and abnormal breath sounds. The nurse is using which of the following assessment techniques?

   a. Percussion

   b. Palpation

   c. Auscultation

   d. Inspection

CHAPTER 5

Legal and Ethical Issues

Learning Objectives

1. Explain the difference between laws and ethics.
2. Categorize sources of U.S. law.
3. Differentiate intentional and unintentional torts.
4. Summarize negligence, malpractice, and liability.
5. Describe measures such as risk management that help limit nurses' liability in malpractice suits.
6. Describe procedures and regulations to protect client information.
7. Discuss informed consent, advance directives, and do-not-resuscitate (DNR) orders.
8. Explain utilitarianism, deontology, duties, and rights.
9. Summarize the characteristics of ethical values.
10. Define six professional values.
11. Describe factors that affect healthcare ethics.
12. Explain an ethical decision-making model.

SECTION I: ASSESSING YOUR UNDERSTANDING

Activity A *Fill in the blanks by choosing the correct word from the options given in parentheses.*

1. One of the two systems or theories that predominate in nursing ethics is _____. *(Autonomy, Deontology, Beneficence)*

2. _____ is the duty to maintain commitments of professional obligations and responsibilities. *(Fidelity, Veracity, Justice)*

3. This type of law guarantees fundamental freedom to all people in the United States. *(Statutory law, Constitutional law, Administrative law)*

4. Negligence involving licensed healthcare workers is referred to as _____. *(Malpractice, Intentional tort, Limiting liability)*

5. _____ is the duty to be fair to all people regardless of age, sex, race, sexual orientation, or other factors. *(Justice, Veracity, Beneficence)*

6. _____ means that the person is legally responsible. *(Liability, Malpractice, Negligence)*

7. _____ is safeguarding the clients' rights and supporting their interests. *(Beneficence, Nonmaleficence, Advocacy)*

8. _____ is the duty to tell the truth, providing factual information so the client can exercise autonomy. *(Advocacy, Beneficence, Veracity)*

Activity B *Mark each statement as either "T" (True) or "F" (False). Correct any false statements.*

1. T F Laws are moral principles and values that guide the behavior of honorable people.

2. T F A tort is an injury that occurred because of another person's intentional or unintentional actions or failure to act.

3. T F One of the primary tools of risk management is liability insurance.

4. T F Good Samaritan laws provide legal immunity for rescuers who provide first aid in an emergency to accident victims outside the hospital setting.

5. **T F** When obtaining an informed consent, the physician must inform the client of acceptable alternatives available.

6. **T F** Criminal law includes misdemeanors, which are minor offenses; and felonies, which are serious offenses.

7. **T F** All hospitalized clients may be restrained if they attempt to leave without medical consent.

8. **T F** If a nurse gives a client the wrong medication, and the client is harmed as a result, the nurse is liable for the harm.

Activity C *Write the correct definition for the descriptions about the legal and ethical issues.*

1. The outcome-oriented approach for decision-making. _____

2. The rules or principles a person uses to make a decision about what is right and wrong. _____

3. The law which applies to disputes that arise between individual citizens. _____

4. The duty to do no harm to the client. _____

5. The client's right to self-determination or the freedom to make choices without any opposition. _____

6. An unofficial, handwritten, personal account of an incident made at the time of occurrence and updated as needed. _____

7. The duty to do good for the clients assigned to the nurse's care. _____

8. Law that is based on precedent, or the court will make new rules if the precedent is outdated. _____

Activity D *Match the terms associated with the legal and ethical issues given in column A with their related explanations or definitions given in Column B.*

Column A

____ 1. Informed consent

____ 2. Living will

____ 3. Medical durable power of attorney

____ 4. Do-not-resuscitate orders

Column B

a. The client designates another person to be the healthcare proxy.

b. A written medical order for end-of-life instructions.

c. A document that states a client's wishes regarding healthcare if he or she is terminally ill.

d. Voluntary permission granted by a client for medical staff to perform an invasive procedure on the client.

Activity E *Compare and contrast the functions of the Nurse Practice Act, The State Board of Nursing, and The ANA Code of Ethics for Nurses.*

	Compare and Contrast the Functions
Nurse Practice Act	
State Board of Nursing	
American Nurses Association Code of Ethics for Nurses	

Activity F *Briefly answer the following questions.*

1. What is tort law?

2. What are intentional torts? Provide examples.

3. What are unintentional torts? Provide examples.

4. What is risk management?

5. What are the advantages of deontology?

6. What are the different types of assault?

_____

_____

_____

SECTION II: APPLYING YOUR KNOWLEDGE

Activity G _Give rationale for the following questions._

1. Why is it essential for the nurse to document forewarning a client about a potential hazard to his or her safety and the client choosing to ignore the warning?

_____

_____

_____

2. Why is it difficult to reconcile nonmaleficence with medical care?

_____

_____

_____

3. Why does the State Board of Nursing have the authority to implement disciplinary procedures?

_____

_____

_____

4. Developments in science and technology now pose serious ethical issues. Explain this concept using examples.

_____

_____

_____

Activity H _Answer the following questions related to legal and ethical issues._

1. What are the responsibilities of a risk manager?

_____

_____

_____

2. Give examples of felonies involving healthcare.

_____

_____

_____

3. What are the nursing interventions required if the nurse must apply restraints and no current medical order exists?

_____

_____

_____

4. What measures should be taken by health professionals to protect the privacy of the clients?

_____

_____

_____

5. What are the principles of the Good Samaritan law?

_____

_____

_____

6. What is the difference between negligence and malpractice? How is malpractice determined?

_____

_____

_____

Activity I _Think over the following questions. Discuss them with your instructor or peers._

1. Use an ethical decision-making process to evaluate the following situation:
   - A 24-year-old client is in a motor vehicle accident and deemed "brain dead." The client's parents are deceased; he has no siblings, and is unmarried.
   - The client has no living will and no instructions on his driver's license indicating a preference for or against organ donation.
   - Two maternal aunts are present, and both indicate that they are opposed to organ donation and have no reason to believe that their nephew would have wished that his organs be donated. They believe the

client would want life support immediately withdrawn.

- His girlfriend is also present; she and the client have been dating for 18 months. She states that she and the client have had conversations about organ donation and his wishes were to donate if possible. She states that the client would want to remain on life support until his organs could be harvested.

_____

_____

_____

2. Does your decision reflect the utilitarian or deontology view of ethics?

_____

_____

_____

SECTION III: GETTING READY FOR NCLEX

Activity J *Answer the following questions.*

1. Which of the following is a medical example of invasion of privacy?
   a. Orally uttering a character attack in the presence of others.
   b. Writing a damaging statement that is read by others.
   c. Allowing unauthorized persons to observe the client during care.
   d. Offering exaggerated negative opinions about the clients.

2. Which of the following is the primary tool of risk management?
   a. Incident report
   b. Advance directives
   c. Living will
   d. Medical durable power of attorney

3. Which of the following must the client be informed of when an informed consent is obtained?
   a. The scope of nursing practice.
   b. The grounds for disciplinary action.
   c. The identification of legal titles for the nurse.
   d. The description of the treatment proposed.

4. Which of the following is a type of advance directive?
   a. Living will
   b. DNR orders
   c. Informed consent
   d. Liability insurance

5. Which of the following is an argument of deontology, a theory of ethics?
   a. Consequences are the only important consideration.
   b. Consequences are good if they bring pleasure.
   c. Duty is equally important.
   d. The greatest good for the greatest number.

6. Which of the following is an issue every time an older adult is asked to agree to a treatment or to execute an advanced directive or living will?
   a. Ability to give informed consent.
   b. Cognitive impairment.
   c. Sanctions to force compliance.
   d. Decision regarding feeding tube.

7. An example of a statutory law in the practice of nursing includes which of the following?
   a. Freedom of speech
   b. Nurse Practice Act
   c. Licensure exams
   d. Breech of duty

8. If person A's failure to act the way a reasonable person would act in a similar situation causes person B harm, person A may be sued for which of the following?
   a. Negligence
   b. Malpractice
   c. Battery
   d. Liability

9. Which of the following measures to limit liability includes providing legal immunity for rescuers who provide first aid in an emergency to accident victims, noting that the emergency must have occurred outside a hospital, not in an emergency department?
   a. Statute of limitations
   b. Assumption of risk
   c. Good Samaritan laws
   d. HIPPA

10. Ethical principles are important in the field of nursing. Which of the following ethical principles relates to the ability to tell the truth?
    a. Fidelity
    b. Nonmaleficence
    c. Autonomy
    d. Veracity

Leadership Roles and Management Functions

1. Differentiate leadership and management.
2. Define three styles of leadership.
3. Outline the purpose of power in the leadership role.
4. Describe the role of the LPN/LVN in managing client care.
5. Distinguish delegation and supervision.
6. Compare responsibility and accountability.
7. Discuss problems that may occur with delegation and supervision.
8. Describe the role of the LPN/LVN in collaboration and advocacy.
9. Explain the role of the LPN/LVN in resource management.
10. Discuss methods of managing time effectively.

SECTION I: ASSESSING YOUR UNDERSTANDING

Activity A *Fill in the blanks by choosing the correct word from the options given in parentheses.*

1. _____ involves qualities related to a person's character and behavior, as well as roles within a group or organization. *(Leadership, Management, Supervision)*

2. _____ means promoting the cause of another person or an organization. *(Collaboration, Advocacy, Acuity)*

3. A team effort to achieve client care outcomes is called _____. *(Collaboration, Advocacy, Resource management)*

Activity B *Mark each statement as either "T" (True) or "F" (False). Correct any false statements.*

1. T F Leaders emphasize control, decision-making, decision analysis, and results.

2. T F Managers typically possess expert power through education and work experience.

3. T F Responsibility means being answerable for the consequences of one's actions or inactions.

4. T F Leaders have the ability to guide and influence others.

Activity C *Write the correct term for each description given below.*

1. The ability to control, influence, or hold authority over an individual or a group. _____

2. Procrastination, inefficient use of time, inability to delegate, and socializing. _____

3. Transferring to a competent individual the authority to perform a selected nursing task in a selected situation. _____

4. The term used to measure the degree of a client's illness and identify the care required to meet the client's needs. _____

Activity D *Match the types of power given in Column A with related examples given in Column B.*

Column A

_____ 1. Reward power

_____ 2. Coercive power

_____ 3. Legitimate power

_____ 4. Expert power

_____ 5. Referent power

_____ 6. Informational power

Column B

a. Power due to knowledge one has that others need to accomplish certain goals.

b. Power attained through the ability to grant favors or rewards.

c. Power that results from knowledge, expertise, or experience.

d. Power exerted through threat of punishment.

e. Power exercised through a designated position.

f. Power due to association with others who are powerful.

Activity E *Compare the leadership styles based on the given criteria.*

	Advantages	**Disadvantages**
Autocratic		
Democratic		
Laissez-faire		

Activity F *Briefly answer the following questions.*

1. LPN/LVNs must have what skills to provide care to clients?

2. What qualities must effective leaders and mangers posses?

3. What are the overall goals of the manager?

4. What are the five rights of delegation?

5. What are the three basic steps for managing time?

SECTION II: APPLYING YOUR KNOWLEDGE

Activity G *Answer the following questions related to leadership roles and management functions.*

1. Explain the role of LPN/LVN as a leader/manager in various healthcare settings.

2. What steps are required by a LPN/LVN to carry out the five rights of delegation?

3. Describe the role of supervision as it relates to delegation.

4. What are the cost-conscious measures the nurse should follow?

5. What are the traits that distinguish the integrated leader/manager from those who are just leaders or managers?

_____

_____

_____

Activity H *Think over the following questions. Discuss them with your instructor or peers.*

1. Prioritize the given tasks, indicating which tasks the LPN should attend to and which tasks the LPN should delegate.
   (i) A client who does not experience adequate pain relief from a prescribed analgesic.
   (ii) A client with diabetes mellitus who requires an insulin injection.
   (iii) A client who is very scared about a surgery scheduled for later in the week.
   (iv) A client who is stable and requests assistance to the bathroom.
   (v) A client who requires a dressing change.

_____

_____

_____

2. An LPN is assigned as the team leader in a long-term care facility. Which type of leadership style would be ideal in this care facility? What issues with delegation and supervision may occur for the LPN as a result of his or her position as the team leader?

_____

_____

_____

SECTION III: GETTING READY FOR NCLEX

Activity I *Answer the following questions.*

1. Which of the following is the advantage of democratic leadership style?
   a. Staff members acknowledge the manager's role.
   b. Staff members share the process of making decisions for the group.
   c. Subordinates contribute to decision-making and policy-making.
   d. Subordinates perform at high level because of their independence.

2. Which of the following roles of a nurse is an example of coercive power?
   a. Director of nursing
   b. Team leader making assignments
   c. Shift supervisor
   d. Head nurse scheduling vacations

3. Which of the following techniques are useful in learning to manage time?
   a. Assess expectations for 24 hours at a time.
   b. Do one thing at a time and avoid multitasking.
   c. Use a worksheet to identify specific tasks.
   d. Avoid delegating tasks.

4. The LPN/LVN may experience some problems with delegation and supervision of tasks. Which of the following is the solution when confronting problems?
   a. Focus on client care needs.
   b. Leave the UAP to perform task independently.
   c. Being friendly with coworkers.
   d. Assign a UAP who is accountable for the evaluation of the result of the tasks.

5. Which of the following is the power a person has because of his or her association with others who are powerful?
   a. Coercive power
   b. Referent power
   c. Legitimate power
   d. Reward power

6. At what point does supervision of an employee begin once a task is delegated to them?
   a. Immediately upon receiving the direction until the task is done.
   b. Upon implementation of the task, throughout procedure, including evaluation.
   c. When the procedure is completed.
   d. For as long as the client is on the unit.

7. An LPN/LVN is taking care of a client and changes a dressing that should not have been changed. The LPN/LVN seeks out the RN and lets her know what transpired. The LPN/LVN demonstrated what trait?
   a. Responsibility
   b. Advocacy
   c. Collaboration
   d. Accountability

8. What type of leadership style features a communication style from top to bottom in the organization?
   a. Laissez-faire
   b. Democratic
   c. Autocratic
   d. Multicratic

9. Which of the following focuses on group process, information gathering, feedback, and empowering others?
   a. Leaders
   b. Managers
   c. Supervisors
   d. Delegators

10. The LPN/LVN is responsible for understanding the rights of all clients, remaining informed about diagnoses, treatments, prognoses, and choices, contributing to the provision of information and education, supporting the client's decisions, and communicating with other professionals. What is another word for these characteristics?
    a. Collaboration
    b. Advocacy
    c. Responsibility
    d. Accountability

CHAPTER 7

Nurse–Client Relationships

Learning Objectives

1. List four roles that nurses perform within the nurse–client relationship.
2. Describe three phases in a nurse–client relationship.
3. Differentiate between verbal, nonverbal, and therapeutic communication.
4. Give examples of therapeutic and nontherapeutic communication techniques.
5. List and explain five components of nonverbal communication.
6. Name and explain the four proxemic zones.
7. Explain what is meant by a client's "comfort zone."
8. Differentiate between task-oriented and affective touch.
9. Explain the learning styles of cognitive, affective, and psychomotor learners.
10. Describe variables that affect learning.
11. Compare informal with formal learning.
12. Discuss guidelines for teaching adult clients.

SECTION I: ASSESSING YOUR UNDERSTANDING

Activity A *Fill in the blanks by choosing the correct word from the options given in parentheses.*

1. A _____ is one who performs health-related activities that a sick person is unable to perform independently. *(Caregiver, Educator, Collaborator)*

2. _____ is an exchange of information. *(Hearing, Communication, Listening)*

3. The _____ processes information best by listening to or reading facts and descriptions. *(Cognitive learner, Affective learner, Psychomotor learner)*

4. An organized arrangement of content in a specific time frame is known as _____. *(Formal teaching, A teaching plan, A learning style)*

5. _____ refers to using verbal and nonverbal communication to promote a person's physical and emotional well-being. *(Therapeutic communication, Touch, Proxemics)*

6. _____ refers to a person's intellectual ability to understand, remember, and apply new information. *(Motivation, Learning capacity, Learning readiness)*

Activity B *Mark each statement as either "T" (True) or "F" (False). Correct any false statements.*

1. T F Task-oriented touch is typically used to demonstrate concern or affection.

2. T F Restoring independence is a motivating force.

3. T F The affective learner prefers to learn by doing.

4. T F Informal teaching typically requires a plan to avoid being haphazard.

5. T F Older adults may have short-term memory impairment but long-term memory remains intact.

Activity C *Write the correct term for each description related to nurse–client relationship given below.*

1. One who works with others to achieve a common goal. _____

2. Manner in which a person best comprehends new information. _____

3. An intuitive awareness of what the client is experiencing to perceive the client's emotional state and need for support.

   _____

4. The skills and concepts that the client and family must acquire to restore, maintain, or promote health. _____

5. This relationship exists during the period when the nurse interacts with clients, sick or well, to promote or restore their health, help them cope with their illness, or assist them to die with dignity. _____

Activity D *Match the terms associated with nurse–client relationships given in Column A with their related explanations or definitions given in Column B.*

Column A

_____ 1. Kinesics

_____ 2. Paralanguage

_____ 3. Proxemics

_____ 4. Touch

_____ 5. Silence

Column B

a. Refers to the use of space when communicating.

b. Tactile stimulus produced by personal contact with another person or object.

c. Vocal sounds that communicate a message.

d. The art of remaining silent.

e. Body language.

Activity E *The nurse–client relationship progresses through three phases. Compare these three phases given below using the given criteria.*

	Nurse–client Interaction	Role(s) of the Nurse
Introductory phase		
Working phase		
Terminating phase		

Activity F *Briefly answer the following questions.*

1. What are the four basic roles of a nurse?

   _____

   _____

   _____

2. Describe the two kinds of touch within the context of nursing.

   _____

   _____

   _____

3. What factors can decrease a client's learning readiness? How should the nurse proceed?

   _____

   _____

   _____

4. What is the role of a nurse as an educator? Give examples.

   _____

   _____

   _____

5. What motivates clients to learn at an accelerated rate? What forces motivate clients to acquire new information?

   _____

   _____

   _____

SECTION II: APPLYING YOUR KNOWLEDGE

Activity G *Give rationale for the following questions.*

1. Why should both the nurse and the client participate in the working phase?

   _____

   _____

   _____

2. What would be the best response by the nurse to a quiet and uncommunicative client?

_____

_____

_____

3. Why is empathetic listening important during nurse–client communication?

_____

_____

_____

4. Why should a nurse use affective touching cautiously?

_____

_____

_____

Activity H *Answer the following questions related to the nurse–client relationship.*

1. Which verbal and nonverbal communication techniques are effective with most American clients?

_____

_____

_____

2. Why is it important to acknowledge the "comfort zone" of a client? How can a nurse relieve a client's anxiety about physical closeness?

_____

_____

_____

3. How should the nurse respond when asked his or her opinion about treatment decisions by the client or their family?

_____

_____

_____

4. What are the factors that interfere with a client's learning capacity? How can receptiveness to learning be increased?

_____

_____

_____

Activity I *Think over the following questions. Discuss them with your instructor or peers.*

1. Identify the options for communication with each type of client:
- A client who has suffered a stroke, has expressive aphasia, and has lost use of their dominant hand.
- A non-English-speaking client.
- A client who has been deaf since birth.
- A client who has experienced significant hearing loss due to an occupational accident.

_____

_____

_____

2. A client diagnosed with a new onset of diabetes requires instruction on how to use a glucometer and self-administer insulin. What information will you need to gather in the learner assessment? How would you accommodate each style of learner: cognitive, affective, and psychomotor?

_____

_____

_____

SECTION III: GETTING READY FOR NCLEX

Activity J *Answer the following questions.*

1. Which of the following describes a "comfort zone"?
- **a.** The area where closeness is not required during nursing care.
- **b.** The area that encompasses up to 5 to 7 feet from the client.
- **c.** The area that, when intruded upon, does not create any kind of anxiety.
- **d.** The area where a client is well draped.

2. Which of the following describes task-oriented touch?
- **a.** It is used to demonstrate concern or affection.
- **b.** It involves the contact required for nursing procedures.
- **c.** The nurse uses task-oriented touch therapeutically when a client is lonesome.
- **d.** It involves the touch used for sensory deprived clients.

3. Which of the following is a therapeutic use of silence?
   a. Encourages a client to use verbal communication.
   b. Facilitates reaching the goals of a client.
   c. Ensures a client's comprehension before self-care.
   d. Avoids overwhelming a client with new information.

4. Which of the following describes the manner in which an affective learner best comprehends new information?
   a. The learner processes information by listening to descriptions.
   b. The learner likes to learn by doing.
   c. The learner processes information best by reading facts.
   d. The learner learns by information that appeals to values.

5. Which of the following helps the nurse to identify goals, tailor the teaching plan, and evaluate outcomes?
   a. Desire to acquire new information.
   b. Assessment of what the client knows.
   c. Purpose or reason for mastering skills.
   d. Restored independence.

6. What should the nurse do while dealing with older adults who lose the ability to hear at high-pitched ranges?
   a. Lower the voice pitch.
   b. Insert a stethoscope in client's ears.
   c. Use a magic slate or chalkboard.
   d. Ensure that the hearing aid is in good working order.

7. There are three phases of the nurse–client relationship. Which of the following phases demonstrates a plan that is constructed mutually to meet goals identified during the assessment of the client?
   a. Termination phase
   b. Working phase
   c. Introductory phase
   d. Transition phase

8. Communication with a client who has Limited English proficiency (LEP) is becoming more common. What is the best strategy for communicating with clients with LEPs?
   a. Ask a family member to translate.
   b. Request a telephonic interpreter.
   c. Request a certified interpreter.
   d. Ask a bilingual staff member to interpret.

9. What is the term that reflects the principles used in teaching adult learners?
   a. Pedagogy
   b. Gerogogy
   c. Cybertexting
   d. Androgogy

10. Which of the following groups of learners were born between 1961 and 1981 and have different learning needs as a result of technology and imposed independence?
   a. Generation Y
   b. Generation Net
   c. Generation X
   d. Baby Boomers

CHAPTER 8

Cultural Care Considerations

Learning Objectives

1. Define terms related to culture.
2. List the five population groups delineated in the United States.
3. Differentiate race from ethnicity and culture.
4. Contrast stereotyping and generalization.
5. Describe how cultural background and practices influence actions and behaviors.
6. Name three views that societies use to explain illness or disease.
7. Discuss biocultural assessment.
8. Describe cultural assessment.
9. Explain the meaning and characteristics of transcultural nursing.
10. List at least five ways to demonstrate culturally competent nursing care.

SECTION I: ASSESSING YOUR UNDERSTANDING

Activity A *Fill in the blanks by choosing the correct word from the options given in parentheses.*

1. _____ provides a means for understanding people's values and beliefs, including those related to health practices. *(Ethnicity, Culture, Ethnocentrism)*

2. _____ refers to the activities governed by the rules of behavior that a particular cultural group avoids, forbids, or prohibits. *(Cultural blindness, Cultural imposition, Cultural taboos)*

3. _____ means the nurse understands his or her own worldview as well as the client's and how these worldviews affect nursing care. *(Cultural competence, Transcultural sensitivity, Cultural assessment)*

4. _____ refers to biological differences in physical features, such as skin color, bone structure, and eye shape. *(Race, Culture, Ethnicity)*

Activity B *Mark each statement as either "T" (True) or "F" (False). Correct any false statements.*

1. T F To deliver culturally competent care, the nurse must view each person as a unique human being who may have a similar or different frame of reference as the nurse.

2. T F The defining characteristics for a minority group are based on numbers.

3. T F Health practices are the actions a person takes to maintain or restore health based on their health beliefs.

4. T F Subculture refers to a particular group that shares characteristics identifying the group as a distinct entity.

5. T F Cultural imposition involves the process of adapting to or taking on the behaviors of another group.

Activity C *Write the correct term for each description below.*

1. Assuming that all people in a particular culture, racial, or ethnic group share the same values and beliefs, behave similarly, and also are basically alike. _____

2. The belief that one's own ethnic heritage is the "correct" one and is superior to others. _____

3. An inability to recognize the values, beliefs, and practices of others because of strong ethnocentric preferences. _____

4. The care that fits a person's cultural values. _____

5. A person's ideas about what causes illness, the role of the sick person, how to restore health, and how one stays healthy. _____

Activity D *In general, societies use three overall views to explain illness or disease. Match these views given in Column A with their related examples given in Column B.*

Column A

____ **1.** Biomedical or scientific perspective

____ **2.** Naturalistic or holistic perspective

____ **3.** Magico-religious perspective

Column B

a. Supernatural forces dominate.

b. Embraces a cause-and-effect philosophy of human body functions.

c. Espouses that human beings are only one part of nature; natural balance or harmony is essential for health.

Activity E *Compare the culturally influenced characteristics for each of the given groups of clients.*

	Eye contact	Verbal communication Patterns	Touch/ space
Anglo-American			
Asian American			
Native American			
Hispanic			

Activity F *Briefly answer the following questions.*

1. What are the basic concepts that characterize culture?

_____

_____

_____

2. How do people demonstrate pride in their ethnic heritage?

_____

_____

_____

3. What is culture generalization? How does culture generalization assist healthcare providers to provide appropriate care?

_____

_____

_____

4. What is transcultural nursing? What are its characteristics?

_____

_____

_____

SECTION II: APPLYING YOUR KNOWLEDGE

Activity G *Give rationale for the following questions.*

1. Why is it important for the nurse not to equate skin color and other physical features with culture?

_____

_____

_____

2. Why is it important to evaluate biocultural ecology when providing healthcare?

_____

_____

_____

3. Why may it pose a challenge to supplement or restrict dietary consumption when providing health related education to clients from culturally diverse populations?

_____

_____

_____

4. Why is caution needed when asking family members to interpret?

_____

_____

_____

5. How will recognizing that clients have different perceptions of time assist the nurse to provide more sensitive care?

_____

_____

_____

Activity H _Answer the following questions related to cultural care considerations._

1. What general appearance and obvious physical characteristic components should the nurse evaluate when completing a biocultural assessment?

_____

_____

_____

2. What cultural elements should a nurse ask about or observe when performing a cultural assessment on a client?

_____

_____

_____

3. What are the recommendations that can help develop culturally sensitive nursing care?

_____

_____

_____

Activity I _Think over the following questions. Discuss them with your instructor or peers._

1. During an assessment on a Navajo client, the nurse is required to obtain the family members' health history. Because Navajos feel that no person has the right to speak for another, the client refuses to comment on family members' health problems. How would you respond?

_____

_____

_____

2. When assessing the health beliefs and practices of an older Hispanic adult, the nurse observes that the client uses a traditional folk healer to manage health problems. How would you respond?

_____

_____

_____

SECTION III: GETTING READY FOR NCLEX

Activity J _Answer the following questions._

1. Why would older Asian adults agree with a nurse even though they do not understand each other?

   a. Because they consider it shameful to express that they did not understand each other.

   b. Because they consider it disrespectful to disagree with the nurse.

   c. Because they believe that disagreeing with the nurse would harm their spirit.

   d. Because they believe that listening to the nurse non judgmentally is polite.

2. Which of the following societal views of illness and disease identifies a cause-and-effect philosophy of human body functions?

   a. Biomedical or scientific perspective

   b. Naturalistic perspective

   c. Magico-religious perspective

   d. Holistic perspective

3. Which of the following communication techniques will help a nurse to communicate with clients who do not speak English?

   a. Repeat the question without changing words.

   b. Look at the translator when asking questions.

   c. Speak slowly, using simple words and short sentences.

   d. Refer to an English or foreign language dictionary for bilingual words.

4. How can a nurse provide culturally competent care to all individuals?

   a. Become familiar with physical differences among ethnic groups.

   b. Learn to speak a second language.

   c. Develop strategies to avoid cultural imposition.

   d. Consult the client about ways to solve health problems.

5. Which of the following techniques facilitate interactions between the nurse and client?

   a. Ask questions that can be answered with "yes" or "no."

   b. Sit within the client's comfort zone.

   c. Avoid making eye contact.

   d. Address clients by their first names.

6. Why is it necessary for a nurse to assess a client's health beliefs and practices?

   a. For possessing knowledge of health problems affecting a particular cultural group.

   b. For accepting each client as an individual.

   c. For providing culturally competent care to the client.

   d. For viewing the situation from the client's perspective.

7. Which of the following terms describes a nurse's inability to differentiate between the beliefs of clients in the same culture?

   a. Generalization

   b. Stereotyping

   c. Ethnocentrism

   d. Cultural imposition

8. There are four basic concepts that characterize culture. Which of the four concepts are the same as continuously evolving?

   a. Learned from birth through language and socialization.

   b. Learned by members of the same cultural group

   c. Influenced by specific conditions related to environment, technology, and availability of resources.

   d. Dynamic and ever-changing.

9. What is the term that best describes biologic differences in physical features, such as skin color, bone structure, and eye shape?

   a. Culture

   b. Ethnicity

   c. Race

   d. Minority

10. A biocultural assessment is made up of four areas. Which of the areas is defined as gait and range of motion?

    a. Physical appearance

    b. Mobility

    c. Behavior

    d. Body structure

CHAPTER 9

Complementary and Alternative Therapies

Learning Objectives

1. Differentiate between the terms *complementary therapy*, *alternative therapy*, and *integrative medicine*.
2. Give five reasons that individuals choose to use complementary and alternative therapies.
3. List five categories of complementary and alternative therapies that the National Center for Complementary and Alternative Medicine investigates.
4. Describe the basic beliefs of three examples of alternative whole medical systems: Ayurvedic medicine, Chinese medicine, and Native American medicine.
5. Identify four examples of practices that use the mind to promote or restore physical health.
6. Describe four examples of biologically based practices.
7. Name anatomic structures that are the focus of manipulative and body-based therapies, and give examples of these therapies.
8. Describe techniques that are used in energy medicine.
9. Discuss the role nurses can play in relation to complementary and alternative therapies.

SECTION I: ASSESSING YOUR UNDERSTANDING

Activity A *Fill in the blanks by choosing the correct word from the options given in parentheses.*

1. _____ therapy is one used in addition to conventional medical treatment. *(Complementary, Alternative, Allopathic)*

2. _____ has its roots in India and is the oldest system of medicine in the world. *(Acupuncture, Homeopathy, Ayurvedic)*

3. Chinese medicine proposes that health is the outcome of balancing _____, opposing forces that must remain equalized to maintain qi (or chi). *(Prana and chakra, Mind and body, Yin and yang)*

4. _____ is one mind–body medicine used to help individuals overcome habits (such as smoking), relieve chronic pain, and extinguish irrational fears. rearrange? *(Humor, Hypnosis, Biofeedback)*

5. _____ is the use of scents to alter emotions and biological responses. *(Apitherapy, Shiatsu, Aromatherapy)*

6. _____ is a complementary health practice in which manual pressure is applied to the feet and hands. *(Reflexology, Massage therapy, Shiatsu)*

Activity B *Mark each statement as either "T" (True) or "F" (False). Correct any false statements.*

1. T F Homeopathy considers disease an aberration in natural healing.

2. T F Imagery is a psychobiological technique that uses the mind to visualize a positive physiological effect.

3. T F In Ayurvedic medicine, one belief is that chakras are the life force.

4. **T F** Yoga and tai chi both incorporate techniques that combine mental and physical exercise for the purpose of integrating body and mind.

5. **T F** Laughter has no effect on the immune system.

Activity C *Write the correct term for each description given below.*

1. The Native Americans' medicine man (or woman) and spiritual figure with the extraordinary ability to heal. _____

2. Practitioners apply pressure to acupoints in various body meridians (energy channels) that correlate with an organ or its function to rebalance the body's energy and restore health. _____

3. Supplements that are microorganisms that exert beneficial health effects. _____

4. The medicinal use of bee venom.

   _____

5. Practitioners who perform spinal manipulation to treat neuromuscular disorders and a host of other diseases. _____

6. A mind–body technique in which the individual voluntarily controls one or more physiologic functions, such as body temperature, heart rate, blood pressure, and brain waves.

   _____

Activity D *Match the complementary and/or alternative therapy given in Column A to the associated feature or example given in Column B.*

Column A

_____ 1. Whole medical system

_____ 2. Mind-body medicine

_____ 3. Biologically based practices

_____ 4. Manipulative and body-based therapies

_____ 5. Energy medicine

_____ 6. Conventional (allopathic) medicine

Column B

a. Use techniques that rely on the power of the brain, emotions, social interactions, and spiritual factors to alter body functions or symptoms such as biofeedback, imagery, and spiritual healing.

b. Healing methods that focus on the structures and systems of the body such as massage therapy, chiropractic, yoga, and tai chi.

c. Practices that embody traditional Western treatment of disease.

d. Techniques are used that claim to manipulate electromagnetic fields in the body such as reiki, acupuncture, and techniques involving magnets and electricity.

e. The belief that one's body has the power to heal itself, and that healing involves the mind, body, and spirit (examples include Ayurvedic medicine, Chinese medicine, and homeopathy).

f. Use natural products such as dietary supplements, aromatherapy, and animal-derived extracts such as bee venom.

Activity E *Compare the whole medical systems based on the given criteria.*

	Goal of treatment/cause of Illness	Common treatment measures
Ayurvedic medicine		
Native American medicine		
Chinese medicine (also includes contributions from Japan, Korea, and other Southeast Asian countries)		

Activity F *Briefly answer the following questions.*

1. Compare and contrast complementary therapy, alternative therapy, and integrated medicine.

   _____

   _____

   _____

2. What are the goals of NCCAM?

_____

_____

_____

3. Why is the use of medicinal plants and herbs for therapy referred to as folk medicine?

_____

_____

_____

4. Which structures and systems of the body are the focuses of manipulative and body-based therapies?

_____

_____

_____

5. Why has the United States Food and Drug Administration warned against the use of Actra-Rx (Yilishen)?

_____

_____

_____

SECTION II: ASSESSING YOUR UNDERSTANDING

Activity G _Provide rationale for the following questions._

1. Why do individuals choose to use complementary or alternative therapies?

_____

_____

_____

2. Why is it important for clients to check labels on over-the-counter medications when taking herbal preparations?

_____

_____

_____

3. Why can't manufacturers of herbal preparations claim that their herbal product prevents or treats a disease?

_____

_____

_____

4. Why might tai chi be preferred by some clients rather than other forms of aerobic exercises?

_____

_____

_____

5. Why should the nurse and other healthcare providers tolerate or even support the use of complementary and alternative therapies if the practice is not dangerous or unhealthy?

_____

_____

_____

Activity H _Answer the following questions related to complementary and alternative therapies._

1. A client asks how massage therapy can be of benefit to them. What information should the nurse provide?

_____

_____

_____

2. A client has heard about an herbal supplement and is considering using it as complementary therapy. The client is currently taking numerous medications. How should the nurse instruct the client?

_____

_____

_____

3. A client wants help in choosing between api-therapy and chiropractic treatments. The client is worried about the safety and the insurance coverage. Compare and contrast the two methods in terms of safety and insurance coverage.

---

4. A client is curious about energy medicine. How would the nurse describe the techniques used in this type of complementary/alternative therapy?

Activity I *Think over the following questions. Discuss them with your instructor or peers.*

1. The smell of the earth after a rain makes you feel happy. After a recent car accident, the smell of gas makes you break into a sweat. The two smells produce two different reactions. How do these smells elicit physiologic and psychological responses?

---

2. Why has it become necessary for nurses to understand complementary and alternative therapies along with the allopathic system of medicine?

SECTION III: GETTING READY FOR NCLEX

Activity J *Answer the following questions.*

1. What is the term that describes a type of therapy or medicine that is used in conjunction with conventional medicine?
   a. Integrative medicine
   b. Alternative therapy
   c. Allopathic medicine
   d. Complementary therapy

2. A nurse interviews a client and learns that the client is using alternative therapy to treat a sore back that has defied conventional therapy. What is one of the reasons that might apply to this client's rationale for using alternative therapy?
   a. Desire to become more active in decision-making and self-care.
   b. Chronic incurable back condition.
   c. Difficulty meeting the rising costs of healthcare.
   d. Client does not share traditional American health beliefs and practices.

3. An LPN is giving an in-service to her fellow colleagues as she is interested in alternative and complementary medicine. Which of the following categories of complementary and alternative medicine involves healing methods that focus on the structures and systems of the body, including the bones and joints, the soft tissues, and the circulatory and lymphatic system?
   a. Energy medicine
   b. Whole medical systems
   c. Manipulative and body-based therapies
   d. Biologically based practices

4. Which of the following categories of complementary and alternative medicine involves healing theory and practice that evolved from other cultures?
   a. Energy medicine
   b. Whole medical systems
   c. Manipulative and body-based therapies
   d. Biologically based practices

5. An LPN goes on a mission trip to India and learns techniques of Ayurvedic medicine. What is the basic premise of this type of medicine?
   a. Views disease as resulting from disharmony with Mother Earth, possession by an evil spirit, or violation of a taboo.
   b. Health is the outcome of balancing yin and yang, opposite forces that must remain equalized to maintain life's energy force.
   c. Help individuals become unified with nature to develop a strong body, clear mind, and tranquil spirit.
   d. Correcting an imbalance between two attributes, such as motion and stillness or hot and cold, restores harmony and health.

6. A nurse is using mind–body techniques in teaching a client how to overcome pain. Which of the following techniques in the mind–body medicine category allows an individual to voluntarily control one or more physiologic functions, such as body temperature, heart rate, blood pressure, and brain waves?

   a. Biofeedback

   b. Hypnosis

   c. Imagery

   d. Humor

7. Which of the following techniques in the biologically based practices is the use of scents to alter emotions and biologic processes?

   a. Herbal supplements

   b. Apitherapy

   c. Probiotics

   d. Aromatherapy

8. Which of the following manipulative and body-based techniques uses pressure that is applied to the feet and hands?

   a. Massage

   b. Reflexology

   c. Shiatsu

   d. Chiropractic technique

9. Which of the following energy medicine techniques promotes healing using electricity, magnets, or both?

   a. Reiki

   b. Acupuncture

   c. Electromagnetic therapy

   d. Chiropractic therapy

10. A nurse learns about the techniques of complementary medicine to assist clients in making informed choices. A client asks the nurse if she can use massage along with chemotherapy treatments for breast cancer. What is the nurse's best answer to the question?

    a. "I would think about this, as it may harm the chemotherapy treatment."

    b. "I think it would be worth trying, especially since you said you ache after chemotherapy."

    c. "There are other therapies out there that might help you better."

    d. "I can't tell you that, as your doctor would have to approve."

10

End-of-Life Care

Learning Objectives

1. Define attitudes of society and healthcare workers toward death.
2. Discuss outcomes of informing a client about a terminal illness.
3. Explain how clients and families can maintain hopefulness during a terminal illness.
4. Name the emotional reactions the dying client experiences.
5. Identify how the dying client can ensure that others carry out his or her wishes for terminal care.
6. Describe physical phenomena that occur during the dying process.
7. Summarize psychological events that dying clients have reported.
8. Describe nursing management of the dying client and the family.

SECTION I: ASSESSING YOUR UNDERSTANDING

Activity A *Fill in the blanks by choosing the correct word from the options given in parentheses.*

1. Physical effects of impending death include _____, in which peristalsis slows, causing gas and intestinal contents to accumulate. This buildup may stimulate the vomiting center, resulting in nausea and vomiting. *(Renal impairment, Gastrointestinal disturbances, Musculoskeletal changes)*

2. The client can use _____ and determination to survive and prolong life, often referred to as the "will to live." *(Will power, Religious faith, Inner resources)*

3. _____ is a painful yet normal reaction that helps clients to cope with loss and leads to emotional healing. *(Grieving, Coping, Accepting)*

4. _____ is one of the first signs of the client's condition worsening and of impending death. *(Cardiac dysfunction, Renal impairment, Central nervous system alteration)*

5. _____ may be prescribed by the physician to relieve the anxiety created by the feeling of suffocation caused by pulmonary edema in the dying client. *(An antidepressant, Pain medication, A sedative)*

Activity B *Mark each statement as either "T" (True) or "F" (False). Correct any false statements.*

1. T F Central nervous system alterations of the dying client include apnea and diminished pain perception.

2. T F The nurse should only offer hospital prescribed meals at breakfast, lunch, and dinner time to the dying client.

3. T F An essential component of quality care is to recognize that nursing care always requires sensitivity and compassion for clients, families, and significant others.

4. T F In a dying client, the reflexes become hyperactive.

5. T F The nurse is usually responsible for informing clients of the nature and gravity of their illness.

Activity C *Write the correct term for each description given below.*

1. Treatment that reduces physical discomfort but does not alter a disease's progression. _____

2. Care that is arranged to provide periodic relief for the primary caregiver of the dying client. _____

3. Some clients seem to forestall dying when they feel that their loved ones are not yet prepared to deal with their death. _____

4. Care for terminally ill clients, who can live out their final days with comfort, dignity, and meaningfulness. _____

Activity D *Match the physical events that occur in a dying client given in Column A with the signs given in Column B.*

Column A	Column B
____ 1. Renal impairment	a. The client loses urinary and rectal sphincter muscle control, causing incontinence of urine and stool.
____ 2. Musculoskeletal changes	
____ 3. Pulmonary function impairment	b. The skin becomes pale or mottled, nail beds and lips may appear blue, and the client may feel cold.
____ 4. Peripheral circulation changes	
	c. Low cardiac output causes volume to diminish and toxic waste products to accumulate.
	d. Failure of the heart's pumping function causes fluid to collect and breath sounds become moist.

Activity E *Given below in random order is a series of five reactions experienced by dying clients when informed about their terminal illness. Write the correct sequence for the stages experienced by dying clients in the boxes given below.*

1. Clients may displace feelings onto others, such as the physician, nurses, family, or even God. They may express feelings in less obvious ways, such as complaining about their care or blaming anyone and everyone for the slightest aggravation.

2. Dying clients accept their fate and make peace spiritually and with those to whom they are close. Clients may begin to detach themselves from activities and acquaintances and seek to be with only a small circle of relatives or friends.

3. A psychological coping mechanism in which a person refuses to believe certain information. Dying clients usually first deny that the diagnosis is accurate.

4. An attempt to postpone death. Usually the clients make a secret bargain with God or some higher power. Clients attempt to negotiate a delay in dying until after a particularly significant event.

5. As clients realize the reality of their situation, they may mourn their potential losses, such as separation from their loved ones, the inability to fulfill their future goals, or loss of control.

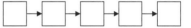

Activity F *Compare institutionally based and home hospice care based on the given criteria.*

	Institutionally based hospice care	Hospice home care
Care provided		
Benefits & disadvantages		

Activity G *Briefly answer the following questions.*

1. What have been the effects of technology and aggressive treatment on the attitude of health-care workers towards death and dying?

_____

_____

_____

2. What is hospice care?

_____

_____

_____

3. What is a living will?

_____

_____

_____

4. What is a durable power of attorney?

_____

_____

_____

5. What factors should the nurse consider when caring for dying clients?

_____

_____

_____

6. How does the nurse facilitate and support the client's final decisions?

_____

_____

_____

SECTION II: ASSESSING YOUR UNDERSTANDING

Activity H *Give rationale for the following questions.*

1. Why does a nurse administer pain medications on a routine schedule for dying clients?

_____

_____

_____

2. Why would a physician prescribe a mild tranquilizer or antidepressant to the dying client?

_____

_____

_____

3. Why is it important for a nurse to be flexible and to interrupt physical care if and when the client indicates a need for companionship, support, and communication?

_____

_____

_____

4. Why does the nurse give oral care and ice chips to a dying client?

_____

_____

_____

5. Why should the nurse to avoid unnecessary assessments and make frequent checks of the dying client?

_____

_____

_____

6. Why must the nurse convey a spirit of hopefulness to the dying client?

_____

_____

_____

Activity I *Answer the following questions related to end-of-life care.*

1. When a family member is dying, how can the nurse promote family coping?

_____

_____

_____

2. What are the outcomes of being truthful with the client and honoring their right to know the seriousness of their condition?

_____

_____

_____

3. How does the nurse address spiritual distress with the dying client?

_____

_____

_____

Activity J *Think over the following questions. Discuss them with your instructor or peers.*

1. How will you prepare yourself to care for dying clients and their families?

_____

_____

_____

2. How would client and family care differ for a client with an acute terminal illness and a chronic terminal illness?

_____

_____

_____

3. How would you respond to a family member experiencing anticipatory grieving who emotionally withdraws from the client?

_____

_____

_____

SECTION III: GETTING READY FOR NCLEX

Activity K _Answer the following questions._

1. Why does a nurse avoid administering glycerin to a dying client?

  a. Because it diminishes the heart's oxygen supply.

  b. Because it causes the skin to be pale or mottled.

  c. Because it tends to pull fluid from the body of the client.

  d. Because it causes skin breakdown.

2. Which of the following nursing interventions will help a nurse minimize the disturbed sleep pattern of a dying client?

  a. Play the client's favorite music.

  b. Mask the continuous hum of equipment.

  c. Provide a glass of warm milk before the client goes to bed.

  d. Shut doors and windows to prevent noise from coming in.

3. Which of the following interventions should a nurse use when the client is unable to cough and raise secretions?

  a. Give the client water to drink.

  b. Pat the client on the back.

  c. Gently suction the client.

  d. Give the client cough syrup.

4. When caring for a dying client, which of the following interventions should a nurse perform to protect the client's skin from breakdown?

  a. Applying oil to the client's body.

  b. Providing plenty of drinking water to hydrate the client's skin.

  c. Giving the client a sponge bath twice a day.

  d. Changing the client's position every 2 hours.

5. Which of the following is an essential component of quality care for dying clients?

  a. Assist the client with personal hygiene.

  b. Inform all the members of healthcare regarding the client's prognosis.

  c. Provide sensitivity and compassion for the client and their family members.

  d. Promote the care of dying clients at home or in hospice settings.

6. Which of the following is the first sign that the condition of a dying client is worsening?

  a. Pulmonary function impairment

  b. Peripheral circulation changes

  c. Central nervous system alterations

  d. Failing cardiac function

7. Which of the following outcomes of being truthful about a terminal illness enhances the nurse–client relationship with regard to the ability to choose what to do when the client is told the truth about their illness?

  a. The client's autonomy and right to determine how to spend the rest of their life is upheld.

  b. Meaningful communication between clients and family members is promoted.

  c. The nurse–client relationship is based on honesty rather than on the false pretense that recovery will occur.

  d. Clients can use inner resources and determination to survive and prolong life, often referred to as the "will to live."

8. Which of the following emotional reactions does the client go through when facing his/her mortality in an attempt to postpone death?
   a. Denial
   b. Bargaining
   c. Acceptance
   d. Depression

9. Which of the following indicates a person who is selected on the client's behalf to make medical decisions when the client cannot?
   a. Durable power of attorney for healthcare
   b. Living will
   c. Advance directive
   d. Informed consent

10. Which of the following settings allows the dying client to have advanced care in an institution due to the necessity to control pain that is unable to be managed at home?
    a. Hospice care
    b. Acute care
    c. Palliative care
    d. Home care

CHAPTER 11

Pain Management

Learning Objectives

1. Define the term *pain*.
2. Compare nociceptive pain with neuropathic pain.
3. Give characteristics distinguishing acute from chronic pain.
4. Describe four phases of pain transmission.
5. Differentiate between pain perception, pain threshold, and pain tolerance.
6. Describe essential components of pain assessment.
7. Explain why assessing pain is difficult.
8. Give examples of tools for assessing the intensity of pain.
9. Discuss the Joint Commission's standards on pain assessment and pain management.
10. Explain pain management, and list five techniques commonly used.
11. Name categories of drugs used to manage pain.
12. Describe methods of administration for analgesic drugs.
13. Discuss the issues of addiction, tolerance, and physical dependence associated with pain medication.
14. List examples of noninvasive techniques used to manage pain.
15. Identify two surgical procedures performed on clients with intractable pain.
16. List at least three nursing diagnoses, besides acute pain and chronic pain, that are common among clients with pain.
17. Discuss the nursing management of clients with pain.
18. Describe information pertinent to teaching clients and family about pain management.

SECTION I: ASSESSING YOUR UNDERSTANDING

Activity A *Fill in the blanks by choosing the correct word from the options given in parentheses.*

1. _____ pain is subdivided into somatic and visceral pain. *(Neuropathic, Nociceptive, Chronic)*

2. It is speculated that some non drug methods relieve pain by releasing _____ such as endorphins and enkephalins, which are natural morphine-like substances in the body that modulate pain transmission by blocking receptors for substance P. *(Endogenous opiates, GABA, Serotonin)*

3. _____ is a pain management technique that delivers bursts of electricity to the skin and underlying nerves. *(PENS, TENS, Acupuncture)*

4. _____ is discomfort that has a short duration (from a few seconds to less than 6 months). It is associated with tissue trauma or some other recent identifiable etiology. *(Acute pain, Nociceptive pain, Neuropathic pain)*

5. _____ meals may help maximize intake in clients with drug-related or pain-related anorexia. *(Heavy, Protein-rich, Small and frequent)*

Activity B *Mark each statement as either "T" (True) or "F" (False). Correct any false statements.*

1. T F Suffering is a privately experienced, unpleasant sensation usually associated with disease or injury.

2. T F Analgesic drugs can only be administered by oral or parenteral (injected) routes.

3. T F Cancer pain may be either nociceptive or neuropathic.

4. T F The linear scale is a better assessment tool for quantifying pain intensity than a numeric or word scale.

5. T F Chronic pain sufferers may have periods of acute pain, which is referred to as breakthrough pain.

6. T F Confused older adults may be unable to report pain, but it may manifest as agitation, aggression, withdrawal, or changes in behavior, positioning or sleep patterns.

Activity C *Write the correct term for each description given below.*

1. The conscious experience of discomfort.
   _____

2. The point at which the pain-transmitting neurochemicals reach the brain, causing conscious awareness. _____

3. Discomfort that lasts longer than 6 months.
   _____

4. The amount of pain a person endures after the threshold has been reached. _____

5. A term used to describe discomfort that is perceived in a general area of the body, but not in the exact site where an organ is anatomically located. _____

Activity D *Match the phases of pain transmission in Column A with the specific action that occurs in each of these phases in Column B.*

Column A

____ **1.** Transduction

____ **2.** Transmission

____ **3.** Perception

____ **4.** Modulation

Column B

a. The phase during which peripheral nerve fibers form synapses with neurons in the spinal cord. The pain impulses move from the spinal cord to sequentially higher levels in the brain.

b. The phase of pain impulse transmission during which the

brain interacts with the spinal nerves in a downward fashion to alter the pain experience.

c. The conversion of chemical information in the cellular environment to electrical impulses that move toward the spinal cord. This phase is initiated by cellular disruption during which affected cells release various chemical mediators.

d. The phase of impulse transmission during which the brain experiences pain at a conscious level.

Activity E *Differentiate between nociceptive pain and neuropathic pain based on the given criteria.*

	Nociceptive pain	Neuropathic pain
Cause		
Source		
Examples		

Activity F *Briefly answer the following questions.*

1. How do opioid and opiate medications differ in their action from non opioid analgesic medications?

   _____

   _____

   _____

2. List the five general techniques for achieving pain management.

   _____

   _____

   _____

3. List examples of adjuvant drugs used to manage pain.

_____

_____

_____

4. Explain why rhizotomy and cordotomy are effective treatments for intractable pain.

_____

_____

_____

Activity G _Label the phases of pain transmission in the given figure._

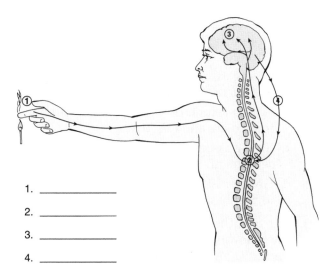

1. _____

2. _____

3. _____

4. _____

SECTION II: APPLYING YOUR KNOWLEDGE

Activity H _Give rationale for the following questions._

1. Why is the Wong-Baker FACES scale assessment tool best for specific types of clients?

_____

_____

_____

2. Why is risk for injury a concern for the client who is receiving narcotic analgesics?

_____

_____

_____

3. Why do older adults avoid taking opioid medications?

_____

_____

_____

4. Why do some nurses fear giving larger doses of narcotic analgesics when the client experiences tolerance?

_____

_____

_____

5. Why are drugs that are known to cause physical dependence discontinued gradually?

_____

_____

_____

Activity I _Answer the following questions related to pain management._

1. What are the essential components of a pain assessment?

_____

_____

_____

2. A client requires an increased amount of opioid analgesic to achieve pain relief and fears addiction. How would the nurse explain the difference between addiction and tolerance?

_____

_____

_____

3. What are the Joint Commission's standards on pain assessment and pain management?

_____

_____

_____

4. Identify nursing responsibilities for pain management.

_____

_____

_____

5. Identify non drug interventions used to help manage pain.

_____

_____

_____

Activity J _Think over the following questions._
Discuss them with your peers or instructor.

1. Discuss negative reactions that others may have to clients experiencing chronic pain.

_____

_____

_____

2. What factors can decrease a client's ability to cope with pain or lower pain tolerance?

_____

_____

_____

3. How does culture play a role in expressions of pain?

_____

_____

_____

4. What nonverbal behaviors may clients demonstrate in response to pain?

_____

_____

_____

5. Besides acute pain or chronic pain, discuss additional nursing diagnoses that are common among clients with pain

_____

_____

_____

SECTION III: GETTING READY FOR NCLEX

Activity K _Answer the following NCLEX-style questions._

1. Although acute pain is severe, why does a client with acute pain cope better with the discomfort in the later stages?
   a. Because the pain is negligible in the later stages.
   b. Because an increased dosage of analgesics is used in the later stages.
   c. Because the client's perception of pain minimizes in the later stages.
   d. Because there is a reinforcing belief that the pain will resolve in time.

2. When caring for a client with pain, which of the following is essential throughout the client's care?
   a. Giving assurance that pain management is a nursing and agency priority.
   b. Giving assurance that pain relief will be immediate and effective.
   c. Giving assurance that pain relief will be permanent.
   d. Giving assurance that pain has a psychological basis and can be easily managed.

3. In a client receiving opiate therapy, which of the following should the nurse closely monitor for in order to minimize the risk for imbalanced nutrition?
   a. Diarrhea
   b. Anorexia and nausea
   c. GI tract infection
   d. Gastric ulcer

4. Fill in the blank: Scheduling the administration of analgesics every __ hours often affords a uniform level of pain relief.

5. A young client who is developing wisdom teeth informs the nurse that he has been using ibuprofen three times per day for 3 months and now wishes to take aspirin instead. What advice should the nurse give this client?

   a. To avoid dairy products if aspirin is administered.

   b. To get the wisdom teeth extracted.

   c. To consult a physician immediately before taking aspirin.

   d. To maintain the same dosage of aspirin as of ibuprofen.

6. Which of the following should the nurse closely monitor for in older adults receiving nonsteroidal anti-inflammatory drugs?

   a. Cardiac problems

   b. Metabolic acidosis

   c. Septic shock

   d. Gastrointestinal problems

7. An LPN is working with a client who has pain. What are the key components of the definition of pain according to the text?

   a. Publicly experienced sensation.

   b. Privately experienced sensation.

   c. Publicly experienced emotion.

   d. Privately experience emotion.

8. A nurse is identifying pain in a client and determines that the pain is processed abnormally by the nervous system. Which of the following terms represents pain from damage to either the pain pathways in peripheral nerves or pain processing centers in the brain?

   a. Neuropathic pain

   b. Nociceptive pain

   c. Somatic pain

   d. Visceral pain

9. Which of the four phases of pain transmission is characterized by the peripheral nerve fibers forming synapses with neurons in the spinal cord and the pain impulses moving away from the spinal cord to the reticular activating system, the limbic system, the thalamus, and finally the cerebral cortex?

   a. Modulation

   b. Transduction

   c. Transmission

   d. Perception

10. A nurse assesses a client's pain level as a 5 out of 10 on the pain scale. The order reads for the client to receive morphine. Which of the following five ways of managing pain does the drug morphine fall under?

   a. Altering pain transmission at the level of the spinal cord

   b. Combining analgesics with adjuvant drugs

   c. Blocking brain perception

   d. Interrupting pain-transmitting chemicals at the site of injury

Infection

Learning Objectives

1. Describe types of infectious agents and list examples.
2. Differentiate between nonpathogens and pathogens.
3. Describe the six components of the chain of infection.
4. List factors that increase susceptibility to infection.
5. Explain the difference between mechanical and chemical defense mechanisms.
6. Describe events during the inflammatory process.
7. Differentiate localized from generalized infections.
8. List reasons why clients in healthcare agencies are at increased risk for infection.
9. Explain nursing actions to prevent or control transmission of infection in the hospital and in the community.
10. Describe measures to take if a needlestick injury occurs.
11. Name diagnostic tests ordered for clients suspected of having an infectious disorder.
12. Discuss the medical management of clients with infectious disorders.
13. Describe nursing care for the client with a potential or actual infection

SECTION I: ASSESSING YOUR UNDERSTANDING

Activity A *Fill in the blanks by choosing the correct word from the options given in parentheses:*

1. _____ are physical barriers that prevent microorganisms from gaining entry or expel microorganisms before they multiply. *(Mechanical defense mechanisms, Chemical defense mechanisms, Electrical defense mechanisms)*

2. _____ bacteria grow and multiply in an atmosphere that lacks oxygen. *(Spirochetes, Aerobic, Anaerobic)*

3. _____ transmit rickettsial diseases. *(Humans, Arthropods, Microscopic worms)*

4. An infection that becomes widespread or systemic is called _____. *(Localized infection, Generalized infection, Opportunistic infection)*

5. WBCs and other cells produce _____ in response to viral infection and other factors. This chemical protein appears to trigger infected cells to manufacture an antiviral protein and inhibit cell reproduction. *(Lysozyme, Immunoglobulins, Interferon)*

6. _____ are nonpathogenic or remotely pathogenic microorganisms that take advantage of favorable situations and overwhelm the host. They commonly occur among immunocompromised clients. *(Nosocomial infections, Opportunistic infections, Reemerging infectious disease)*

Activity B *Mark each statement as either "T" (True) or "F" (False). Correct any false statements.*

1. T F Nonpathogens have a high potential to cause infectious disease.

2. T F All humans and animals infected with a microorganism will show evidence of infectious disease.

3. **T F** Some viral infections are minor and self-limiting.

4. **T F** Helminths cause transmissible spongiform encephalopathies (TSEs).

5. **T F** Fungi are divided into two basic groups; yeasts and molds.

6. **T F** Nosocomial infections are infections acquired while receiving care in a healthcare agency that were not active, incubatory, or chronic at admission.

Activity C *Write the correct term for each description.*

1. Destroy or incapacitate microorganisms with naturally produced biologic substances. Examples include enzymes, antibody substances, and secretions._____

2. If microorganisms gain entry, sneezing, coughing, and vomiting can forcefully expel them. _____

3. Their primary function is phagocytosis, the ingestion of cells and foreign material including microorganisms. _____

4. The ability of some bacteria to remain unaffected by antimicrobial drugs. _____

5. Occasionally, this type of microorganism is dormant in a living host, reactivates periodically, and causes infection to reoccur.

_____

6. A bactericidal enzyme, capable of splitting the cell wall of some gram-positive bacteria. Present in tears, saliva, mucus, skin secretions, and some internal body fluids. _____

7. Infections acquired in the community setting that are infectious communicable diseases. In addition to general signs of systemic infection, these infections produce clusters of signs and symptoms that reflect dysfunction of the organs or tissues that the microorganisms have invaded._____

Activity D *Match the six components of the chain of infection given in Column A with their characteristics given in Column B.*

Column A

_____ 1. Infectious agent

_____ 2. Reservoir

_____ 3. Portal of exit

_____ 4. Means of transmission

_____ 5. Portal of entry

_____ 6. Susceptible host

Column B

a. The route by which the infectious agent escapes from the reservoir. Examples include the respiratory, GI, or genitourinary tract; the skin and mucous membranes; and blood and other body fluids.

b. The person on or in whom the infectious agent will reside. Whether infection occurs depends on duration of exposure to the infectious agent and the person's ability to be compromised by or infected with disease.

c. Characteristics that must be present include the ability to move or be moved from one place to another, power to produce disease, an adequate number of agents, and the ability to invade a host.

d. The environment in which the infectious agent can survive and reproduce. It may be human, animal, or nonliving, such as contaminated food and water.

e. How the infectious agent is transferred or moved from its reservoir to the susceptible host. The five potential means are contact, droplet, airborne, vehicle, and vector.

f. How an infectious agent gains entrance into a susceptible host. Staphylococci, for example, can cause disease via the respiratory tract (pneumonia), skin (boils), blood (internal abscesses), or GI tract (food poisoning).

Activity E *Provide the description and give examples of the following types of microorganisms.*

	Description	Examples
Bacteria		
Viruses		
Fungi		
Rickettsiae		
Protozoans		
Mycoplasmas		
Helminths		

Activity F *Briefly answer the following questions.*

1. Which types of individuals are at increased risk for infection because their defenses are compromised in one or more ways?

2. Describe how the skin and mucous membranes provide the first line of defense against microorganisms.

3. How do antibodies work with other WBCs to defend the body from microorganisms?

4. What is the difference between an emerging and reemerging infectious disease?

5. Fever, which is the body's attempt to destroy the pathogen with heat, occurs in most people as an infection worsens. Which types of individuals may be an exception?

SECTION II: APPLYING YOUR KNOWLEDGE

Activity G *Give rationale for the following questions.*

1. Why are emerging and reemerging infectious diseases of serious concern?

2. Why do nurses and other health care providers take precautions to control infection when caring for all clients regardless of diagnosis or infection status?

3. Why is a WBC with a differential a more valuable source of information than a WBC without a differential?

4. Why are hospitalized clients more susceptible to nosocomial infections?

Activity H *Answer the following questions related to infection.*

1. What information will the nurse gather when performing an assessment on a client with a potential or actual infection?

2. What are the postexposure recommendations following a needlestick injury?

3. What actions will the nurse take to control the transmission of infection and prevent complications?

_____

_____

_____

4. Describe the medical management of a client with an infectious disorder.

_____

_____

_____

5. The initial localized reaction to an invading microorganism activates the inflammatory process; describe this process.

_____

_____

_____

6. What is the purpose of a culture and sensitivity test?

_____

_____

_____

Activity I *Think over the following questions. Discuss them with your instructor or peers.*

1. What community-acquired infections have you observed in your community?

_____

_____

_____

2. What were the signs and symptoms?

_____

_____

_____

3. How were these infections spread?

_____

_____

_____

4. Were some individuals more susceptible than others?

_____

_____

_____

SECTION III: GETTING READY FOR NCLEX

Activity J *Answer the following questions.*

1. Why is the potential for death from infections with multidrug-resistant microorganisms increased?
   a. Such microorganisms remain unaffected by antimicrobial drugs.
   b. Such microorganisms react adversely with antimicrobial drugs.
   c. Antimicrobial drugs used for treatment cause severe adverse effects.
   d. Antimicrobial drugs used for treatment are not readily available.

2. A client has periodic outbreaks of cold sores long after the initial infection of herpes simplex virus. Why does this occur?
   a. The client has low resistance.
   b. The client has not received proper treatment.
   c. The viruses are dormant in the client.
   d. The viruses are immune to the therapy.

3. A client is diagnosed with superficial mycotic infections. Which of the following should the nurse closely monitor in this client for infection?
   a. Eyes and ears
   b. Skin, hair, and nails
   c. Subcutaneous tissues
   d. Mouth and teeth

4. A nurse is teaching a client about intestinal ova and parasites. Which of the following instructions should a nurse provide clients suspected of having intestinal ova and parasites?
   a. Avoid beef products.
   b. Take precautions to avoid direct sunlight.
   c. Increase the intake of between-meal supplements.
   d. Perform scrupulous handwashing.

5. Which of the following aspects should a nurse pay particular attention to when assessing a client with a potential or actual infection?

   a. The client's age and sex

   b. The client's lifestyle and drinking habits

   c. The client's recent travel to a foreign country

   d. The client's diet and preference for meat

6. Fill in the blank. After administering injections of penicillin, the nurse should ask the client to wait at least _____ minutes before allowing the client to leave the healthcare facility.

7. A licensed practical nurse works in a physician's office and has just taken a client back to a room to see the doctor. The client has recently been to Europe and has eaten meat in the country. What type of infectious agent may the client have been exposed to according to the text?

   a. Fungi

   b. Bacteria

   c. Protozoa

   d. Prions

8. A client is concerned about the recent commercials regarding yogurt having something in it that actually helps to aid in digestion. What is the term that best describes an item that is a microorganism or prion that is generally harmless to humans?

   a. Nonpathogenic

   b. Pathogenic

   c. Infection

   d. Helminth

9. Which of the following steps in the chain of infection refers to how a pathogen is transferred or moved from its reservoir to the susceptible host?

   a. Reservoir

   b. Portal of entry

   c. Means of transmission

   d. Susceptible host

10. A client is learning how to best protect himself from disease. In the process of the class, the client learns that his body has several mechanical defenses as a first line of defense. What is the best answer that describes a mechanical defense in a client?

   a. Enzymes

   b. Antibodies

   c. Skin and mucous membranes

   d. Secretions

CHAPTER 13

Intravenous Therapy

Learning Objectives

1. Explain common indications for intravenous (IV) therapy.
2. Differentiate between crystalloid and colloid solutions and give examples of each.
3. Describe the difference between isotonic, hypotonic, and hypertonic solutions.
4. Explain the difference between whole blood, packed cells, blood products, and plasma expanders.
5. Describe nursing responsibilities for preparing intravenous solutions, selecting tubing, and selecting an infusion technique.
6. Identify nursing responsibilities when preparing the client for IV therapy.
7. Describe nursing actions involved in performing a venipuncture, including sites and devices commonly used.
8. Explain the equipment that must be replaced during IV therapy.
9. List complications of IV therapy and signs and symptoms for which the nurse monitors.
10. Explain how the nurse discontinues IV therapy.
11. Discuss the purpose of a medication lock.
12. Describe the nursing process for the client requiring IV therapy.
13. Discuss the purpose of total parenteral nutrition, and name one solution often administered concurrently.
14. Explain special considerations for blood transfusion therapy, including the equipment used, blood compatibility, and complications.

SECTION I: ASSESSING YOUR UNDERSTANDING

Activity A *Fill in the blanks by choosing the correct word from the options given in parentheses.*

1. The nurse will select _____ to administer 1000mL of 0.9% normal saline over 12 hours. *(Primary tubing, Secondary tubing, Y-administration tubing)*

2. The diameter of the venipuncture device always should be _____ that of the vein into which it will be inserted to reduce the potential for occluding blood flow. *(Larger than, Smaller than, Equal to)*

3. Microdrip tubing, regardless of the manufacturer, delivers a standard volume of _____ drops (gtt)/mL. *(10, 15, 60)*

4. When an electronic infusion device is used to deliver IV solution, the rate is calculated in _____. *(mL/hr, gtts/mL, gtts/min)*

5. _____ are nonblood solutions that pull fluid into the vascular space. They are used as an economical and virus-free substitute for blood and blood products when treating clients with hypovolemic shock. *(Plasma expanders, Packed red blood cells, Blood products)*

6. Used when the client no longer needs continuous infusions, needs intermittent IV medication administration, or may need emergency IV fluids or medications. *(Macrodrip tubing, Microdrip tubing, Medication lock)*

Activity B *Mark each statement as either "T" (True) or "F" (False). Correct any false statements.*

1. T F The nurse should select secondary tubing for the administration of whole blood.

2. T F The nurse should discontinue the IV infusion and remove the venipuncture device if signs and symptoms of infection exist.

3. T F When infusing solutions by gravity the nurse determines the drop factor, which is important in calculating the gravity infusion rate, by reading the package label.

4. T F Blood products are administered to clients who need specific blood substances but not all the fluid and cellular components in whole blood.

5. T F Vented tubing does not draw air into the container of the solution and is used for solutions packaged in plastic bags.

6. T F All nurses can administer intravenous therapy.

Activity C *Write the correct term for each description given below.*

1. The nurse will select this type of tubing to administer a small volume of solution in a relatively short time through a port in the primary tubing. _____

2. A device that exerts positive pressure to infuse solutions. _____

3. The method for gaining access to the venous system by piercing a vein with one of a variety of devices. _____

4. The veins that are used for infusing IV fluids in infants. _____

5. The type of infusions that deliver solutions into a large central vein such as the vena cava. _____

6. Administered when clients need fluid restoration as well as blood cells. _____

Activity D *Match the type of IV solution in Column A with their description in Column B.*

Column A

____ 1. Isotonic solutions

____ 2. Crystalloid solutions

____ 3. Hypotonic solutions

____ 4. Hypertonic solutions

____ 5. Colloid solutions

Column B

a. This type of solution is more concentrated (contains more dissolved substances) than plasma. Consequently, it draws fluid into the intravascular compartment from the more dilute areas in the cells and interstitial spaces.

b. This type of solution is used to replace circulating blood volume because the suspended molecules in the solutions pull fluid from other fluid compartments in the body. Examples include blood (whole blood and packed cells), blood products such as albumin, and solutions known as plasma expanders.

c. This type of solution contains fewer dissolved substances compared with plasma. Because the solution is dilute, the water in the solution passes through the semipermeable membrane of blood cells, causing them to swell.

d. This type of solution contains the same concentration of dissolved substances as is normally found in plasma. Because of its equal concentration to plasma, the solution causes no appreciable redistribution of body fluid on administration.

e. This type of solution consists of water and uniformly dissolved crystals such as salt (sodium chloride) or sugar (glucose, dextrose). Examples include 0.9% normal saline, 0.45% normal saline, and 10% dextrose in water.

Activity E *Identify the percentage of the population and compatibility types of the blood groups listed.*

	Percentage of Population	Compatible Blood Types
A		
B		
O		
AB		
Rh+		
Rh−		

Activity F *Briefly answer the following questions.*

1. Describe the indications for intravenous therapy.

_____

_____

_____

2. What are the nursing responsibilities for preparing intravenous solutions?

_____

_____

_____

3. When is filtered tubing used?

_____

_____

_____

4. What are the selection criteria for a venipuncture site?

_____

_____

_____

5. What circumstances would require a central venous access devices insertion? Why is a chest x-ray required following insertion?

_____

_____

_____

6. What is the purpose of total parenteral nutrition?

_____

_____

_____

SECTION II: APPLYING YOUR KNOWLEDGE

Activity G *Give rationale for the following questions.*

1. Why do tubing manufacturers design the drop size to deliver large-size drops (macrodrip tubing) and small-sized drops (microdrip tubing)?

_____

_____

_____

2. Why must the nurse elevate the solution 18 to 24 inches above the infusion site when infusing an IV solution by gravity?

_____

_____

_____

3. Why is venipuncture in the foot avoided?

_____

_____

_____

4. Why are midline and midclavicular catheters considered peripheral venous access devices?

_____

_____

_____

5. Why are packed red blood cells preferred over whole blood in clients with congestive heart failure?

_____

_____

_____

6. Why is a lipid emulsion sometimes administered concurrently with total parenteral nutrition?

_____

_____

_____

Activity H _Answer the following questions related to intravenous therapy._

1. Identify the nursing responsibilities when preparing a client for IV therapy.

_____

_____

_____

2. Which healthcare providers may insert a central venous access device?

_____

_____

_____

3. Identify the appropriate time frames to replace IV equipment.

_____

_____

_____

4. What complications should the nurse monitor for when caring for a client with IV therapy?

_____

_____

_____

5. What are the possible complications of a blood transfusion?

_____

_____

_____

Activity I _Think over the following questions. Discuss them with your peers or instructor._

1. Discuss the nursing interventions indicated for a client receiving IV therapy with a nursing diagnosis of risk for imbalanced fluid volume related to the rate of infusion exceeds circulatory capacity.

_____

_____

_____

2. Discuss the nursing interventions indicated for a client receiving IV therapy with a nursing diagnosis of risk for infection secondary to venipuncture and presence of a venous access device.

_____

_____

_____

3. Discuss the nursing care required for a client receiving total parenteral nutrition.

_____

_____

_____

SECTION III: GETTING READY FOR NCLEX

Activity J _Answer the following NCLEX-style questions._

1. Why should the nurse closely monitor older adults when they are receiving IV therapy?

   a. Because their defense mechanisms are less efficient.

   b. Because they are prone to fluid overload.

   c. Because they are prone to increased renal efficiency.

   d. Because they have inadequate intake of dietary fiber.

2. When a client is receiving blood, which of the following nursing actions is essential to determine if chilling is the result of an emerging complication or of infusing cold blood?

   a. Monitoring the client's temperature before, during, and after the transfusion.

   b. Documenting the client's temperature after the transfusion.

   c. Documenting the temperature of the blood before the transfusion.

   d. Comparing the client's temperature with the temperature of the blood.

3. Why should the nurse closely monitor a client to ensure that the venous access device remains in the vein during a transfusion?

   a. It minimizes the risk of phlebitis.

   b. It minimizes the risk of pulmonary embolism.

   c. It minimizes the risk of circulatory overload.

   d. It minimizes the risk of localized edema.

4. Fill in the blank: IV tubing can be used for up to _____ hours provided solution is continuously infusing through it.

5. In which of the following circumstances should a nurse avoid using midline and midclavicular sites for IV therapy?

   a. To administer solutions with a pH greater than 5 and less than 9.

   b. To administer antineoplastic chemotherapy.

   c. To administer slow, low-volume infusions.

   d. To administer solutions with an osmolality less than 500 mOsm/L.

6. Deaths have occurred when potassium chloride has been used incorrectly to flush a lock or central venous catheter. Which of the following precautions should a nurse take to minimize this risk?

   a. Use a dilute form of potassium chloride before flushing locks.

   b. Warm the potassium chloride before flushing locks.

   c. Read labels carefully on vials containing flush solutions for locks.

   d. Replace the existing locks with new ones to avoid flushing.

7. Which type of intravenous fluid draws fluid into the intravascular compartment from the more dilute areas in the cells and interstitial spaces?

   a. Isotonic fluid

   b. Hypertonic fluid

   c. Hypotonic fluid

   d. Colloid fluid

8. A nurse hangs microdrip tubing on a client who needs an IV. How many gtts per mL is delivered with microdrip tubing?

   a. 20 gtts per mL

   b. 10 gtts per mL

   c. 15 gtts per mL

   d. 60 gtts per mL

9. A client receives a central venous catheter. Which of the following is the best reason for a client to receive a central venous catheter?

   a. Client is receiving 0.9 normal saline

   b. Client is receiving total parenteral nutrition (TPN)

   c. Client is receiving short term IV therapy.

   d. Client has had one infiltrated IV.

10. A client is receiving a blood transfusion and the nurse notes that the client has the universal donor blood type. Which blood type does the client have?

    a. B

    b. A

    c. O

    d. AB

CHAPTER 14

Perioperative Care

Learning Objectives

1. Describe why surgical procedures may be performed.
2. Differentiate the phases of perioperative care.
3. Outline preoperative assessments needed to identify surgical risk factors.
4. List components of a preoperative teaching plan.
5. Describe physical preparation of the client for surgery.
6. List preoperative medications that may be ordered.
7. Discuss psychosocial preparation of the client for surgery, including strategies for alleviating clients' preoperative anxiety.
8. Compare types of anesthesia.
9. Describe the roles and functions of the surgical team members.
10. Describe nursing management of the intraoperative client.
11. Discuss assessments needed to prevent postoperative complications.
12. Describe standards of care, nursing diagnoses, and common interventions for general surgical clients in the later postoperative period.

SECTION I: ASSESSING YOUR UNDERSTANDING

Activity A *Fill in the blanks by choosing the correct word from the options given in parentheses.*

1. The _____ begins with admission to the recovery area and continues until the client receives a follow-up evaluation at home or is discharged to a rehabilitation unit. *(Preoperative phase, Intraoperative phase, Postoperative phase)*

2. The _____ is a physician who has completed 2 years of residency in anesthesia. *(Anesthesiologist, Anesthetist, First assistant)*

3. Healing by _____ occurs when the wound layers are sutured together so that wound edges are well approximated. This type of incision usually heals in 8 to 10 days, with minimal scarring. *(Primary intention, Secondary intention, Tertiary intention)*

4. Interruption of blood supply secondary to prolonged pressure, nerve injury related to prolonged pressure, postoperative hypotension, dependent edema, and joint injury may result from _____ in the OR. *(Hypothermia, Poor body alignment, Malignant hyperthermia)*

5. Postoperative pain reaches its peak between _____ hours after surgery. *(6 and 12, 12 and 36, 36 and 48)*

6. Occurs when the wound completely separates and organs protrude. *(Wound infection, Wound evisceration, Wound dehiscence)*

7. The _____ assists the surgical team by handing instruments to the surgeon and assistants, preparing sutures, receiving specimens for laboratory examination, and counting sponges and needles. *(Scrub nurse, Circulating nurse, Anesthetist)*

Activity B *Mark each statement as either "T" (True) or "F" (False). Correct any false statements.*

1. T F The intraoperative phase includes the entire surgical procedure until transfer of the client to the recovery area.

2. T F The surgeon is responsible for determining the surgical procedure required, obtaining the client's consent, performing the procedure, and following the client after surgery.

3. T F An anesthetist may be a medical doctor who administers anesthesia but has not completed a residency in anesthesia, a dentist who administers limited types of anesthesia, or a Certified Registered Nurse Anesthetist.

4. T F Medical asepsis prevents contamination of surgical wounds.

5. T F Healing by secondary intention occurs when granulating tissue fills in the wound for the healing process. The skin edges are not approximated. This method is used for ulcers and infected wounds. This type of wound healing is slow, although new products promote healing.

6. T F Complications as a result of fluid volume excess/deficit are monitored in the OR by recording client intake of IV fluid and urine output.

7. T F Malignant hyperthermia is related to the low temperature in the OR, administration of cold IV fluids, inhalation of cool gases, exposure of body surfaces for the surgical procedure, opened incisions/wounds, and prolonged inactivity.

Activity C *Write the correct term for each description given below.*

1. Danger of aspiration from saliva, mucus, vomitus, or blood exists until the client is fully awake and can swallow without difficulty. This equipment must be kept at the client's bedside until the danger of aspiration no longer exists._____

2. This phase begins with the decision to perform surgery and continues until the client reaches the operating area. _____

3. This member of the surgical team may be an RN, a licensed practical or vocational nurse (LPNs/LVNs), or a surgical technologist who assist the surgeon and first assistant. _____

4. The approximation of wound edges is delayed secondary to infection. When the wound is drained and cleaned of infection, the wound edges are sutured together. The resulting scar is wider than that with primary intention. _____

5. Separation of wound edges without the protrusion of organs. _____

6. This member of the surgical team assists in the surgical procedure and may be involved with the client's preoperative and postoperative care. He or she may be another physician, a surgical resident, or an RN who has appropriate approval and endorsement from the American Operating Room Nurses (AORN) and the American College of Surgeons. _____

Activity D *Match the preoperative medications given in Column A with the corresponding benefits given in Column B*

Column A	Column B
____ **1.** Anticholinergics	**a.** Decrease gastric acidity and volume.
____ **2.** Antianxiety drugs	**b.** Decrease respiratory tract secretions, dry mucous membranes, and interrupt vagal stimulation.
____ **3.** Histamine-2 receptor antagonists	**c.** Reduce nausea, prevent emesis, and enhance preoperative sedation.
____ **4.** Narcotics	**d.** Reduce preoperative anxiety, slow motor activity, and promote induction of anesthesia.
____ **5.** Sedatives	
____ **6.** Tranquilizers	**e.** Decrease the amount of anesthesia needed, help reduce anxiety and pain, and promote sleep.
	f. Promote sleep, decrease anxiety, and reduce the amount of anesthesia needed.

Activity E *Differentiate between the various types of surgery based on purpose and provide examples.*

Type of Surgery	Purpose	Examples
Diagnostic		
Exploratory		
Curative		
Palliative		
Cosmetic		
Preventive or prophylactic		
Reconstructive		

Activity F *Consider the following figure.*

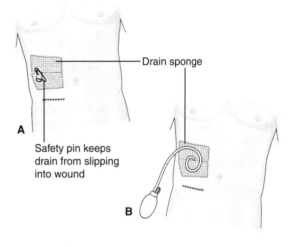

Drain sponge

A

Safety pin keeps drain from slipping into wound

B

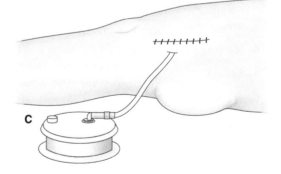

C

1. Identify the types of surgical drains.

   A._____ B._____ C._____

2. What are the assessments a nurse should perform when assessing a wound?

   _____

   _____

   _____

Activity G *Briefly answer the following questions.*

1. Identify the basic elements of a nursing pre-operative assessment.

   _____

   _____

   _____

2. The nurse identifies if the client is a risk for complications during or after surgery based on what general risk factors?

   _____

   _____

   _____

3. What is the purpose of adequate preoperative teaching/learning?

   _____

   _____

   _____

4. What is included in the physical preparation of a client for surgery?

   _____

   _____

   _____

5. What is procedural sedation?

   _____

   _____

   _____

6. Describe the responsibilities of the circulating nurse.

   _____

   _____

   _____

7. What factors may lead to hypoxia postoperatively?

   _____

   _____

   _____

SECTION II: APPLYING YOUR KNOWLEDGE

Activity H *Give rationale for the following questions:*

1. Why is it best to teach clients about their surgical procedure and expectations during the preoperative period?

2. Why should a client sign a surgical consent form or operative permit before surgery; what does it indicate?

3. Why is the air filtered and a positive pressure maintained in the surgical suite?

4. Why must shock be detected early and treated promptly in the postoperative phase?

5. Why are antiembolism stockings used postoperatively?

6. Why must the nurse inspect dressings frequently and check under the bedding of the client postoperatively?

Activity I *Answer the following questions related to perioperative care.*

1. What assessments will the nurse perform on a client admitted for surgery?

2. What information will the nurse include in preoperative teaching?

3. Describe the differences between general anesthesia and regional anesthesia.

4. Describe psychosocial preparation for the client.

5. Describe nursing management of the intraoperative client.

6. Identify the minimum standards of care for the general surgical client.

Activity J *Think over the following questions. Discuss them with your instructor or peers.*

1. A client complains of discomfort and does not want to perform deep breathing and coughing exercises, use the incentive spirometer, or ambulate. How will you proceed? What education will you provide?

_____

_____

_____

2. A client who has undergone surgery is unable to expel gas or have a bowel movement. What nursing interventions would you implement? If the nursing interventions are not effective what would you do?

_____

_____

_____

3. A client is receiving pain medication postoperatively. What safety measures would you implement to prevent client injury?

_____

_____

_____

4. A client is being discharged following a surgical procedure. What information will you need to provide to the client and/or the family?

_____

_____

_____

SECTION III: GETTING READY FOR NCLEX

Activity K *Answer the following questions.*

1. A client is hospitalized for a surgery. During the assessment, the nurse assesses that the client has not carried out a specific portion of the preoperative instructions. Which of the following nursing interventions should the nurse perform?

    a. Suggest an alternative recommendation to the instruction.

    b. Notify the surgeon.

    c. Document on the client's chart.

    d. Ask the client to implement the instructions and appear for the surgery later.

2. Which of the following are the responsibilities of a circulating nurse?

    a. Obtaining and opening wrapped sterile equipment.

    b. Preparing sutures.

    c. Handing instruments to the surgeon and assistants.

    d. Assisting with putting the client to sleep.

3. Which of the following factors may promote anxiety for a client undergoing a surgical procedure?

    a. Decreased mobility

    b. Unfamiliar environment

    c. Unclear expectations

    d. Decreased alertness

4. A nurse needs to care for a client during the immediate postoperative period. Which of the following factors predispose the client to hypoxia?

    a. Pooling of secretions in the lungs

    b. Fluid and electrolyte loss

    c. Physical and psychological trauma

    d. Increased mobility

5. Why should a nurse practice caution when changing the wound dressings of a client who underwent surgery?

    a. To avoid damaging new tissue.

    b. To avoid causing pain to the client.

    c. To fasten the wound healing.

    d. To avoid wound infection.

6. What does weight gain during the postoperative period signify?

    a. Urine retention

    b. Fluid accumulation

    c. Healthy recovery

    d. Paralytic ileus

7. Which of the following preoperative medications cause a decrease in respiratory tract secretions, dry mucous membranes, and interrupt vagal stimulation?

    a. Histamine$_2$-receptor antagonists

    b. Antianxiety drugs

    c. Anticholinergics

    d. Sedatives

8. Which type of anesthesia describes a state in which the client is free of pain, fear, and anxiety and can tolerate unpleasant procedures while maintaining independent cardiorespiratory function and the ability to respond to verbal commands and tactile stimulation?

   a. General

   b. Regional

   c. Epidural

   d. Procedural sedation

9. Which of the following postoperative complications results from saliva, mucus, vomitus, or blood making its way into the lungs as a result of difficulty in swallowing or a client's inability to rid himself/herself of oral secretions?

   a. Aspiration

   b. Hypoxia

   c. Shock

   d. Hemorrhage

10. Which of the following stages of wound healing lasts from 21 days to several months and even 1 to 2 years and allows the strength of the wound to increase through synthesis of collagen by fibroblasts and lysis by collagenase enzymes?

    a. Inflammatory stage

    b. Proliferative phase

    c. Maturation phase

    d. Approximation phase

Disaster Situations

1. Define *disaster* and give two general examples.
2. Identify three categories of human disasters that may result from acts of terrorism.
3. Name three methods by which a radiologic disaster could be created.
4. Explain the difference between external and internal radiation contamination.
5. Name three substances used to prevent or reduce radiologic organ damage.
6. List possible indications of a bioterrorism attempt.
7. Name three biologic agents likely to be used as weapons of mass destruction.
8. List possible indications of a chemical terrorism attempt.
9. Name four types of chemical agents that may be used to create a human disaster.
10. List four triage categories that emergency workers use to prioritize victims' need for treatment.
11. Provide examples of collaborative problems and nursing diagnoses that the nurse may be required to manage following a disaster.

SECTION I: ASSESSING YOUR UNDERSTANDING

Activity A *Fill in the blanks by choosing the correct word from the options given in parentheses.*

1. _____ is a disaster caused by pathogens or their toxins that cause harm to humans and other living species. (*Biological disaster, Radiologic disaster, Chemical disaster*)

2. _____ is a disease that develops from the neurotoxin produced by *Clostridium botulinum*, which is generally food-borne. There have been no reports of person-to-person transmission. (*Anthrax, Botulism, Smallpox*)

3. Laboratory studies suggest that _____, a new antiviral agent, may be effective against smallpox. (*Cidofovir, Doxycycline, Ciprofloxacin*)

4. Detection of _____ is difficult because most agents are liquids that vaporize quickly with either no odors or odors that may be attributed to other substances. (*Biological disasters, Radiologic disasters, Chemical disasters*)

5. Exposure to _____ leads to tearing, coughing, broncho- and laryngospasms with airway obstruction from localized swelling. (*Biological toxins, Respiratory toxins, Radiologic toxins*)

6. _____ occurs from exposure to fallout on the skin, hair, and clothing. (*Prussian blue, External radiologic contamination, Internal radiologic contamination*)

Activity B *Mark each statement as either "T" (True) or "F" (False). Correct any false statements.*

1. T F There are essentially two types of disasters: biological disasters and chemical disasters.

2. T F The smallpox vaccine is effective in preventing infection if administered within 12 hours of exposure to smallpox.

3. T F Blistering agents, also known as vesicants, are chemicals that damage

exposed skin and mucous membranes on contact. Inhalation of the vesicant is almost sure to cause death within 24 hours from airway obstruction with blisters within the respiratory passages.

4. **T F** Nursing skills are an essential component in the Department of Homeland Security's plan for preparing and defending the United States against the global threat of terrorism.

5. **T F** The most serious form of anthrax develops with ingestion.

Activity C *Write the correct term for each description given below.*

1. The American Red Cross define this as "A threatening ... event of such destructive magnitude and force as to dislocate people, separate family members, damage or destroy homes, and injure or kill people".
_____

2. A spore-forming bacterium known as *Bacillus anthracis*, which causes disease when inhaled, ingested, or introduced into nonintact skin. It is treated fairly successfully with fluoroquinolones. _____

3. A solid salt or volatile liquid chemical that causes death in minutes. The gas that forms with release is colorless and may have a faint odor of "bitter almonds." _____

4. This type of contamination occurs when fallout enters an open wound, is inhaled via contaminated air, or is consumed through contaminated food and water._____

5. The greatest potential for lethality occurs with paralysis of the respiratory muscles. If large numbers of people were to become acutely ill simultaneously as a consequence of bioterrorism, the numbers of ventilators available in any particular agency would likely become exhausted quickly. _____

6. A highly contagious disease caused by the variola virus. _____

Activity D *Match the antidotes or medications given in Column A, with the conditions they treat in Column B.*

Column A

___ 1. Prussian blue

Column B

a. Prevents radioactive iodine from reaching

___ 2. Pralidoxime chloride

___ 3. Potassium iodide

___ 4. Diethylenetriamine pentaacetate (DTPA)

___ 5. Atropine sulfate

___ 6. Amyl nitrite, sodium nitrite, and sodium thiosulfate

the thyroid gland by saturating the gland with nonradioactive iodine. The person must take it as soon as possible up to 24 hours after exposure. It limits or protects only the thyroid gland; it does not interfere with radiologic effects on other organs.

b. Reactivates acetylcholinesterase with exposure to nerve agents.

c. A dye used to treat internal contamination with ingested radioactive cesium. The dye promotes the excretion of cesium by trapping it in the intestine and preventing its absorption.

d. An injectable salt or inhalant spray that contains calcium (Ca-DTPA) or zinc (Zn-DTPA) and is used to treat internal contamination with radioactive substances such as plutonium.

e. May be administered alone or together as an antidote for cyanide poisoning.

f. Counteracts excess acetylcholine at muscarinic sites with exposure to nerve agents.

Activity E *Identify the triage categories based on the given criteria.*

Category	Color Coordinate	Description	Examples
Immediate			
Delayed			
Minimal			
Expectant			

Activity F *Briefly answer the following questions.*

1. Identify three types of human disasters.

_____

_____

_____

2. How can radiologic disasters occur?

_____

_____

_____

3. What are indications of bioterrorism?

_____

_____

_____

4. How can smallpox be distinguished from chickenpox?

_____

_____

_____

5. What are the indications of a chemical terrorism?

_____

_____

_____

6. What are the early signs of botulism?

_____

_____

_____

SECTION II: APPLYING YOUR KNOWLEDGE

Activity G *Give rationale for the following questions.*

1. Why do terrorists exploit actual or potential human disasters?

_____

_____

_____

2. How can radiologic disasters cause life-threatening consequences when injury is not caused by penetrating or blunt trauma?

_____

_____

_____

3. Why are anthrax, botulism, and smallpox likely to be used in bioterrorist warfare?

_____

_____

_____

4. Why are tetracyclines not used initially to treat anthrax infections?

_____

_____

_____

5. How could a person who was not directly exposed to a radiologic disaster exhibit signs and symptoms of radiologic contamination?

_____

_____

_____

Activity H *Answer the following questions related to disaster situations.*

1. What is the most immediate concern when dealing with a radiologic disaster?

_____

_____

_____

2. Describe the isolation precautions for smallpox.

_____

_____

_____

3. What are the supportive measures that should be taken with exposure to a nerve agent?

_____

_____

_____

4. Describe the signs and symptoms of cyanide poisoning.

_____

_____

_____

5. What measures should be taken with exposure to chlorine or phosgene?

_____

_____

_____

6. Describe the decontamination process for exposure to a vesicant.

_____

_____

_____

Activity I *Think over the following questions. Discuss them with your instructor or peers.*

1. There has been an accidental explosion at a chemical plant near your facility. You have been assigned to triage the victims. Describe the precautions you would take and the care you would provide to each of the following victims:

- Casualty A – this victim was close to the blast and has sustained partial and full-thickness burns over 85% of their body, respirations are shallow, and pulse is thready.
- Casualty B – this victim has an obvious fracture to the left forearm and some tearing from exposure to the chemicals. This victim has no coughing and states they have no difficulty breathing.
- Casualty C – this victim has no tearing, coughing or difficulty breathing. The victim has some minor lacerations and is emotionally distraught; casualty A is this person's spouse.
- Casualty D – this victim was not exposed to the blast but was exposed to the chemicals escaping from the receptacles. The victim has no obvious signs of trauma but is repeatedly coughing and gasping for breath.

_____

_____

_____

SECTION III: GETTING READY FOR NCLEX

Activity J *Answer the following questions:*

1. When caring for a client exposed to cyanide, which of the following antidotes that the nurse administers is an inhalant to convert cyanide into a nontoxic substance?
- **a.** Methemoglobin
- **b.** Sodium nitrite
- **c.** Amyl nitrite
- **d.** Sodium thiosulfate

2. Why is it important for a nurse to move a victim of a common respiratory toxin to higher ground immediately?
- **a.** The toxins flow to the lower ground.
- **b.** The toxic vapors stay close to the ground.
- **c.** The toxins are always released close to the ground.
- **d.** The heavy and the solid toxins cannot move to a height.

3. What type of contamination is the nurse trying to eliminate when he or she requests people to remove all garments before entering a house or shelter?
- **a.** Internal radiologic contamination
- **b.** External vesicant contamination
- **c.** External radioactive contamination
- **d.** Cross-contamination

4. A client who is under treatment for cesium contamination complains about blue feces. How should the nurse explain the reason to the client?
- **a.** Radiation tends to cause the change in color.
- **b.** Cesium is blue when eliminated from the body.
- **c.** Prussian blue causes the blue feces.
- **d.** It is a sign of intestinal radiation poisoning.

5. Anthrax is not transmitted from human to human. Yet why does the nurse advise a client with painless lesions, after exposure to anthrax, to avoid contact with others?
- **a.** So the client is not exposed to pathogens.
- **b.** Because the sight of the lesions may cause distress and panic.

  c. Because the lesions may release more spores.

  d. Skin infection is one form of anthrax that spreads by direct contact.

6. What is the main drawback of the botulism antitoxin that the nurse should be aware of?

  a. It causes 9% hypersensitivity.

  b. It requires monthly booster dosages.

  c. It is not available from the CDC.

  d. It is not available as a pre-exposure vaccine.

7. What is one of the ways to limit external contamination?

  a. Stay indoors and go to a centrally located room or basement with as few windows as possible.

  b. Cover the mouth and nose with a scarf, handkerchief, or other cloth.

  c. Drink only bottled water.

  d. Consume canned, dried, and packaged food products.

8. Which of the following biological agents has a vaccine readily available but it is only used for military and at risk civilians?

  a. Botulism

  b. Anthrax

  c. Smallpox

  d. Influenza

9. Which type of agent does sulfur mustard fall under?

  a. Nerve agents

  b. Blistering agents

  c. Respiratory toxins

  d. Cyanide poisonings

10. Which of the following triage assessments prioritizes the client's need for treatment as the need to be seen now?

  a. Delayed

  b. Immediate

  c. Minimal

  d. Expectant

CHAPTER 16

Caring for Clients with Fluid, Electrolyte, and Acid-Base Imbalances

Learning Objectives

1. List three chemical substances that are components of body fluid.
2. Name the two main fluid locations in the human body and two subdivisions.
3. Give the average fluid intake per day for adults.
4. List four ways in which the body normally loses fluid.
5. Identify five processes by which water and dissolved chemicals are relocated in the body.
6. Name three mechanisms that help regulate fluid and electrolyte balance.
7. List two types of fluid imbalance.
8. Explain the difference between hypovolemia and dehydration.
9. Explain hemoconcentration and hemodilution.
10. Identify assessment findings of and nursing interventions for hypovolemia.
11. List and identify the differences in three types of edema.
12. Identify assessment findings of and nursing interventions for hypervolemia.
13. Explain third-spacing and medical techniques for relocating this fluid.
14. List factors that contribute to electrolyte loss and excess.
15. Name four electrolyte imbalances that pose a major threat to well-being.
16. Discuss the nursing management of clients with electrolyte imbalances.
17. Discuss the role of acids and bases in body fluid.
18. Explain pH and identify the normal range of plasma pH.
19. Identify two chemicals and two organs that play major roles in regulating acid-base balance.
20. Give the names of two major acid-base imbalances and subdivisions of each.
21. List three components of arterial blood gas findings used to determine acid-base imbalances.
22. Discuss the nursing management of clients with acid-base imbalances.

SECTION I: ASSESSING YOUR UNDERSTANDING

Activity A *Fill in the blanks by choosing the correct word from the options given in parentheses.*

1. _____ can occur with severe renal failure; severe burns; administration of potassium-sparing diuretics; overuse of potassium supplements, salt substitutes or some diet sodas, or potassium-rich foods; crushing injuries; Addison's disease; and rapid administration of parenteral potassium salts.
(Hypercalemia, Hypernatremia, Hyperkalemia)

2. _____ are substances that carry an electrical charge when dissolved in fluid. *(Electrolytes, Acids, Bases)*

3. About 60% of the adult human body is water. Most body water is located in _____. *(Intravascular fluid, Intracellular fluid, Interstitial fluid)*

4. The power to draw water toward an area of greater concentration is referred to as _____. *(Filtration, Tonicity, Osmotic pressure)*

5. Hypovolemia results in _____, a high ratio of blood components in relation to watery plasma, which increases the potential for blood clots and urinary stones and compromises the kidney's ability to excrete nitrogen wastes. *(Hemodilution, Hypervolemia, Hemoconcentration)*

6. _____ is associated with parathyroid gland tumors, multiple fractures, Paget's disease, hyperparathyroidism, excessive doses of vitamin D, prolonged immobilization, some chemotherapeutic agents, and certain malignant diseases. *(Hypercalcemia, Hyperkalemia, Hypernatremia)*

7. In healthy adults, oral fluid intake averages about 2500 mL/day; however, it can range between _____ with a similar volume of fluid loss. *(1800 to 3000mL/day, 2000 to 3000mL/day, 1500 to 3500mL/day)*

8. Normal plasma pH is _____, or slightly alkaline. *(7 which is neutral, 7.35 to 7.45, 1 to 14)*

Activity B *Mark each statement as either "T" (True) or "F" (False). Correct any false statements.*

1. T F Causes of hypocalcemia include vitamin D deficiency, hypoparathyroidism, severe burns, acute pancreatitis, certain drugs such as corticosteroids, rapid administration of multiple units of blood that contain an anticalcium additive, intestinal malabsorption disorders, and accidental surgical removal of the parathyroid glands.

2. T F Bases are substances that release hydrogen into fluid.

3. T F Extracellular fluid is body water outside the cells and includes the water between cells (interstitial fluid) and in the plasma (intravascular fluid).

4. T F The heart and lungs facilitate the ratio of bicarbonate to carbonic acid.

5. T F Hemodilution, a reduced ratio of blood components to watery plasma, is a diagnostic finding with hypervolemia.

6. T F Edema in body areas most affected by gravity, such as the feet, ankles, and sacrum (or buttocks in clients confined to bed), is referred to as generalized edema.

7. T F An imbalance in acids or bases is life-threatening. Death occurs quickly if plasma pH is outside the range of 6.8 to 8.0.

Activity C *Write the correct term for each description given below.*

1. Positively or negatively charged substances. _____

2. As excess fluid volume is distributed to the interstitial space, indentations in the skin after compression may be noted. This type of edema usually does not occur, however, until there is a 3-liter excess in the intravascular volume. _____

3. The concentration of substances in blood. _____

4. Causes include profuse watery diarrhea, excessive salt intake without sufficient water intake, high fever, decreased water intake, excessive administration of solutions that contain sodium, excessive water loss without an accompanying loss of sodium, and severe burns. _____

5. Positively charged ion. _____

6. This electrolyte imbalance may result from renal failure, Addison's disease, excessive use of antacids or laxatives that contain magnesium, and hyperparathyroidism. _____

7. The main tool for measuring blood pH, CO_2 content ($PaCO_2$), and bicarbonate. _____

8. Negatively charged ion. _____

Activity D *Match the terms given in Column A with their related descriptions given in Column B.*

Column A

_____ **1.** Osmosis

_____ **2.** Filtration

_____ **3.** Passive diffusion

_____ **4.** Facilitated diffusion

_____ **5.** Active transport

Column B

a. Promotes the movement of fluid and some dissolved substances through a semipermeable membrane according to pressure differences.

b. Certain dissolved substances require assistance from a carrier molecule to pass through a semipermeable membrane.

c. The movement of water through a semipermeable membrane from a dilute area to a more concentrated area.

d. Requires an energy source, a substance called adenosine triphosphate (ATP), to drive dissolved chemicals from an area of low concentration to an area of higher concentration.

e. A physiologic process by which dissolved substances (e.g., electrolytes) move from an area of high concentration to an area of lower concentration through a semipermeable membrane.

Activity E *Identify the mechanisms of fluid and electrolyte regulation based on the given criteria.*

Mechanism	How Change is Detected	Regulating Action
Osmoreceptors		
Baroreceptors		
Renin-Angiotensin-Aldosterone System		
Natriuretic peptides		

Activity F *Briefly answer the following questions.*

1. What are the mechanisms of fluid loss?

_____

_____

_____

2. Describe the difference between hypovolemia and dehydration.

_____

_____

_____

3. Describe conditions that place the client at risk for developing hyponatremia?

_____

_____

_____

4. What are causes of hypervolemia?

_____

_____

_____

5. What is third-spacing? What is it associated with?

_____

_____

_____

6. What is responsible for electrical potentials that develop across cell membranes and perhaps for the degree of cell membrane permeability?

_____

_____

_____

7. What two signs can be used to assess for hypocalcemia?

_____

_____

_____

SECTION II: APPLYING YOUR KNOWLEDGE

Activity G *Give rationale for the following questions.*

1. Why is dehydration the most common fluid imbalance in older adults?

_____

_____

_____

2. How do colloids contribute to fluid concentration and act as a force for attracting water?

_____

_____

_____

3. Why is the forehead or sternum used to assess fluid status in older adults?

_____

_____

_____

4. Why should potassium never be administered in a concentrated strength by IV?

_____

_____

_____

5. Why are older adults at risk for developing electrolyte imbalances?

_____

_____

_____

6. Why is the client closely monitored when administering magnesium sulfate IV?

_____

_____

_____

Activity H *Answer the following questions related to fluid, electrolyte, and acid-base imbalances.*

1. How do chemical regulators in the body maintain acid-base balance?

_____

_____

_____

2. What conditions place the client at risk for developing hypomagnesemia?

_____

_____

_____

3. How do the lungs and kidneys facilitate the ratio of bicarbonate to carbonic acid?

_____

_____

_____

4. Describe the medical management of third-spacing.

_____

_____

_____

5. What conditions place the client at risk for developing hypokalemia?

_____

_____

_____

6. Identify the types and subtypes of acid-base imbalances.

_____

_____

_____

Activity I *Think over the following questions. Discuss them with your instructor or peers.*

1. Laboratory results for your client include elevated hematocrit and blood cell counts, and the urine specific gravity is high. Your client has been experiencing excessive thirst. What do these assessment findings indicate? What nursing assessments and interventions are indicated?

_____

_____

_____

2. Assessment of your client reveals an elevated BP, an increased breathing effort, and pitting edema. Laboratory results include a decreased blood cell count, a decreased hematocrit, and the urine specific gravity is low. What nursing assessments and interventions are indicated?

_____

_____

_____

SECTION III: GETTING READY FOR NCLEX

Activity J *Answer the following questions:*

1. For which of the following conditions would the use of salt tablets be considered?
   a. Mild deficits of serum sodium
   b. Severe deficits of serum magnesium
   c. Severe deficits of serum potassium
   d. Severe deficits of serum calcium

2. If a client's parathyroid glands were accidentally removed during a procedure, which condition should the nurse prepare for?
   a. Hypomagnesemia
   b. Hyperkalemia
   c. Hypernatremia
   d. Hypocalcemia

3. Which of the following vitamins does a client lack if there is a problem with the absorption of calcium?
   a. Vitamin A
   b. Vitamin B
   c. Vitamin C
   d. Vitamin D

4. Which of the following points should a nurse include in the teaching plan for clients who have a potential for hypovolemia?
   a. Avoid alcohol and caffeine.
   b. Increase intake of dried peas and beans.
   c. Increase intake of milk and dairy products.
   d. Avoid table salt or food containing sodium.

5. A pregnant client with hypertension and cardiac dysrhythmias is admitted in the hospital. Which of the following imbalances should the nurse check for?
   a. Metabolic acidosis
   b. Hypomagnesemia
   c. Hypernatremia
   d. Hypercalcemia

6. Which of the following values pertaining to different clients shows the normal range of plasma pH?
   a. 7.35 to 7.45
   b. 6.35 to 6.45
   c. 7 to 8
   d. 8.35 to 8.45

7. Which of the following processes is defined as the movement of fluid and some dissolved substances through a semipermeable membrane according to pressure differences?
   a. Osmosis
   b. Diffusion
   c. Active Transport
   d. Filtration

8. Which of the following symptoms is the first one to occur in hypovolemia?
   a. Hypotension
   b. Thirst
   c. Central venous pressure below 2 to 3 mmHg
   d. Urine specfic gravity high

9. Which of the following nursing diagnoses is appropriate for a client on a fluid restriction?
   a. Excess fluid volume related to intake that exceeds fluid loss
   b. Altered comfort: dry mouth and thirst related to restricted oral fluid
   c. Risk for impaired skin integrity related to compromised circulation secondary to edema
   d. Fluid volume deficit secondary to dehydration

10. Which of the following can be a cause of hyperkalemia?
    a. Severe burns
    b. Renal stones
    c. Overuse of salt
    d. Underuse of potassium supplements

Caring for Clients in Shock

1. Define shock.
2. Name four general categories of shock.
3. Identify the subcategories of distributive shock.
4. List pathophysiologic consequences of shock.
5. Name the three stages of shock.
6. Identify three physiologic mechanisms that attempt to compensate for shock.
7. Discuss signs and symptoms manifested by clients in shock.
8. Name three diagnostic measurements used when monitoring clients in shock.
9. Give three medical approaches for treating shock.
10. List complications of shock.
11. Discuss the nursing management of clients with shock.

SECTION I: ASSESSING YOUR UNDERSTANDING

Activity A *Fill in the blanks by choosing the correct word from the options given in parentheses.*

1. The most common type of shock; the volume of extracellular fluid is significantly diminished, primarily because of lost or reduced blood or plasma. *(Hypovolemic shock, Distributive shock, Cardiogenic shock)*

2. In shock the partial pressure of oxygen in arterial blood falls below _____. *(40 mm Hg, 60 mm Hg, 80 mm Hg)*

3. _____ is the pressure of the blood in the right atrium or venae cavae. It distinguishes relationships among hemodynamic variables in shock: venous return, quality of right ventricular function, and vascular tone. *(Pulmonary artery pressure, Arterial blood gas, Central venous pressure)*

4. Drugs with this activity increase peripheral vascular resistance and raise BP. _____ *(Alpha-adrenergic activity, Beta-adrenergic activity, IV fluids)*

5. In shock, the pulse pressure tends to _____ as the falling systolic pressure nears the diastolic pressure. *(Widen, Narrow, Falter)*

6. Capillary filling longer than three seconds and cyanosis, especially of the nailbeds, lips, and earlobes, indicates _____. *(Fluid deficiency, Electrolyte deficiency, Oxygen deficiency)*

Activity B *Mark each statement as either "T" (True) or "F" (False). Correct any false statements.*

1. T F Obstructive shock occurs when heart contraction is ineffective, which reduces cardiac output (the volume of blood ejected from the left ventricle per minute).

2. T F The irreversible stage of shock occurs when significant cells and organs become damaged. The client no longer responds to medical interventions and multiple systems begin to fail.

3. T F Arterial blood gas (ABG), central venous pressure, and pulmonary artery pressure measurements can support a diagnosis of shock and are also used to monitor response to treatment.

4. T F An IV fluid ratio of 2:1; that is, 2 liters of fluid is administered for every 1 liter of fluid lost, is usually administered to restore intravascular volume.

5. T F With the possible exception of septic shock, subnormal body temperature is a characteristic of the different types of shocks.

6. T F Mechanical devices used in the treatment of cardiogenic shock include the intra-aortic balloon pump (IABP) and ventricular assist device (VAD).

Activity C *Write the correct term for each description given below.*

1. A life-threatening condition that occurs when arterial blood flow and oxygen delivery to tissues and cells are inadequate. This condition develops as a consequence of one of three events: (1) blood volume decreases, (2) the heart fails as an effective pump, or (3) peripheral blood vessels massively dilate.

_____

2. This type of shock is sometimes called normovolemic shock because the amount of fluid in the circulatory system is not reduced, yet the fluid circulation does not permit effective tissue perfusion. _____

3. This diagnostic measurement is used because left ventricular function is more pertinent to circulation than the right. Knowing fluid pressures on the left side of the heart is more meaningful. _____

4. These drugs are the main medications used to treat shock. _____

5. Any condition that fills this cavity with fluid, air, or tissue can lead to obstructive shock.

_____

6. Drugs with this type of activity increase heart rate and improve the force of heart contraction. _____

Activity D *Match the physiologic mechanisms of compensation in Column A with their specific effects in Column B:*

Column A

____ 1. Catecholamines (epinephrine and norepinephrine)

____ 2. Aldosterone

____ 3. Glucocorticoids

____ 4. Angiotensin II

____ 5. Antidiuretic hormone (also known as vasopressin)

Column B

a. Helps the body respond to stress.

b. Eventually produced via the renin-angiotensin-aldosterone system; which is a potent vasoconstrictor that raises blood pressure.

c. Low blood volume stimulates the pituitary to secrete this hormone; which promotes reabsorption of water that the kidneys would ordinarily excrete.

d. Neurotransmitters that increase in heart rate and myocardial contractility. Venous return to the right atrium subsequently increases, as does blood sent to the lungs. Bronchial dilatation increases the amount of oxygenated air entering the lungs, followed by a more efficient exchange of oxygen and carbon dioxide (CO_2).

e. Angiotensin II stimulates the hypothalamus to signal the adrenal cortex via the pituitary gland to release this mineralocorticoid; which promotes reabsorption of sodium and water by the kidney, which serves to increase blood volume.

Activity E *The steps of cellular hypoxia are in random order. Arrange the steps in proper sequence.*

1. Sodium and water enter the cells, potassium exits the cell and the cells eventually rupture.

2. Pyruvic and lactic acid increases, causing metabolic acidosis.

3. A decreased amount of oxygen reaches the cells.

4. Lysosomes leak enzymatic fluid and contribute to further cellular destruction.

5. Hypoxic cells are forced to switch to anaerobic metabolism.

6. Without an energy source the sodium-potassium pump is ineffective.

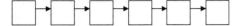

Activity F *Differentiate among the types of distributive shock based on the given criteria.*

	Occurrence	Causes	Physiologic Response
Neurogenic Shock			
Septic Shock			
Anaphylactic Shock			

Activity G *Briefly answer the following questions.*

1. What situations can cause hypovolemic shock?

_____

_____

_____

2. Following cellular hypoxia, as the decompensation stage progresses, coagulation defects occur. Describe these events.

_____

_____

_____

3. What are often the first sign of inadequate oxygen delivery to the tissues?

_____

_____

4. What cardiovascular changes occur during the decompensation phase of shock?

_____

_____

_____

5. How are respirations affected during shock?

_____

_____

_____

SECTION II: APPLYING YOUR KNOWLEDGE

Activity H *Give rationale for the following questions.*

1. Why is administration of whole blood or packed RBCs best in cases of hemorrhage or if the hemoglobin level is 70 g/L or less?

_____

_____

_____

2. Why is the use of PASGs and MAST controversial?

_____

_____

_____

3. Why does the systolic and diastolic blood pressure fall during shock?

_____

_____

_____

4. Why is activity restricted to total rest during shock?

_____

_____

_____

5. Why would a client's recovery from shock be tenuous?

_____

_____

_____

Activity I *Answer the following questions that related to caring for clients in shock.*

1. How are pulse rate, volume, and rhythm used to identify the severity of shock and estimate the approximate reduction in blood volume?

_____

_____

_____

2. What factors lead to decreased urine output during shock?

_____

_____

_____

3. What changes are seen in the skin during shock?

_____

_____

_____

4. Describe nursing management of clients with impending or actual shock.

_____

_____

_____

5. What are the criteria for diagnosing systemic inflammatory response syndrome?

_____

_____

_____

Activity J *Think over the following questions. Discuss them with your peers or instructors.*

1. A client is brought into the emergency department with acute hemorrhagic blood loss. Blood pressure is 85/45, heart rate 118, respirations 30, oxygen saturation 93%, temperature 97.7. Skin is cool; the client drifts in and out of consciousness. A foley catheter is inserted, there is no urine return.

   a. What type of shock is the client experiencing?

   b. What stage of shock is the client experiencing?

   c. What are the priority medical interventions?

   d. What are the priority nursing diagnoses?

   e. What are the priority nursing interventions?

SECTION III: GETTING READY FOR NCLEX

Activity K *Answer the following questions.*

1. A client in shock has been prescribed dopamine or a vasopressor and IV fluid therapy. Which of the following would be the best time for the administration of dopamine?

   a. Before fluid therapy

   b. After fluid therapy

   c. When the client's PAP ranges from 20 to 30 mm Hg systolic

   d. When the client's PCWP ranges from 4 to 12 mm Hg

2. During the assessment of a client in shock, the nurse observes the conditions of hypotension, bradycardia, confusion, lethargy, decreased urine production, cold, pale skin, and reduced peristalsis. In which stage of shock is the client?

   a. Initial stage

   b. Compensatory stage

   c. Decompensation stage

   d. Irreversible stage.

3. Which of the following is an important nursing assessment specific to cases of suspected cardiogenic shock?

   a. Measure the client's urine output.

   b. Auscultate the client's chest for abnormal lung and heart sounds.

   c. Check the client's laboratory test results for evidence of low RBCs and hemoglobin.

   d. Check the client's laboratory test results for evidence of elevated white blood cell count.

4. Fill in the blank: If the SpO$_2$ level is above 90%, it can be assumed that the PaO$_2$ is ___ mm Hg or above.

5. Which of the following characteristics is the reason why older adults are more likely to develop hypovolemic shock?
   a. Low-activity lifestyle
   b. Altered cardiac function
   c. Decreased percentage of body water
   d. Decline in muscle strength and bone mass

6. What kind of condition could predispose a client to shock?
   a. The kidneys work improperly.
   b. The heart fails as an effective pump.
   c. Peripheral blood vessels massively constrict.
   d. Blood volume increases.

7. In hypovolemic shock, what volume of fluid loss causes a client to undergo marked deterioration?
   a. 30% to 40% (1500 mL to 2000 mL)
   b. 15% to 30% (750 mL to 1500 mL)
   c. 10% to 15% (500 mL to 750 mL)
   d. More than 40% (more than 2000 mL)

8. Which of the following types of shock has the highest mortality rate?
   a. Neurogenic shock
   b. Anaphylactic shock
   c. Hypovolemic shock
   d. Septic shock

9. Which of the following drugs are used to treat shock in MI, trauma, septicemia, renal failure, and cardiac decompensation?
   a. Dopamine
   b. Digoxin
   c. Epinephrine
   d. Dobutamine

10. Which of the following are life threatening complications of shock?
    a. Catheter infection
    b. Pulmonary edema
    c. Kidney failure
    d. Stasis ulcers

CHAPTER 18

Caring for Clients with Cancer

Learning Objectives

1. Discuss the pathophysiology and etiology of cancer.
2. Compare benign and malignant tumors.
3. Name factors that contribute to the development of cancer.
4. Identify the warning signs of cancer.
5. Describe ways to reduce risks of cancer.
6. Explain methods for diagnosing cancer.
7. Describe systems for staging and grading malignant tumors.
8. Differentiate various treatments and methods for managing cancer.
9. Discuss various adverse effects that occur with cancer treatments and methods used to treat those effects.
10. Describe emotions associated with the diagnosis of cancer.
11. Use the nursing process as a framework for caring for clients with cancer.

SECTION I: ASSESSING YOUR UNDERSTANDING

Activity A *Fill in the blanks by choosing the correct word from the options given in parentheses.*

1. The _____ is the area where malignant cells first form. *(Primary site, Secondary site, Tertiary site)*

2. A surgical procedure when the entire tumor cannot be removed but as much of it as possible is removed is referred to as _____. *(Cytoreductive surgery, Primary treatment, Salvage surgery)*

3. _____ carcinogens include prolonged exposures to sunlight, radiation, and pollutants. *(Chemical, Environmental, Unavoidable)*

4. _____ surgery may be done after extensive surgery to correct defects caused by the original surgery. *(Mohs, Laser, Reconstructive)*

Activity B *Mark each statement as either "T" (True) or "F" (False). Correct any false statements.*

1. T F Benign tumors usually do not cause death unless their location impairs the function of a vital organ, such as the brain.

2. T F Prophylactic or preventive surgery is done when there is a local recurrence of cancer.

3. T F Breast, lung, and colon cancer most commonly affect men.

4. T F Viruses and bacteria are implicated in many cancers. The cell changes that a virus incorporates into the genetic information may cause cancerous cells to form.

5. T F Cancer is the third leading cause of death in the United States; one half of all women and one fourth of all men will develop cancer during their lives.

6. T F Cryosurgery uses electric current to destroy tumor cells.

Activity C *Write the correct term for each description given below.*

1. When tumors are confined and have not invaded vital organs, the surgery is more likely to be curative. _____

2. These types of carcinogens are believed to account for 75% of all cancers. Examples include tobacco, asbestos, coal dust, pesticides and formaldehydes. _____

3. When radioisotopes are used to treat cancer, what three safety principles must always be kept in mind? _____

4. Surgery that helps to relieve uncomfortable symptoms or prolong life. _____

5. Specialized tests that identify specific proteins, antigens, hormones, genes, or enzymes that cancer cells release. _____

6. A type of surgery that involves shaving off one thin layer of skin, layer-by-layer. Each layer is examined microscopically. Surgery ends when all cells look normal. _____

Activity D *Match the terms in column A with their related descriptions in Column B.*

Column A

_____ **1.** Neoplasm (tumor)

_____ **2.** Carcinoma

_____ **3.** Lymphoma

_____ **4.** Leukemia

_____ **5.** Sarcoma

_____ **6.** Benign

_____ **7.** Malignant

Column B

a. Cancers originating from organs that fight infection.

b. Not invasive or spreading; remain at their site of development.

c. New growths of abnormal tissue.

d. Invasive and capable of spreading; likely to metastasize.

e. Cancers originating from organs that form blood.

f. Cancers originating from epithelial cells.

g. Cancers originating from connective tissue, such as bone or muscle.

Activity E *Compare the non-surgical treatments of cancer based on the given criteria.*

Treatment	Location/ Source	Method	Outcome
External Radiation Therapy			
Internal Radiation Therapy			
Chemotherapy			
Stem Cell Transplantation			
Immunotherapy			
Hyperthermia			
Photodynamic Therapy			
Gene Therapy			
Apoptosis			

Activity F *Briefly answer the following questions.*

1. Describe the difference between normal and abnormal cell growth.

_____

_____

_____

2. How can malignant cancers metastasize?

_____

_____

_____

3. How do cancer cells develop?

_____

_____

_____

4. What is laser surgery?

_____

_____

_____

5. What is the TNM classification grading system?

_____

_____

_____

6. Explain cell differentiation and how it relates to prognosis.

_____

_____

_____

SECTION II: APPLYING YOUR KNOWLEDGE

Activity G _Give rationale for the following questions._

1. How are genetic factors linked to cancer?

_____

_____

_____

2. When a malignant tumor is removed, why is a lymph node dissection usually done, along with a wide excision of the tumor?

_____

_____

_____

3. Why are the lungs, liver, and kidneys most affected by chemical carcinogens?

_____

_____

_____

4. How is diet related to cancer?

_____

_____

_____

5. Why are epithelial tissue, hair follicles, and bone marrow most susceptible to the adverse effects of chemotherapy? Which common adverse effects are associated with this susceptibility?

_____

_____

_____

Activity H _Answer the following questions related to caring for the client with cancer._

1. How is the immune system a factor in the prevention or development of cancer?

_____

_____

_____

2. What are the seven warning signals of cancer?

_____

_____

_____

3. What are healthy lifestyle habits that reduce the risk of cancer?

_____

_____

_____

4. What types of diagnostic findings contribute to the diagnosis of cancer?

_____

_____

_____

5. What are the expected side effects of radiation therapy? Why do clients experience chronic or long-term side effects after completing therapy?

_____

_____

_____

6. What is the focus of client and family teaching for the client diagnosed with cancer?

_____

_____

_____

7. What nursing management is involved in caring for terminally ill client?

_____

_____

_____

Activity I *Think over the following questions. Discuss them with your instructor or peers.*

1. A client is receiving sealed brachytherapy. What precaution would you take to protect the client, yourself, and others who may come in contact with the client?

   _____

   _____

   _____

2. A client is receiving chemotherapy. What are priority nursing diagnoses for this client? What will you include in client and family teaching?

   _____

   _____

   _____

3. A client has been diagnosed with cancer and has a poor prognosis. What psychosocial nursing diagnoses would you anticipate? What nursing interventions would you use to provide support for the client and the client's family?

   _____

   _____

   _____

SECTION III: GETTING READY FOR NCLEX

Activity J *Answer the following questions.*

1. Which of the following diet modification may be recommended to reduce the risk of cancer?
   a. Increased intake of red meat
   b. Decreased intake of fiber
   c. Increased intake of processed meat
   d. Increased intake of vegetables such as broccoli and cabbage

2. Which of the following instructions does the nurse provide to clients receiving radiation therapy?
   a. Report when there is difficulty with swallowing
   b. Report when there are mood swings
   c. Report when there is a loss of appetite
   d. Report when there are sleep disorders

3. Which of the following types of surgery uses liquid nitrogen to freeze tissue and destroys cells?
   a. Electrosurgery
   b. Laser
   c. Cryosurgery
   d. Chemosurgery

4. Which of the following is a nursing intervention when managing clients receiving radiation therapy?
   a. Monitor clients for signs of bone marrow suppression.
   b. Monitor clients for dehydration.
   c. Monitor clients for insufficient urine output.
   d. Monitor clients for signs of bone marrow depression.

5. Which of the following safety measures must the nurse implement to minimize radiation effects when working with clients who have just undergone radiation therapy?
   a. Wear a special uniform to block radiation.
   b. Do not attend the client for the first 14 hours.
   c. Wear a face mask and gloves.
   d. Limit time spent with the client.

6. Which of the following is an important nursing intervention when managing clients receiving a bone marrow transplant?
   a. Monitor clients for signs of elevated urine specific gravity.
   b. Monitor clients for signs of infection.
   c. Monitor clients for signs of elevated blood urea nitrogen.
   d. Monitor clients for signs of elevated blood pressure.

7. Which of the following tumor classification cancers originate from connective tissue, such as bone or muscle?
   a. Lymphomas
   b. Leukemias
   c. Carcinomas
   d. Sarcomas

8. A client comes to the nurse practitioner's office with some concerns that have persisted over the course of the last six months. The nurse practitioner is concerned that the client has not had regular check ups as a means of catching any abnormalities early. Which of the following are early warning signs and symptoms of cancer?

   a. Fibrocystic breast disease

   b. Yeast infection

   c. Stasis ulcers

   d. A change in a wart or mole

9. Which of the following diagnostic tests done for clients with cancer provides three-dimensional cross-sectional views of tissues to determine tumor density, shape, size, volume, and location, as well as highlighting blood vessels that feed the tumor?

   a. Nuclear scans

   b. Computed tomography

   c. Ultrasound

   d. Fluoroscopy

10. Which of the following stages of cancer do not provide a good prognosis for the client?

    a. Stage II

    b. Stage 0

    c. Stage IV

    d. Stage III

CHAPTER 19

Introduction to the Respiratory System

Learning Objectives

1. Describe the structures of the upper and lower airways.
2. Explain the normal physiology of the respiratory system.
3. Differentiate respiration, ventilation, diffusion, and perfusion.
4. Describe oxygen transport.
5. Define forces that interfere with breathing, including airway resistance and lung compliance.
6. Identify elements of a respiratory assessment.
7. List diagnostic tests that may be performed on the respiratory tract.
8. Discuss preparation and care of clients having respiratory diagnostic procedures

SECTION I: ASSESSING YOUR UNDERSTANDING

Activity A *Fill in the blanks by choosing the correct word from the options given in parentheses.*

1. _____ secreted from the nasal mucosa traps small particles. *(Mucus, Conchae, Cilia)*

2. The _____ transports air from the laryngeal pharynx to the bronchi and lungs. *(Trachea, Oropharynx, Nasopharynx)*

3. Stimulating the carina causes _____. *(Sneezing, Coughing, Aspiration)*

4. The _____ are extensions of the nasal cavity located in the surrounding facial bones. *(Frontal sinuses, Sphenoidal sinuses, Paranasal sinuses)*

5. The _____ contains the adenoids and openings of the eustachian tubes. *(Nasopharynx, Oropharynx, Laryngeal pharynx)*

6. The _____ are paired elastic structures enclosed by the thoracic cage which contain the alveoli. *(Bronchi, Lungs, Vocal cords)*

7. _____ are discrete sounds that result from the delayed opening of deflated airways. *(Crackles, Wheezes, Friction rubs)*

Activity B *Mark each statement as either "T" (True) or "F" (False). Correct any false statements.*

1. T F The vascular and ciliated mucous lining of the nasal cavities warms and humidifies inspired air.

2. T F Immunoglobulin A (IgA) antibodies in the mucus protect the upper respiratory tract from infection.

3. T F The turbinates have a large, moist, and warm mucous-membrane surface that can trap almost all dust and microorganisms. They also contain sensitive nerves that detect odors or induce sneezing to remove irritating particles, such as dust or soot.

4. **T F** The tonsils and adenoids protect the lower airway from foreign objects because they facilitate coughing.

5. **T F** Type II cells present in the epithelium of the alveoli produce elastic and collagen fibers.

6. **T F** Disturbances in pH that involve the lungs are considered metabolic.

7. **T F** Wheezes result from air passing through narrowed or partially obstructed air passages and are heard in clients with increased secretions.

Activity C *Write the correct term for each description given below.*

1. These fine hairs move the mucus to the back of the throat. This movement helps prevent irritation to and contamination of the lower airway. _____

2. This is an important structure in the larynx; it is a cartilaginous valve flap that covers the opening to the larynx during swallowing.
_____

3. These cells are located within the epithelium of the alveoli; they destroy foreign material such as bacteria. _____

4. Bones that change the flow of inspired air to moisturize and warm it better. _____

5. The area of the pharynx that contains the tongue. _____

6. The ratio that indicates the effectiveness of airflow within the alveoli and the adequacy of gas exchange within the pulmonary capillaries. _____

7. Adventitious breath sounds heard as crackling or grating sounds on inspiration or expiration. They occur when the pleural surfaces are inflamed and do not change if the client coughs. _____

Activity D *Match the diagnostic tests in column A with the corresponding descriptions in column B.*

Column A

____ **1.** Arterial blood gases

____ **2.** Pulmonary function studies

____ **3.** Sputum studies

____ **4.** Pulse oximetry

____ **5.** Pulmonary angiography

____ **6.** Lung scans

____ **7.** Radiography

____ **8.** Bronchoscopy

Column B

a. Examined for pathogenic microorganisms and cancer cells. Culture and sensitivity tests are done to diagnose infections and prescribe antibiotics.

b. A radioisotope study that allows the physician to assess the arterial circulation of the lungs, particularly to detect pulmonary emboli.

c. Measure the functional ability of the lungs.

d. Determine the blood's pH, oxygen-carrying capacity, and levels of oxygen, CO_2, and bicarbonate ion.

e. Allows for direct visualization of the larynx, trachea, and bronchi.

f. Used for diagnostic purposes, such as: to diagnose lung cancer, COPD, Pulmonary edema, and evaluate malignancies.

g. A noninvasive method that uses a light beam to measure the oxygen content of hemoglobin (SaO_2).

h. Screen for asymptomatic disease and to diagnose tumors, foreign bodies, and other abnormal conditions.

Activity E *Identify elements of respiratory physiology based on the criteria given.*

	Definition	Mechanics
Respiration		
Ventilation		
Diffusion		
Perfusion		

Activity F *Answer the following questions using the figure given below.*

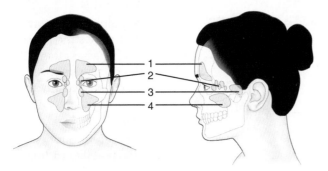

1. Identify and label the paranasal sinuses shown on the figure.

   1. _____

   2. _____

   3. _____

   4. _____

2. Which sinuses are the largest and the most accessible to treatment?

   _____

Activity G *Briefly answer the following questions.*

1. Describe the flow of air once it enters the right and left mainstem bronchi.

   _____

   _____

   _____

2. Where is the site of oxygen and CO_2 exchange?

   _____

   _____

   _____

3. What does alveolar respiration determine?

   _____

   _____

   _____

4. How do the lungs and kidneys compensate for acid-base imbalances?

   _____

   _____

   _____

5. What would be the indications for a thoracentesis?

   _____

   _____

   _____

6. Describe the difference between sibilant and sonorous wheezes.

   _____

   _____

   _____

SECTION II: APPLYING YOUR KNOWLEDGE

Activity H *Give rationale for the following questions:*

1. Why is aspiration of foreign objects more likely in the right mainstem bronchus and right upper lung?

   _____

   _____

   _____

2. Why are older adults at a greater risk from respiratory disease?

   _____

   _____

   _____

3. Why may it be necessary to collect sputum on successive days?

   _____

   _____

   _____

4. Why must the nurse determine if the client has any allergies, particularly to iodine, shellfish, or contrast dye with a pulmonary angiography?

   _____

   _____

   _____

Activity I *Answer the following questions related to caring for clients with respiratory disorders.*

1. What forces can interfere with breathing including airway resistance and lung compliance?

   _____

   _____

   _____

2. Describe the transport of gases.

   _____

   _____

   _____

3. What are the neurological control mechanisms of ventilation?

   _____

   _____

   _____

4. What is included in the assessment of the client's respiratory history?

   _____

   _____

   _____

5. What is included in a physical assessment of the respiratory system?

   _____

   _____

   _____

Activity J *Think over the following questions. Discuss them with your instructor or peers.*

1. You are preparing a client for a therapeutic thoracentesis at the bedside. Describe the pre-procedural and post-procedural nursing care required.

   _____

   _____

   _____

2. You are preparing a client for a bronchoscopy. Describe the pre-procedural and post-procedural nursing care required.

   _____

   _____

   _____

3. You are performing a physical assessment on a client and detect crackles that were not noted on the previous assessment. You ask to client to cough and listen again. The crackles are still present. What does this indicate? What further nursing assessments and interventions would you initiate?

   _____

   _____

   _____

SECTION III: GETTING READY FOR NCLEX

Activity K *Answer the following questions.*

1. In an older client, the alveolar walls become thinner and contain fewer capillaries. What does this condition lead to?
   a. Loss of elasticity in the lungs
   b. Decreased gas exchange
   c. Increased stiffness in lungs
   d. Decreased numbers of alveoli

2. During the physical examination of a client, which of the following methods does the examiner use to palpate for tactile or vocal fremitus?
   a. The examiner uses the palmar surface of the fingers and hands.
   b. The examiner asks client to repeat "11" while moving his or her hands.
   c. The examiner performs percussion of the neck wall.
   d. The examiner observes vibrations when the client remains quiet.

3. How is a client positioned for a thoracentesis?
   a. The client sits at the side of the bed.
   b. The client lies on the affected side.
   c. The client lies flat on the back.
   d. The client lies down with the head raised.

4. Sputum specimens are examined to detect which of the following?
   a. Foreign bodies
   b. Cancer cells
   c. Pulmonary emboli
   d. Inflammation

5. During the physical examination of a client, the nurse auscultates breath sounds. Which of the following are normal breath sounds?
   a. Sounds heard over the trachea - medium pitch
   b. Sounds heard between the trachea and upper lungs - loud
   c. Sounds heard over the lung fields - quiet and low-pitched
   d. Sounds that are discrete - continuous and musical

6. When examining the posterior pharynx and tonsils, which of the following objective data does the nurse note?
   a. Difficulty in sneezing
   b. Suppressed gag reflex
   c. Deformities
   d. Inflammation

7. The sinuses lighten the weight of the skull and give resonance to the voice. There are four pairs of these bony cavities. Which of the following sinuses are located on either side of the nose?
   a. Ethmoidal sinuses
   b. Frontal sinuses
   c. Maxillary sinuses
   d. Sphenoidal sinuses

8. Which of the following neurological controls of ventilation responds to changes in the pH and levels of oxygen and CO_2 in the blood?
   a. Central chemoreceptors in the medulla
   b. Peripheral chemoreceptors in the aortic arch and carotid arteries
   c. Respiratory centers in the medulla oblongata and pons
   d. Central chemoreceptors in the spinal cord

9. In general, when looking at acid base balance, how does the body compensate with metabolic acidosis?
   a. Lungs "blow off" CO_2 to raise pH
   b. Lungs retain CO_2 to lower pH
   c. Kidneys retain more HCO_3 to raise the pH
   d. Kidneys excrete more HCO_3 to lower pH

10. Which of the following nursing activities is most important when a client comes back from a respiratory test if they have respiratory problems?
    a. Allow the client to rest.
    b. Assess the client's airway.
    c. Teach the client important information.
    d. Teach the family about respiratory disease.

Caring for Clients with Upper Respiratory Disorders

1. Describe nursing care for clients experiencing infectious or inflammatory upper respiratory disorders.
2. Discuss assessment data required to provide nursing care to clients with structural disorders of the upper airway.
3. Describe airway problems a client may experience following trauma or obstruction to the upper airway.
4. Identify risk factors that contribute to the development of laryngeal cancer.
5. Identify the earliest symptom of laryngeal cancer.
6. Discuss treatments for laryngeal cancer.
7. Describe measures used to promote alternative methods of communication for clients with a laryngectomy.
8. Discuss psychosocial issues that clients may experience following a laryngectomy.
9. Relate treatment modalities for clients experiencing short-term or long-term problems with airway management.
10. Identify possible reasons for and nursing management of a tracheostomy.
11. Explain why a client may require endotracheal intubation.

SECTION I: ASSESSING YOUR UNDERSTANDING

Activity A *Fill in the blanks by choosing the correct word from the options given in parentheses.*

1. Chronic adenoidal infections can result in acute or chronic infections in the _____. (*Middle ear, Inner ear, Outer ear*)

2. If drainage of clear fluid is observed following a nasal fracture, a Dextrostix is used to determine the presence of glucose, which is diagnostic for _____ and suggests a fracture in the cribriform plate. (*Hemorrhage, Mucus, Cerebrospinal fluid*)

3. Expectoration of bloody sputum is called _____. (*Hemoptysis, Epistaxis, Rhinorrhea*)

4. _____ is usually the earliest symptom of laryngeal cancer. (*A lump in the throat, Persistent hoarseness, Dysphagia*)

5. The physician specifies the amount of air to be injected into the cuffed tracheostomy tube, usually to achieve a pressure between _____. (*10 and 15 mm H_2O, 20 and 25 mm H_2O, 30 and 35 mm H_2O*)

6. _____ is a nursing intervention frequently used to promote maximum lung expansion and improve oxygen exchange. (*Application of oxygen, Positioning in semi-Fowler's, Monitoring ABGs*)

Activity B *Mark each statement as either "T" (True) or "F" (False). Correct any false statements.*

1. T F Laboratory results for hematocrit, platelet count, and clotting time should be closely monitored for the client

undergoing a tonsillectomy and adenoidectomy because of the high risk for postoperative hemorrhage.

2. T F   Hypertrophied turbinates are grapelike swellings that arise from the nasal mucous membranes.

3. T F   Obstructive sleep apnea results from a reduced diameter of the upper airway, which may develop when the upper airway collapses secondary to the normally reduced muscle tone during sleep.

4. T F   To determine the nature of the sleep apnea, clients undergo polysomnography, which consists of tests that monitor the client's respiratory and cardiac status while he or she is asleep.

5. T F   Cancer of the larynx always has a poor prognosis.

6. T F   Esophageal speech uses a throat vibrator held against the neck that projects sound into the mouth; words are formed with the mouth.

Activity C   *Write the correct term for each description given below.*

1. A deviated septum, nasal polyps, and hypertrophied turbinates are common causes of this condition. _____

2. The universal sign for choking. _____

3. A high-pitched, harsh sound during respiration, indicative of airway obstruction.

   _____

4. Characterized by frequent, brief episodes of respiratory standstill during sleep.

   _____

5. Spasm of the laryngeal muscles, resulting in narrowing of the larynx. _____

6. These two devices are kept at the bedside at all times following a tracheostomy.

   _____

Activity D   *Match the terms in column A with their related descriptions in Column B.*

Column A

____ 1. Tracheotomy

____ 2. Tracheostomy

____ 3. Endotracheal tube

Column B

a. Inserted through the mouth or nose into the trachea to provide a patent airway for clients who cannot

____ 4. Positive pressure ventilator

____ 5. Negative pressure ventilator

____ 6. Airway pressure release ventilation

maintain an adequate airway on their own.

b. Exert a pulling or sucking force on the external chest.

c. A surgical opening into the trachea into which a tracheostomy or laryngectomy tube is inserted.

d. Promotes spontaneous breathing in a ventilated client. This is accomplished through the use of extended periods of CPAP.

e. The surgical procedure that makes an opening into the trachea.

f. Inflate the lungs by pushing air into the airway.

Activity E   *Compare the upper airway illnesses below using the given criteria:*

Description	Cause	Symptoms	Treatment
Rhinitis			
Sinusitis			
Pharyngitis			
Tonsillitis and Adenoiditis			
Peritonsillar abscess			
Laryngitis			

Activity F   *Briefly answer the following questions.*

1. What observations and assessments will the nurse make that are specific for the client following sinus surgery?

   _____

   _____

   _____

2. What complications can occur following pharyngitis caused by streptococci A?

   _____

   _____

   _____

3. What interventions may the nurse initiate independently to control bleeding for epistaxis?

_____

_____

_____

4. What are the symptoms of obstructive sleep apnea?

_____

_____

_____

5. Which carcinogens are associated with laryngeal cancer?

_____

_____

_____

6. What are indications for an endotracheal tube?

_____

_____

_____

SECTION II: APPLYING YOUR KNOWLEDGE

Activity G *Give rationale for the following questions:*

1. Why should clients taking prescription medications consult their physician before taking over-the-counter medications?

_____

_____

_____

2. Why should the head of the bed be elevated 45° when the client is fully awake after a tonsillectomy and adenoidectomy?

_____

_____

_____

3. How does sleep apnea cause serious side effects that affect the cardiopulmonary system?

_____

_____

_____

4. What are the benefits of ice packs or ice collars?

_____

_____

_____

5. How can the creation of a new opening following a tracheostomy cause a life-threatening situation?

_____

_____

_____

Activity H *Answer the following questions related to caring for clients with upper respiratory disorders.*

1. What are the risk factors for sleep apnea?

_____

_____

_____

2. Describe the physical changes associated with a total laryngectomy.

_____

_____

_____

3. Why is a humidified mist collar usually necessary following a tracheostomy?

_____

_____

_____

4. What is the nursing management for the client with an endotracheal tube?

_____

_____

_____

5. Describe a tracheoesophageal puncture.

_____

_____

_____

Activity I *Think over the following questions. Discuss them with your instructor or peers.*

1. A client who has undergone a total laryngectomy is disturbed by the appearance of the tracheostomy and is refusing visitors. What interventions could you use to facilitate the client's acceptance of body changes and promote social interaction?

_____

_____

_____

2. The client with a tracheostomy has copious secretions. What guidelines will you follow to perform suctioning?

_____

_____

_____

3. You are in a restaurant when the person at the next table stands up and clutches their throat. What actions will you take?

_____

_____

_____

SECTION III: GETTING READY FOR NCLEX

Activity J *Answer the following questions:*

1. Which of the following is an important preventive factor that the nurse should teach a client with rhinitis?
   a. Not to blow the nose
   b. Consume small doses of ice chips
   c. Not to lift objects weighing more than 5 to 10 lbs
   d. Wash hands frequently

2. Which of the following signs may be revealed in a client with tonsillar infection by a visual examination if group A streptococci is the cause?
   a. White patches on the tonsils
   b. Hemorrhage in the tonsils
   c. Hypertrophied tonsils
   d. Bleeding in the tonsils

3. Why may an ice collar be ordered for a client who is undergoing drainage of a peritonsillar abscess?
   a. To reduce swelling and pain
   b. To help the client drink fluids
   c. To prevent respiratory obstruction
   d. To prevent excessive bleeding

4. Which of the following conditions is evident by persistent hoarseness?
   a. Bacterial infection
   b. Laryngeal cancer
   c. Aphonia
   d. Peritonsillar abscess

5. What does a nurse assess postoperatively in a client with a nasal fracture?
   a. Allergic reaction
   b. Airway obstruction
   c. Extreme sense of smell
   d. Stridor

6. Which of the following symptoms should a nurse assess in a client when implementing interventions for trauma to the upper airway?
   a. Pain when talking
   b. Burning in the throat
   c. Increased nasal swelling
   d. Presence of laryngospasm

7. Which of the following are risk factors of laryngeal cancer?
   a. Acute laryngitis
   b. Tobacco use
   c. Caffeine use
   d. Sleep apnea

8. What is the least successful treatment for laryngeal cancer?
   a. Surgical treatment
   b. Radical neck dissection
   c. Radiation therapy with surgery
   d. Chemotherapy

9. Which of the following methods of speech following laryngectomy involves a throat vibrator held against the neck that projects sound into the mouth causing words to be formed with the mouth?
   a. Tracheoesophageal puncture (TEP)
   b. Esophageal speech

c. Artificial (electric) larynx

d. Speech therapy

10. Which of the following nursing interventions regarding nutrition is used until the suture line heals, usually 10 to 14 days postoperatively?

a. Enteral feedings

b. Meticulous mouth care every 4 hours

c. Gradual advancement of the diet

d. Reassurance that the sense of taste will return

CHAPTER 21

Caring for Clients with Lower Respiratory Disorders

Learning Objectives

1. Describe infectious and inflammatory disorders of the lower respiratory airway.
2. Identify critical assessments needed for a client with an infectious disorder of the lower respiratory airway.
3. Define disorders classified as obstructive pulmonary disease.
4. Discuss strategies for preventing and managing occupational lung diseases.
5. Describe the pathophysiology of pulmonary hypertension.
6. List risk factors associated with the development of pulmonary embolism.
7. Discuss conditions that may lead to acute respiratory distress syndrome.
8. Differentiate acute and chronic respiratory failure.
9. Explain the difficulties associated with early diagnosis of lung cancer.
10. Describe nursing assessments required for a client who experiences trauma to the chest.
11. Explain the purpose of chest tubes after thoracic surgery.
12. Describe preoperative and postoperative nursing management for clients undergoing thoracic care.

SECTION I: ASSESSING YOUR UNDERSTANDING

Activity A *Fill in the blanks by choosing the correct word from the options given in parentheses.*

1. Inflammation that lines the major bronchi and its branches characterizes _____. *(Pneumonia, Acute bronchitis, Pleurisy)*

2. _____ is an abnormal collection of fluid between the visceral and parietal pleurae. *(Pleurisy, Pleural effusion, Lung abscess)*

3. _____ is an acute respiratory disease of relatively short duration. *(Lung abscess, Empyema, Influenza)*

4. _____ is a bacterial infectious disease primarily caused by *M. tuberculosis*. *(Primary tuberculosis, Secondary tuberculosis, Tertiary tuberculosis)*

5. _____ usually involves reactivation of the initial infection. The person already has had an immune response, and thus the lesions that form tend to remain in the lungs. *(Primary tuberculosis, Secondary tuberculosis, Tertiary tuberculosis)*

6. _____ is collapse of alveoli. It may involve a small portion of the lung or an entire lobe. When alveoli collapse, they cannot perform their function of gas exchange. *(Bronchiectasis, Atelectasis, Chronic bronchitis)*

7. _____ is an inherited multisystem disorder that affects infants, children, and young adults. It obstructs the lungs, leading to major lung infections, as well as obstructing the pancreas. *(Emphysema, Asthma, Cystic fibrosis)*

8. _____ is associated with factors such as upper respiratory infections, emotional upsets, and exercise. *(Nonallergic asthma, Allergic asthma, Mixed asthma)*

9. _____ are a common injury which may result from a hard fall or a blow to the chest. The injuries are not usually considered serious, unless accompanied by other injuries. *(Rib fractures, Penetrating wounds, Blast injuries)*

10. Gunshot and stab wounds are common types of _____ to the lungs; they can potentially affect cardiopulmonary function and may be life-threatening. *(Fracture injuries, Blast injuries, Penetrating wounds)*

11. When symptoms occur, they include chest pain, chest wall bulging, difficulty swallowing, dyspnea, and orthopnea. Symptoms are related to pressure on other chest structures. *(Lung cancer, Mediastinal tumors, Flail chest)*

Activity B *Mark each statement as either "T" (True) or "F" (False). Correct any false statements.*

1. T F Fungal infections and chemical irritants may cause acute bronchitis.

2. T F Pneumonia is an inflammation of the bronchioles and alveoli.

3. T F A lung abscess is a general term used to denote pus in a body cavity. It usually refers, however, to pus or infected fluid in the pleural cavity.

4. T F Tubercle bacilli are susceptible to darkness, which destroy the spores in a few hours.

5. T F A positive tuberculin skin test result is evidence that a TB infection has existed at some time somewhere in the body, but does not necessarily indicate active disease.

6. T F Inflammation of the airway and hyperresponsiveness of the airway to internal or external stimuli characterize emphysema.

7. T F Therapeutic breathing exercises helps to control the respiratory rate and depth and slows expiration.

8. T F Occupational lung diseases result in pneumoconiosis, a fibrous inflammation or chronic induration of the lungs after prolonged exposure to dust or gases.

9. T F Tumors and growths affecting the respiratory system usually are malignant.

10. T F Compression of the chest by an explosion (blast injuries) can seriously damage the lungs by rupturing the alveoli. Death often results from hemorrhage and asphyxiation.

11. T F A cough productive of mucopurulent or blood-streaked sputum is a cardinal sign of lung cancer.

12. T F Subcutaneous emphysema is a common finding with blast injuries because the lungs or air passages have sustained an injury and crepitation is heard or felt upon palpation and may be caused by air leaking around the chest wound.

Activity C *Write the correct term for each of the following descriptions below.*

1. Most commonly gives rise to acute bronchitis. _____

2. This lower respiratory disorder refers to an acute inflammation of the parietal and visceral pleurae. _____

3. Applications may provide some topical comfort for pleurisy. _____

4. Type of pneumonias referred to as *typical pneumonias.* _____

5. Found in clients with COPD and is characterized by chronic infection and irreversible dilatation of the bronchi and bronchioles. _____

6. Prolonged (or extended) inflammation of the bronchi, accompanied by a chronic cough and excessive production of mucus for at least 3 months per year for 2 consecutive years. _____

7. This type of asthma occurs in response to allergens, such as pollen, dust, spores, and animal danders. _____

8. Components include chest physical therapy (including postural drainage, percussion, and vibration) two to four times daily, deep-breathing and coughing exercises, nebulized treatments, and medications. _____

9. Silicosis and asbestosis are in a category of these lower respiratory disorders, which result in the lungs having a decreased volume and inability to expand completely. _____

10. Occurs when two or more adjacent ribs fracture in multiple places and the fragments are free-floating. This affects the stability of the chest wall and results in impairment of chest-wall movement. _____

11. The name for the three conditions that predispose a person to clot formation: venostasis, disruption of the vessel lining, and hypercoagulability. _____

12. It remains the number one cause of cancer-related deaths among men and women in the United States. _____

Activity D *Given in column A are obstructive pulmonary diseases. Match these disorders with their associated assessment findings in column B.*

Column A

____ 1. Bronchiectasis

____ 2. Atelectasis

____ 3. Chronic bronchitis

____ 4. Emphysema

____ 5. Asthma

____ 6. Cystic fibrosis

Column B

a. The earliest symptom is a chronic cough productive of thick, white mucus, especially when rising in the morning and in the evening. Bronchospasm may occur during severe bouts of coughing.

b. Typified by paroxysms of shortness of breath, wheezing, and coughing as well as the production of thick, tenacious sputum.

c. Shortness of breath with minimal activity is called exertional dyspnea and often is the first symptom. As the disease progresses, breathlessness occurs even at rest. A chronic cough invariably is present and productive of mucopurulent sputum. Inspiration is difficult because of the rigid chest cage, and the chest is characteristically barrel shaped.

d. Clients experience a chronic cough with expectoration of copious amounts of purulent sputum and possible hemoptysis. The coughing worsens when the client changes position. Clients also experience fatigue, weight loss, anorexia, and dyspnea.

e. The three major reasons to suspect this disorder in children are respiratory symptoms, failure to thrive, and foul-smelling, bulky, greasy stools.

f. Small areas may cause few symptoms. With larger areas, cyanosis, fever, pain, dyspnea, increased pulse and respiratory rates, and increased pulmonary secretions may be seen. Although crackling may be auscultated over the affected areas, usually breath sounds are absent.

Activity E *To determine peak flow, the nurse instructs the client. The steps are in a jumbled order. Indicate the correct order of instruction by filling the boxes with the correct sequence.*

1. Form a tight seal around the mouthpiece with lips.

2. Note the reading.

3. Sit upright in bed or chair, or stand and inhale as deeply as possible.

4. Exhale forcefully and quickly.

5. Monitor the peak flow readings according to the three zones.

6. After 2 to 3 weeks of asthma therapy, determine your best or usual individual peak flow.

7. Repeat these steps two more times; write the highest of the three numbers in the asthma record.

8. Depending on the zone, take actions as

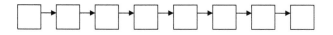

instructed by healthcare providers.

Activity F *Compare the following disorders based on the criteria below.*

Disorder	Definition	Pathophysiology
Pulmonary arterial hypertension		
Pulmonary embolism		
Pulmonary edema		
Respiratory failure		
Acute respiratory distress syndrome		

Activity G *Briefly answer the following questions.*

1. Describe the signs and symptoms of acute bronchitis.

_____

_____

_____

2. What are the causes of pneumonia in addition to microorganism infection?

_____

_____

_____

3. What are the signs and symptoms of pneumonia?

_____

_____

_____

4. What are the assessment findings for a lung abscess?

_____

_____

_____

5. How is TB most commonly transmitted? Does exposure always result in illness?

_____

_____

_____

6. Describe the surgical treatment of tuberculosis.

_____

_____

_____

7. Describe the treatment for bronchiectasis.

_____

_____

8. Describe the nursing interventions indicated for management of chronic bronchitis.

_____

_____

_____

9. What are the dietary indications when cystic fibrosis affects the digestive system?

_____

_____

_____

10. Identify the assessment findings for pulmonary arterial hypertension.

_____

_____

_____

11. What is the treatment for respiratory failure?

_____

_____

_____

SECTION II: APPLYING YOUR KNOWLEDGE

Activity H *Give rationale for the following questions.*

1. Why is a sputum culture and sensitivity ordered with lower respiratory infections?

_____

_____

_____

2. Why is pleurisy so painful?

_____

_____

_____

3. Why are clients susceptible to the influenza virus once they have recovered from an episode and have developed antibodies?

_____

_____

_____

4. Why is treatment of tuberculosis with medication less than ideal? How are these issues addressed?

_____

_____

_____

5. How does emphysema prevent the proper exchange of oxygen and CO_2 during respiration?

_____

_____

_____

6. Why is oxygen cautiously administered to clients with emphysema?

_____

_____

_____

7. How does absence of the protein CF transmembrane conductance regulator result in the symptoms of cystic fibrosis?

_____

_____

_____

8. Why are anticoagulants used in the treatment of pulmonary emboli?

_____

_____

_____

9. What are thrombolytics used in the treatment of pulmonary emboli?

_____

_____

_____

10. Why has the incidence of lung cancer markedly increased since the early 1980s?

_____

_____

_____

11. Why does lung cancer have a high mortality rate?

_____

_____

_____

12. Why are all penetrating wounds to the chest considered serious?

_____

_____

_____

Activity I *Answer the following questions related to caring for clients with lower respiratory disorders.*

1. Describe the pathophysiology of pneumonia.

_____

_____

_____

2. What are typical assessment findings with pleurisy?

_____

_____

_____

3. What are the typical assessment findings with a pleural effusion?

_____

_____

_____

4. Describe the medical and surgical management of empyema.

_____

_____

_____

5. What are the signs and symptoms of tuberculosis?

_____

_____

_____

6. Nursing management of atelectasis focuses on prevention; what are the nursing interventions indicated to assist with the prevention of atelectasis?

_____

_____

_____

7. Describe the pathophysiology of asthma.

_____

_____

_____

8. Describe the medical management for primary pulmonary arterial hypertension. Describe the medical management for secondary pulmonary arterial hypertension.

_____

_____

_____

9. What are the symptoms of pulmonary edema? What type of treatment does pulmonary edema require?

_____

_____

_____

10. What signs and symptoms are seen with impending respiratory failure?

_____

_____

_____

11. Why would a thoracotomy be performed?

_____

_____

_____

12. Describe the care for a chest tube.

_____

_____

_____

Activity J _Think over the following questions and then discuss them with your instructor or peers._

1. Your client is diagnosed with bacterial pneumonia. What nursing assessments and interventions are indicated?

_____

_____

_____

2. You have volunteered to administer the influenza vaccine at a local clinic. Which types of clients will you advise against receiving the vaccine?

_____

_____

_____

3. Your client is diagnosed with asthma. What education will you provide to assist them in managing the symptoms?

_____

_____

_____

4. Your client is diagnosed with emphysema. What strategies will you teach the client to slow the disease progression?

_____

_____

_____

SECTION III: GETTING READY FOR NCLEX

Activity K *Answer the following questions.*

1. Which of the following is an initial sign or symptom of acute bronchitis?
   a. Nonproductive cough
   b. Labored breathing
   c. Anorexia
   d. Gastric ulceration

2. Which of the following should the nurse include in the teaching plan of a client with acute bronchitis?
   a. Not coughing frequently
   b. Consuming adequate calories
   c. Washing the hands frequently
   d. Encouraging a semi-Fowler's position

3. How does nosocomial pneumonia occur?
   a. In a healthcare setting
   b. In the immunocompromised host
   c. In a community setting
   d. Within 48 hours of admission to a health-care facility

4. Which of the following would be the most appropriate nursing intervention when caring for a client with a fractured rib?
   a. Apply immobilization device after examination by physician
   b. Discourage taking deep breaths if breathing is painful
   c. Advice against using analgesics and regional nerve blocks
   d. Encourage increased fluid intake if pulmonary contusion exists

5. Which of the following does the examiner note when auscultating the lungs of a client with pleural effusion?
   a. Pronounced breath sounds
   b. Friction rub
   c. Expiratory wheezes
   d. Fluid in the involved area

6. Which of the following interventions are implemented for a client with empyema?
   a. Teach the client breathing exercises.
   b. Offer assurance that empyema takes less time to resolve.
   c. Recommend that the client eat a balanced but light diet.
   d. Emphasize the completion of the entire course of drug therapy.

7. Which of the following nursing interventions are involved when caring for a client with influenza?
   a. Maintain airborne transmission precautions
   b. Complete bed rest
   c. Oxygen administration
   d. Immediate recognition of respiratory distress

8. Which of the following factors predispose a client to the development of TB?
   a. Exposure to toxic gases
   b. Obstruction by tumor
   c. Congenital abnormalities
   d. Malnutrition

9. Which of the following is a sign or symptom characteristic of the later stages of TB?
   a. Fatigue
   b. Hemoptysis
   c. Anorexia
   d. Weight loss

10. Which of the following is a sign or symptom of asthma?
    a. Production of abnormally thick, sticky mucus in lungs
    b. Faulty transport of sodium in lung cells
    c. Paroxysms or shortness of breath
    d. Altered electrolyte balance in the sweat glands

Introduction to the Cardiovascular System

Learning Objectives

1. Describe the normal anatomy and physiology of the cardiovascular system.
2. Identify and describe focus assessment criteria when caring for a client with cardiovascular problems.
3. List common diagnostic tests used to evaluate the client with suspected heart disease.
4. Discuss the nursing management of a client undergoing cardiovascular diagnostic tests.

SECTION I: ASSESSING YOUR UNDERSTANDING

Activity A *Fill in the blanks by choosing the correct word from the options given in parentheses.*

1. The _____ consists of muscle tissue and is the force behind the heart's pumping action. *(Epicardium, Myocardium, Endocardium)*

2. During a _____ state, the myocardial cells are at rest. This occurs during diastole, before an impulse is generated. *(Polarized, Depolarized, Repolarized)*

3. _____ carry oxygenated blood from the heart. *(Arteries, Veins, Valves)*

4. _____ refers to contraction of the atria and ventricles during the cardiac cycle. *(Systole, Conduction, Diastole)*

5. The heart rate _____ when receptors are stimulated by the cholinergic neurotransmitter acetylcholine released from parasympathetic nerve fibers. *(Increases, Pauses, Decreases)*

6. Taking blood pressure with the client in the lying, sitting, and standing positions is referred to as _____. *(Pulse deficit, Pulse pressure, Orthostatic vital signs)*

7. The normal heart sound, referred to as _____, is heard with the closing of the mitral and tricuspid valves. *(S_1, S_2, S_3)*

8. _____ are caused by turbulent blood flow through diseased heart valves. *(Murmurs and clicks, Atrial and ventricular gallops, Friction rubs)*

Activity B *Mark each statement as either "T" (True) or "F" (False). Correct any false statements.*

1. T F The epicardium is composed of a thin, smooth layer of endothelial cells. Folds of epicardium form the heart valves.

2. T F During depolarization the electrical impulse spreads from cell membrane to cell membrane, causing a transfer of ions. The positive ions move inside the myocardial cell membranes, and the negative ions move outside.

3. T F A valve separates the right side of the heart from the left side.

4. T F The valves of the heart ensure that blood passes through the heart in a two-way (forward and backward) direction.

5. T F Cardiac output is the amount of blood pumped out of the left ventricle each minute. The formula to calculate cardiac output is: Cardiac output = heart rate × stroke volume.

6. T F Fever is characteristic in some types of heart disease. It can accompany the inflammatory response when myocardial cells are damaged after an acute MI (heart attack) or infections such as rheumatic fever and bacterial endocarditis.

7. T F An S_3 is an extra sound just before S_1; it is called an atrial gallop and often associated with hypertensive heart disease.

8. T F A friction rub may cause a rough, grating, or scratchy sound that is indicative of pericarditis.

Activity C *Write the correct term for each description below.*

1. Ions realign themselves in their original position and wait for another electrical impulse. _____

2. These vessels return deoxygenated blood to the heart. _____

3. Refers to relaxation of the atria and ventricle during the cardiac cycle. _____

4. The heart rate and force of contraction increase when receptors are stimulated by adrenergic neurotransmitter released by this type of nerve fiber. _____

5. The amount of blood pumped per contraction of the heart. _____

6. The characteristics that are assessed when the nurse palpates a pulse. _____

7. The heart sound associated with the closing of the aortic and pulmonic valves. _____

8. This occurs when blood is not pumped efficiently. When blood has nowhere else to go and the extra fluid enters the tissues. _____

9. Distention of this vein usually indicates increased fluid volume and pressure in the right side of the heart. _____

Activity D *Match the heart valves given in Column A to their related location or function given in Column B.*

Column A

____ **1.** Atrioventricular (AV) valves

____ **2.** Tricuspid valve

____ **3.** Bicuspid valve

____ **4.** Semilunar valves

____ **5.** Pulmonic valve

____ **6.** Aortic valve

Column B

a. The valve between the right ventricle and pulmonary artery.

b. The valve between the right atrium and right ventricle.

c. The two valves that prevent blood from flowing back into the ventricles after the heart contracts.

d. The two valves that separate the atria from the ventricles. They prevent blood from returning to the atria when the ventricles contract.

e. The valve between the left atrium and left ventricle (also known as the mitral valve).

f. The valve between the left ventricle and aorta.

Activity E *The cardiopulmonary circulation is given below in a jumbled order. Indicate the correct order of events by filling the boxes with the correct sequence.*

1. Blood travels into the right ventricle and is pumped into the pulmonary artery.

2. The left ventricle pumps the blood through the aorta to all the body's cells and tissues.

3. The pulmonary veins bring the oxygenated blood into the left atrium.

4. The lungs exchange the oxygen in inspired air for the CO_2 in the venous blood. The CO_2 is transferred into the alveoli and exhaled.

5. The right atrium fills with blood, and the tricuspid valve opens.

6. The oxygenated blood flows out of the left atrium through the bicuspid (mitral) valve and into the left ventricle.

7. The largest veins, the inferior vena cava and superior vena cava, bring venous (deoxygenated) blood from all areas of the body into the right atrium.

8. The pulmonary artery branches to deliver venous blood to the right and left lungs.

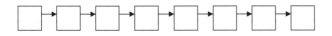

Activity F *Compare the following diagnostic tests based on the given criteria.*

Diagnostic test	Description	Purpose
Radiography		
Radionuclide studies		
Magnetic resonance imaging (MRI)		
Echocardiography		
Transesophageal echocardiography (TEE)		
Electrocardiography		
Ambulatory ECG (Holter monitoring)		
Exercise electrocardiography (Stress test)		
Cardiac catheterization		
Arteriography		
Angiocardiography		
Aortography		
Peripheral arteriography		

Activity G *The conduction system sustains the electrical activity of the heart. Label the locations of each part of the conduction system.*

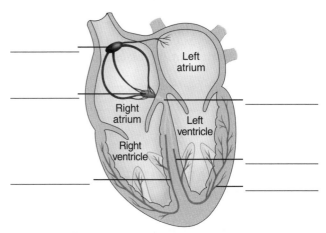

Electrical conduction system of the heart.

Activity H *Briefly answer the following questions.*

1. Describe the structure and function of the pericardium.

_____

_____

_____

2. Describe the function of the chordae tendineae and papillary muscles.

_____

_____

_____

3. Describe the structure and function of capillaries.

_____

_____

_____

4. What type of pain may be indicative of cardiovascular problems?

_____

_____

_____

5. How is a pulse deficit determined?

_____

_____

_____

6. What characteristics of respiration are included in the nursing assessment?

_____

_____

_____

SECTION II: APPLYING YOUR KNOWLEDGE

Activity I *Give rationale for the following questions.*

1. Why is the myocardium the first tissue of the body to receive oxygen-rich blood?

_____

_____

_____

2. Why are cells resistant to electrical stimulation during the refractory period?

_____

_____

_____

3. Why is the family medical history an important feature of the health history?

_____

_____

_____

4. How does the client's general appearance, non-verbal behaviors, and body position contribute to assessment of the cardiovascular system?

_____

_____

_____

5. Why is it important to compare the information on a heart monitor with palpation of the pulse and/or auscultation of the apical heart rate?

_____

_____

_____

6. Why are cardiovascular problems exhibited as crackles in the lungs?

_____

_____

_____

7. Why is the client's weight an important factor in the cardiovascular nursing assessment?

_____

_____

_____

Activity J *Answer the following questions related to the cardiovascular system.*

1. What is the normal sequence of events in the conduction system of the heart?

_____

_____

_____

2. What information is obtained during a history assessment of the cardiovascular system?

_____

_____

_____

3. What information is obtained during the nursing assessment of the skin?

_____

_____

_____

4. How are mental status changes related to cardiovascular problems?

_____

_____

_____

5. How do baroreceptors regulate the heart rate?

_____

_____

_____

6. How do chemoreceptors regulate the heart rate?

_____

_____

_____

Activity K _Think over the following questions._
Discuss them with your instructor or peers.

1. A client is scheduled for an MRI. What questions will you need to ask the client to make sure they are a candidate for this type of procedure? How will you prepare the client for this diagnostic test? What medications may you need to administer?

_____

_____

_____

2. A client is scheduled for a cardiac catheterization. What preprocedure care activities will you perform? What are the postprocedure guidelines will you follow? What discharge instructions will you provide?

_____

_____

_____

SECTION III: GETTING READY FOR NCLEX

Activity L _Answer the following questions._

1. Why does the nurse assess for allergy to seafood during the initial assessment of a client with a disorder of the cardiovascular system?
   a. It can contribute to cardiac symptoms
   b. It may indicate an allergy to iodine
   c. It can contribute to drug interactions
   d. It indicates a genetic predisposition to cardiac disorders

2. What is a classic sign of ischemia?
   a. Increased blood supply
   b. Fever

   c. Thready pulse
   d. Pain

3. Cardiac disorders are often associated with changes in BP. Which type of cuff does the nurse choose to ensure an accurate assessment?
   a. Cuff width appropriate for continuous bedside monitoring
   b. Cuff width suitable for assessing BP during position changes
   c. Cuff width appropriate for the diameter of the client's arm
   d. Cuff width greater than the diameter of the client's right arm

4. When assessing the mental status of a client with cardiac disorders, what does confusion indicate?
   a. Blood congestion in neck veins
   b. Left-sided heart failure
   c. Absence of pulses
   d. Cerebral ischemia

5. Which of the following nursing interventions will eliminate the feeling of being cared for by strangers in a client scheduled for diagnostic procedures of the cardiovascular system?
   a. Allowing for rest periods
   b. Greeting the client by name
   c. Increasing bright lights
   d. Asking the client to paraphrase information

6. Why are repeated explanations and reassurances throughout all phases of the nursing process indicated when dealing with older clients?
   a. Decreased perfusion to the brain
   b. Renal impairment due to advanced age
   c. Nausea during all diagnostic procedures
   d. Absence of delayed conduction in the heart

7. Which of the following heart chambers has the highest pressure in order to pump oxygenated blood to the tissues?
   a. Right atrium
   b. Right ventricle
   c. Left ventricle
   d. Left atrium

8. Which of the following veins is the largest and carries back deoxygenated blood from the tissues in the lower extremities and enters the heart proximally?
   a. Pulmonary artery
   b. Inferior vena cava
   c. Pulmonary vein
   d. Superior vena cava

9. Which of the following structures of the heart is called the pacemaker of the heart?
   a. AV junction
   b. SA node
   c. AV node
   d. Purkinje fibers

10. What test involves the nurse instructing the client to avoid eating or drinking until sensation and the gag reflex return, which may take 1 hour or longer?
    a. Transesophageal echocardiography (TEE)
    b. Magnetic resonance imaging (MRI)
    c. Echocardiography
    d. Cardiac catheterization

Caring for Clients with Infectious and Inflammatory Disorders of the Heart and Blood Vessels

1. Identify three organisms that cause infectious conditions of the heart.
2. List four inflammatory conditions of the heart.
3. Describe treatment for inflammatory and infectious heart disorders.
4. Discuss the nursing management of clients with infectious or inflammatory heart disorders.
5. Name three types of cardiomyopathy.
6. Differentiate between thrombophlebitis and thromboangiitis obliterans.
7. List three interventions that reduce the risk of thrombophlebitis.
8. Discuss the nursing management of clients with inflammatory disorders of peripheral blood vessels.

SECTION I: ASSESSING YOUR UNDERSTANDING

Activity A *Fill in the blanks by choosing the correct word from the options given in parentheses.*

1. The inflammatory symptoms of _____ are believed to be induced by antibodies originally formed to destroy the group A beta-hemolytic streptococcal microorganisms. *(Rheumatic carditis, Infective endocarditis, Myocarditis)*

2. Treatments for _____ involve initially prescribed high doses of an intravenous (IV) antibiotic to which the organism is susceptible. Antibiotic therapy extends at least 2 to 6 weeks. If a heart valve has been severely damaged and drug therapy does not adequately support the failing heart, valve replacement may be necessary. *(Infective endocarditis, Pericarditis, Myocarditis)*

3. The _____ is the most common location of vegetations and microbial deposits. *(Mitral valve, Aortic valve, Pulmonary valve)*

4. Treatment of _____ depends on the underlying cause. A myocardial infarction must be ruled out. Rest, analgesics, antipyretics, nonsteroidal anti-inflammatory drugs, and sometimes corticosteroids are prescribed. Pericardiocentesis may be necessary when cardiac output is severely reduced. *(Rheumatic carditis, Infective endocarditis, Pericarditis)*

5. Black longitudinal lines called _____ can be seen in the nails; a sign associated with infective endocarditis. *(Roth's spots, Janeway lesions, Splinter hemorrhages)*

6. _____ myocarditis has symptoms of exertional dyspnea, dependent edema in the legs, ascites, and hepatomegaly. *(Dilated, Hypertrophic, Restrictive)*

7. Most commonly, blood clots develop deep in the lower extremities; they are referred to as _____. *(Thromboangiitis obliterans, Buerger's disease, Deep vein thrombosis)*

8. Monitoring of prothrombin time (PT) is important for clients taking the oral anticoagulant, warfarin (Coumadin), for venous thrombosis; PT should be _____ times the control value (12–15 seconds) to achieve the therapeutic effect of anticoagulant therapy. *(1.5 to 2.5, 3.0 to 3.5, 3.5 to 4.5)*

Activity B *Mark each statement as either "T" (True) or "F" (False). Correct any false statement.*

1. T F   Myocarditis is inflammation of the inner layer of heart tissue as a result of an infectious microorganism.

2. T F   Pulsus paradoxus develops because of a greater reduction in the volume capacity of the left ventricle during inspiration, combined with an impaired ability of the left ventricle to expand because of the rigid pericardium.

3. T F   The treatment of myocarditis includes treating the underlying cause and preventing complications. Antibiotics are prescribed if the infecting microorganism is bacterial. In severe cases of cardiomyopathy, a heart transplant is necessary.

4. T F   Cardiomyopathy is an acute condition characterized by structural changes in the pericardium.

5. T F   Dilated cardiomyopathy, the most common type, is accompanied by dyspnea on exertion and when lying down. The client feels fatigued and his or her legs swell. He or she may experience palpitations and chest pain.

6. T F   Janeway lesions are white areas in the retina surrounded by areas of hemorrhage.

7. T F   Calf pain that increases on dorsiflexion of the foot is referred to as a negative Homans' sign.

8. T F   Heparin is measured in units and the dosage is regulated by venous clotting time determinations, such as a partial thromboplastin time (PTT) or activated partial thromboplastin time (aPTT).

Activity C *Write the correct term for each description below.*

1. Inflammation can be a primary condition or a secondary condition. The inflammation can occur with or without effusion. _____

2. Treatment of this condition generally involves IV antibiotics. Penicillin is the drug of choice for group A streptococci, unless contraindicated because of an allergy. Bed rest may be indicated depending on the client's condition. Aspirin is used to control the formation of blood clots around heart valves. Steroids are used to suppress the inflammatory response. _____

3. This type of cardiomyopathy is associated with syncope or near-syncopal episodes, which the client may describe as "graying out." Clients also may feel fatigued, become short of breath, and develop chest pain. _____

4. This atypical heart sound may be the first abnormal sign detected in any type of cardiomyopathy. _____

5. Thrombi in the extremity that becomes mobile and moves in the venous circulation to the lungs. _____

6. Painful nodules that may appear on the pads of the fingers and toes with infective endocarditis. _____

7. Inflammation of blood vessels associated with clot formation and fibrosis of the blood vessel wall. It affects primarily the small arteries and veins of the legs. It occasionally involves the arms. _____

Activity D *Match the inflammatory disorders in column A with their symptoms in column B.*

Column A	Column B
____ 1. Rheumatic carditis	a. Clients may complain of sharp stabbing or squeezing chest discomfort that
____ 2. Infective endocarditis	

_____ **3.** Myocarditis

_____ **4.** Pericarditis

resembles a myocardial infarction; however, sitting up relieves the pain. Accompanying manifestations include a low-grade fever, tachycardia, dysrhythmias, dyspnea, malaise, fatigue, and anorexia.

b. The heart rate is rapid and the rhythm may be abnormal. A red, spotty rash referred to as erythema marginatum appears on the trunk but disappears rapidly, leaving irregular circles on the skin. Joints may become swollen, warm, red, and painful. Central nervous system manifestations result in chorea.

c. The client is dyspneic or complains of heaviness in the chest. One chief characteristic is precordial pain. Moving and breathing deeply worsen the pain; sitting upright and leaning forward relieve it. A pericardial friction rub, a scratchy, high-pitched sound, is a diagnostic sign. Heart sounds are difficult to hear because the accumulating fluid muffles them.

d. A heart murmur may be present from malfunctioning valves. Petechiae, tiny, reddish hemorrhagic spots on the skin and mucous membranes, are signs of embolization. Pronounced weakness, anorexia, and weight loss are common.

Activity E *Compare the following procedures based on the given criteria.*

Procedure	Purpose of Procedure
Ventriculomyomectomy	
Pericardiocentesis	
Pericardiostomy	
Pericardiectomy	
Decortication	
Venography	
Impedance plethysmography (IPG)	
Thrombectomy	
Vena caval filter	
Vena caval plication	

Activity F *The steps to perform an assessment of pulsus paradoxus are listed below in a jumbled order. Write the correct sequence for the assessment in the boxes provided below.*

1. Note when the first BP sound (Korotkoff's) is heard.

2. Measure the difference in mm Hg between the first BP sound heard during expiration and the first BP sound heard during both inspiration and expiration.

3. Ask the client to breathe normally throughout the assessment.

4. Deflate the cuff slowly, noting that sounds are audible during expiration but not inspiration.

5. Continue to deflate the cuff until BP sounds are heard during both inspiration and expiration.

6. Inflate the BP cuff 20 mm Hg above systolic pressure.

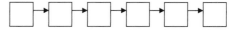

Activity G *Briefly answer the following questions.*

1. How does a blood clot form? Why do signs of swelling, redness, warmth, and tenderness develop?

_____

_____

_____

2. What factors predispose clients to clot formation?

_____

_____

_____

3. Describe the medical and surgical treatment of thrombophlebitis.

_____

_____

_____

4. Describe methods for preventing venous stasis and thrombophlebitis

_____

_____

_____

5. What is involved in the medical and surgical management of thromboangiitis obliterans?

_____

_____

_____

6. Which type of microorganisms cause infective endocarditis? Where are these microorganisms commonly found?

_____

_____

_____

Activity H *Give rationale for the following questions.*

1. Why does rheumatic carditis lead to cardiac complications such as a heart murmur, congestive heart failure, and pericarditis?

_____

_____

_____

2. Why are clients with a history of rheumatic fever told to take prophylactic antibiotics before any invasive procedure, including dental work?

_____

_____

_____

3. Why does infective endocarditis lead to complication such as a murmur, congestive heart failure, and emboli?

_____

_____

_____

4. Why does myocarditis result in complications such as congestive heart failure, tachycardia, and dysrhythmias?

_____

_____

_____

5. Why does pericarditis result in cardiac tamponade and respiratory symptoms?

_____

_____

_____

6. Why has infective endocarditis among older adults increased?

_____

_____

_____

SECTION II: APPLYING YOUR KNOWLEDGE

Activity I *Answer the following questions related to caring for clients with infection and inflammatory disorders of the heart and blood vessels.*

1. What information will the nurse include in teaching for clients with infectious and inflammatory heart disorders?

_____

_____

_____

2. How will the nurse instruct a client required to perform Buerger-Allen exercises?

_____

_____

_____

3. What information is included in teaching for clients with cardiomyopathy?

_____

_____

_____

4. Describe the nursing assessments indicated for a client with thrombophlebitis.

_____

_____

_____

5. What are possible assessment findings for a client with thromboangiitis obliterans?

_____

_____

_____

6. What information is included in teaching for clients with thrombophlebitis?

_____

_____

_____

Activity J _Think over the following questions. Discuss them with your instructor or peers._

1. Your client has been diagnosed with thrombophlebitis. What nursing interventions will you use to prevent complications and promote comfort? What precautions will you need to take with the interventions you identified?

_____

_____

_____

2. Your client is diagnosed with pericarditis. Describe the nursing assessments and intervention to detect and limit the effects of decreased cardiac output. What equipment will you keep at the bedside in the event of cardiac tamponade? What nursing assessments and interventions are indicated following a pericardiocentesis?

_____

_____

_____

SECTION III: GETTING READY FOR NCLEX

Activity K _Answer the following questions._

1. Which of the following is the result of central nervous system manifestations?

a. Congestive heart failure

b. Chorea

c. Valve damage

d. Pericarditis

2. Which of the following nursing interventions should a nurse perform to relieve tachycardia that may develop in a client with myocarditis from hypoxemia?

a. Maintain the client on bed rest.

b. Administer a prescribed antipyretic.

c. Elevate the client's head.

d. Administer supplemental oxygen.

3. Which of the following may be the first abnormal sign detected in a client with cardiomyopathy?

a. Ascites

b. Heart murmur

c. Chest pain

d. Dyspnea

4. Which of the following blood vessels is commonly affected by thrombophlebitis?

a. Veins deep in the upper extremities

b. Veins deep in the lower extremities

c. Popliteal vein of the leg

d. Veins connected to the heart

5. Why are older adults with heart and blood vessel diseases susceptible to thrombophlebitis?

a. Older adults are less mobile.

b. Older adults have more activities.

c. Older adults take more IV drugs and chemicals.

d. Older adults have more diet restrictions.

6. Which of the following is the diagnostic sign for pericarditis?

a. Precordial pain

b. Hypotension

c. Pericardial friction rub

d. Rapid and labored respirations

7. Which of the following cardiomyopathies is accompanied by dyspnea on exertion when lying down, fatigue, and edema in the lower extremities, as well as palpitations and chest pain?
   a. Dilated cardiomyopathy
   b. Hypertrophic cardiomyopathy
   c. Restrictive cardiomyopathy
   d. Arrhythmogenic right ventricular cardiomyopathy

8. A nurse is taking care of a client with an inflammatory cardiac condition. What is the rationale for a nurse asking a client to move frequently instead of staying in one position for too long?
   a. To keep the client from noticing pain
   b. To prevent thrombophlebitis
   c. To provide activity to keep the client from being bored
   d. To prevent stasis ulcers

9. What organism causes endocarditis in 55% of cases?
   a. Staphylococci
   b. Enterococci
   c. Streptococci
   d. HACEK Group

10. Why does the nurse administer non-narcotic analgesics to a client with thrombophlebitis?
    a. To inhibit prostaglandin
    b. To interfere with platelet aggregation
    c. Release of endorphins
    d. Release of cellular chemicals

Caring for Clients with Valvular Disorders of the Heart

1. List five disorders that commonly affect heart valves.
2. Discuss assessment findings common among clients with valvular disorders.
3. Name three diagnostic tests used to confirm valvular disorders.
4. Identify consequences of valvular disorders.
5. Name five categories of drugs used to treat valvular disorders.
6. Give two examples of treatments other than drug therapy to correct valvular disorders.
7. Discuss nursing management of clients with valvular disorders.

SECTION I: ASSESSING YOUR UNDERSTANDING

Activity A *Fill in the blanks by choosing the correct word from the options given in parentheses.*

1. _____ is a narrowing of the opening in the aortic valve when the valve cusps become stiff and rigid. It is a common valvular disorder in the United States, especially among older adults. *(Aortic stenosis, Aortic regurgitation, Mitral stenosis)*

2. Medical management of mitral stenosis may include a daily _____, dipyridamole (Persantine), or other oral anticoagulant to avoid clot formation. *(Aspirin, Beta blocker, Cardiac glycoside)*

3. _____occurs when the mitral valve does not close completely. *(Mitral stenosis, Mitral regurgitation, Aortic stenosis)*

4. If pulmonary congestion occurs with mitral regurgitation, the client will develop _____ *(Shortness of breath and moist lung sounds, Edema of the feet and ankles, Nausea and vomiting)*

5. _____ occurs when valve cusps enlarge, become floppy, and bulge backward into the left atrium. *(Mitral stenosis, Aortic stenosis, Mitral valve prolapse)*

Activity B *Mark each statement as either "T" (True) or "F" (False). Correct the false statement.*

1. T F The pulmonic and tricuspid valves are most commonly affected with valvular disorders.

2. T F In older adults without predisposing cardiac conditions, narrowing of the aortic valve is an age-related degenerative change from progressive calcium deposits in valve cells.

3. **T F**   When blood is pumped through the incompetent aortic valve, some leaks backward into the left ventricle. This backflow reduces cardiac output and causes fluid overload in the left ventricle.

4. **T F**   Digitalis, calcium channel blockers, beta blockers, or other antidysrhythmic drugs are often prescribed with mitral regurgitation to control tachycardia.

5. **T F**   Mitral valve prolapse is considered to be a benign disease for most affected people.

6. **T F**   All symptoms of mitral valve prolapse syndrome are attributed to valvular disease alone.

Activity C *Write the correct term for each description below.*

1. In young adults, aortic stenosis usually is a later consequence of this type of defect in which the valve has two instead of three cusps. _____

2. Can result from damage to the valve cusps or papillary muscles. _____

3. Occurs when the aortic valve does not close tightly and blood can leak backwards into the left ventricle. _____

4. Mitral stenosis is primarily a sequela of this inflammatory heart condition. _____

5. Medical management of mitral regurgitation often includes this type of medication which reduces afterload. _____

Activity D *Match the diagnostic tests in column A with their descriptions in Column B.*

Column A

_____ 1. Chest radiograph

_____ 2. Echocardiogram

_____ 3. Electrocardiogram

_____ 4. Left-sided cardiac catheterization

Column B

a. Reflects the large mass and force of the contracting muscle.

b. Ventricular enlargement is evident.

c. The pressure of blood in the left ventricle is higher than usual.

d. Validates the ventricular thickening and diminished transvalvular size.

Activity E *Compare the following procedures based on the given criteria.*

Procedure	Purpose of procedure
Balloon valvuloplasty	
Annuloplasty	
Intra-aortic balloon pump	
Cardioversion	
Commissurotomy	
Implantation of a biologic or prosthetic valve	

Activity F *Briefly answer the following questions.*

1. In addition to age-related changes and congenital defects, what are other causes of aortic stenosis?

   _____

   _____

   _____

2. A stiff, calcified aortic valve cannot open properly and needs more force to push blood through its narrowed opening. What is the body's response? How can this lead to left-sided heart failure?

   _____

   _____

   _____

3. Describe the medical and surgical management of aortic regurgitation.

   _____

   _____

   _____

4. What are pharmacological considerations with administration of beta blockers?

   _____

   _____

   _____

5. How does mitral stenosis result in pulmonary hypertension and the potential for pulmonary edema? What are the effects on the client?

   _____

   _____

6. What changes in heart sounds occur in mitral stenosis?

_____

_____

_____

SECTION II: APPLYING YOUR KNOWLEDGE

Activity G *Give rationales for the following questions.*

1. Why do clients with aortic stenosis develop symptoms of dyspnea and fatigue with activity, dizziness, fainting, and angina? Why is heart pulsation displaced and carotid pulse weak?

_____

_____

_____

2. Why do clients with aortic regurgitation experience angina?

_____

_____

_____

3. How can mitral stenosis lead to pulmonary emboli?

_____

_____

_____

4. Why do some clients with mitral regurgitation remain asymptomatic or develop symptoms gradually over years?

_____

_____

_____

5. Why do clients with mitral regurgitation develop hypertension and tachycardia?

_____

_____

_____

6. Why are clients with mitral valve prolapse syndrome advised to avoid caffeine and alcohol? What dietary recommendations are made?

_____

_____

_____

Activity H *Answer the following questions related to caring for clients with valvular disorders of the heart.*

1. Describe the medical and surgical management of aortic stenosis.

_____

_____

_____

2. What are signs and symptoms of aortic regurgitation?

_____

_____

_____

3. How can mitral stenosis lead to right-sided heart failure?

_____

_____

_____

4. What happens when the mitral valve becomes incompetent?

_____

_____

_____

5. Describe the assessment finding for mitral valve prolapse.

_____

_____

_____

6. Describe the medical management of mitral valve prolapse.

_____

_____

_____

Activity I *Think over the following questions. Discuss them with your instructor or peers.*

1. Your client is diagnosed with aortic stenosis. What nursing assessments and interventions are indicated to ensure adequate cardiac output and tissue perfusion?

   _____

   _____

   _____

2. Your client is at risk for developing signs and symptoms of pulmonary congestion. What nursing assessments and interventions are indicated to detect and reduce the effects of pulmonary congestion?

   _____

   _____

   _____

SECTION III: GETTING READY FOR NCLEX

Activity J *Answer the following questions.*

1. Which of the following is an early indication of mitral valve stenosis?
   a. Changes in heart sounds
   b. Crackles in the bases of the lungs
   c. Heart palpitations
   d. Dyspnea

2. Which of the following adverse symptoms should a nurse observe when administering quinidine to a client with valvular disorder of the heart?
   a. Ringing of the ears
   b. Stiff neck
   c. Bradycardia
   d. Bluish discoloration of the palms

3. A client with a valvular disorder of the heart is experiencing activity intolerance. Which of the following nursing interventions should the nurse perform to help the client manage self-care and moderate activity?
   a. Assist the client to lie flat.
   b. Caution the client against lifting heavy objects.

   c. Intersperse periods of activity with rest.
   d. Instruct the client to avoid competitive sports.

4. Which of the following symptoms is the first sign of aortic regurgitation?
   a. Water-hammer pulse
   b. Tachycardia
   c. Flushed skin
   d. Heart murmur

5. Which of the following are the reasons a nurse discourages the consumption of alcohol for a client with mitral valve prolapse?
   a. Tachycardia
   b. Cinchonism
   c. Hypertension
   d. Cardiac stimulation

6. Which of the following are the consequences of fluid and electrolyte imbalances resulting from diuretic therapy in older adults?
   a. Fatigue
   b. Dyspnea
   c. Chest pain
   d. Heart palpitations

7. What condition is characterized by a water hammer pulse?
   a. Aortic regurgitation
   b. Mitral valve stenosis
   c. Mitral regurgitation
   d. Aortic stenosis

8. Which of the following conditions is identified by a P wave notch in the ECG of a client?
   a. Aortic stenosis
   b. Mitral regurgitation
   c. Aortic regurgitation
   d. Mitral stenosis

9. What does the nurse teach the client who has had a mechanical valve placed?
   a. The PT must remain below 1.5 times the control value.
   b. The PTT must be higher than 2.5 times the control value.
   c. The INR must be maintained between 2.5 and 3.5 for anticoagulant monitoring
   d. The INR must be maintained below 2.5 for anticoagulant monitoring.

10. What procedure is used cautiously or not at all in elderly clients who have aortic stenosis because stretching may fracture the aortic valve if it is calcified, as is often the case in older clients?

a. Balloon valvuloplasty

b. Cardiac catheterization

c. Coronary artery bypass grafting

d. Valvular heart surgery

Caring for Clients with Disorders of Coronary and Peripheral Blood Vessels

Learning Objectives

1. Distinguish between arteriosclerosis and atherosclerosis.
2. List risk factors associated with coronary artery disease and discuss which can be modified.
3. Describe the symptoms, diagnosis, treatment, and nursing management of coronary artery disease.
4. Discuss the symptoms, diagnosis, treatment, and nursing management of myocardial infarction.
5. Discuss the symptoms, diagnosis, treatment, and nursing management of Raynaud's disease, thrombosis, phlebothrombosis, embolism, and venous insufficiency.
6. Discuss the symptoms, diagnosis, and treatment of varicose veins.
7. Describe nursing management of clients undergoing surgery for varicose veins.
8. Discuss the symptoms, diagnosis, treatment, and nursing management of clients with an aortic aneurysm.

SECTION I: ASSESSING YOUR UNDERSTANDING

Activity A *Fill in the blanks by choosing the correct word from the options given in parentheses.*

1. _____ refers to the loss of elasticity or hardening of the arteries that accompanies the aging process. *(Atheroma, Arteriosclerosis, Atherosclerosis)*

2. _____ is an area of tissue that dies from inadequate oxygenation. *(Ischemia, An infarct, A thrombosis)*

3. _____ is characterized by periodic constriction of the arteries that supply the extremities. The disorder is most common in young women; symptoms often develop after exposure to cold. *(Raynaud's disease, A thrombus, An embolus)*

4. _____ is the development of a clot within a vein without inflammation. *(A thrombus, Phlebothrombosis, An embolus)*

5. Mild fever and pain, swelling, and tenderness of the affected extremity and possibly a positive Homans' sign are signs and symptoms of _____. *(An arterial occlusion, A deep vein thrombosis, An embolus)*

6. _____ is a peripheral vascular disorder in which the flow of venous blood is impaired through deep or superficial veins (or both). The condition usually affects the lower extremities, most often the medial aspect of the leg or around the ankle. *(Venous insufficiency, Varicose veins, Aneurysm)*

7. Legs feel heavy and tired, particularly after prolonged standing; activity or elevation of the legs relieves the discomfort. This is a symptom of _____. *(An aneurysm, A thrombus, Varicose veins)*

Activity B *Mark each statement as either "T" (True) or "F" (False). Correct any false statements.*

1. T F As cells in arterial tissue layers degenerate with age, calcium is deposited in the cytoplasm. The calcium causes the arteries to lose elasticity, resulting in arteriosclerosis.

2. T F Research indicates that infection and inflammation may be implicated in the development of atherosclerosis.

3. T F Coronary artery disease refers to arteriosclerotic and atherosclerotic changes in the coronary arteries supplying the myocardium.

4. T F The size of the necrotic area caused by a myocardial infarction is insignificant; damage to the heart muscle is the same regardless of the type.

5. T F Each coronary artery supplies all areas of the heart. If one coronary artery is occluded, the other coronary arteries will compensate.

6. T F Older adults and diabetics may experience little or no pain with a myocardial infarction and never know they had an MI until an ECG detects it.

7. T F Pain from a myocardial infarction can be relieved with rest and sublingual nitrates.

8. T F An embolus is a stationary clot.

9. T F Vein ligation is a procedure where the ligated veins are severed and removed.

Activity C *Write the correct term for each description given below.*

1. A condition in which the lumen of arteries fill with fatty deposits called plaque. _____

2. Refers to arteriosclerotic and atherosclerotic changes in the coronary arteries supplying the myocardium. _____

3. A radiologic test that produces x-rays of the coronary arteries using an electron beam. _____

4. Occurs when there is prolonged total occlusion of coronary arterial blood flow. _____

5. The most common cause of a myocardial infarction. _____

6. A medically supervised program which combines exercise and educational activities to speed recovery and reduce or prevent recurring episodes following a significant cardiac event. _____

7. Dilated, tortuous veins. _____

8. A stretching and bulging of an arterial wall. _____

Activity D *Match the diagnostic tests of peripheral blood vessels in Column A to their descriptions in Column B.*

Column A

___ 1. Phlebography
___ 2. Doppler ultrasonography
___ 3. Plethysmography
___ 4. Photoplethysmography
___ 5. Air plethysmography

Column B

a. Measures volume changes in the venous or arterial system.

b. Used to detect abnormalities in peripheral blood flow.

c. A diagnostic test for venous pathology, measures light that is not absorbed by hemoglobin and consequently is reflected back to the machine.

d. Measures venous pressure by filling a cuff with air after it is applied to the calf while the client is supine with the legs elevated. When the client stands, the pressure is measured again and venous pressure increases, indicating an increased volume of venous reflux.

e. Uses a contrast dye to identify the point of obstruction.

Activity E *Compare the following procedures based on the following criteria.*

Procedure	Purpose	Description
Percutaneous transluminal coronary angioplasty (PTCA)		
Atherectomy		
Coronary artery bypass graft (CABG)		
Transmyocardial revascularization (TMR)		

Activity F *Briefly answer the following questions.*

1. What are contributing factors to hyperlipidemia?

_____

_____

_____

2. How can atherosclerosis contribute to the development of a blood clot?

_____

_____

_____

3. What are typical symptoms associated with coronary artery disease?

_____

_____

_____

4. Describe the treatment for coronary artery disease.

_____

_____

_____

5. What interventions will the nurse perform to relieve symptoms of angina?

_____

_____

_____

6. What activities may assist the client in aborting an attack associated with Raynaud's disease?

_____

_____

_____

7. Describe the treatment for a venous thrombus.

_____

_____

_____

8. What types of treatments may be ordered to promote venous circulation for a client with venous insufficiency?

_____

_____

_____

9. What is the treatment for an aneurysm?

_____

_____

_____

SECTION II: APPLYING YOUR KNOWLEDGE

Activity G *Provide the rationale for the following questions.*

1. Why are women who have coronary artery disease (CAD) often misdiagnosed?

_____

_____

_____

2. Why do clients with CAD experience angina pectoris?

_____

_____

_____

3. Why are coronary stents usually placed following a percutaneous transluminal coronary angioplasty?

_____

_____

_____

4. Why is troponin considered the gold standard for determining heart damage in the early stages of a myocardial infarction? What other isoenzymes are cardiac specific?

_____

_____

_____

5. Why is the goal for administering thrombolitics a "door to needle" time of 30 minutes? What is the alternative for clients who are not candidates for thrombolitic therapy?

_____

_____

_____

6. Why do symptoms of localized edema, dermatitis, discoloration, and venous stasis ulcers occur with venous insufficiency?

_____

_____

_____

7. How can an aneurysm lead to shock or death?

_____

_____

_____

Activity H *Answer the following questions related to disorders of coronary and peripheral blood vessels.*

1. Describe the significance of low-density lipoproteins and high-density lipoproteins in coronary artery disease.

_____

_____

_____

2. What events follow a myocardial infarction that restores some of the lost blood flow and damage to the myocardial tissue?

_____

_____

_____

3. What treatment is indicated in the symptomatic management following a myocardial infarction?

_____

_____

_____

4. What conditions or situations commonly precipitate the development of a thrombosis in the venous system?

_____

_____

_____

5. What are the signs and symptoms of an arterial thrombus?

_____

_____

_____

6. What is the treatment for an arterial thrombus?

_____

_____

_____

7. How do varicose veins develop?

_____

_____

_____

Activity I *Think over the following questions. Discuss them with your instructor or peers.*

1. Your client states they are at risk for coronary artery disease because of heredity factor and asks what behavior changes they can make to reduce their risk. What educational information would you provide?

_____

_____

_____

2. A client is diagnosed in the emergency department with an acute myocardial infarction. You took the client's medical history and know that thrombolitic therapy is absolutely

contraindicated. What are the possible reasons this client can not receive thrombolitics?

_____

_____

_____

3. Your client is ready for discharge following percutaneous transluminal coronary angioplasty. What discharge information will you provide?

_____

_____

_____

4. Your client has been admitted with a deep vein thrombosis. What are the nursing assessments and interventions indicated?

_____

_____

_____

SECTION III: GETTING READY FOR NCLEX

Activity J *Answer the following questions.*

1. Which of the following determine the possibility of the client having coronary artery disease?
   a. Tachycardia
   b. Hair loss
   c. Chest Pain
   d. Numbness and tingling

2. Why should a nurse assess a client's mental status after a TMR (Transmyocardial Revascularization) procedure?
   a. Cerebral hemorrhage may occur.
   b. Severe headache may occur.
   c. Loss of consciousness may occur.
   d. Cerebral emboli may occur.

3. Which of the following is the correct manner of estimating a cardiac risk?
   a. Divide total serum cholesterol level by the HDL level; result greater than five suggests a potential for CAD.
   b. Multiply total serum cholesterol level by the HDL level; result greater than five suggests a potential for CAD.

   c. Divide total serum cholesterol level by the LDL level; result greater than five suggests a potential for CAD.
   d. Divide total serum cholesterol level by the HDL level; result greater than seven suggests a potential for CAD.

4. A male client, age 72, complains of swollen and heavy legs. The client also informs the nurse that activity or elevation of the leg relieves the pain in his legs. Which of the following conditions will the nurse suspect from the symptoms mentioned by the client?
   a. Coronary artery disease
   b. Myocardial infraction
   c. Varicose veins
   d. Thrombosis

5. Which of the following is an appropriate nursing intervention for clients with varicose veins?
   a. The nurse assesses the appearance of the ankles and the quality of circulation extending downward.
   b. The nurse assesses the skin, distal circulation, and peripheral edema.
   c. The nurse obtains the family history and identifies the characteristics of the pain.
   d. The nurse assesses the characteristics of chest pain.

6. Which of the following should the nurse monitor for clients with aneurysms to determine the signs of hemorrhage or dissection?
   a. Nurse monitors for swelling and heaviness of the legs.
   b. Nurse monitors for chest pain and elevated LDL levels.
   c. Nurse monitors the BP, hourly urine output, skin color, and level of consciousness.
   d. Nurse monitors for mild fever and swelling of extremities.

7. Which of the following diets should the nurse recommend for clients with hypercholesterolemia under the physician's guidance?
   a. The food guide pyramid
   b. The step one diet
   c. The General Motors diet
   d. The Fad diet

8. An elderly client is diagnosed with a condition in which calcium causes the arteries to lose elasticity. As the left ventricle contracts, sending oxygenated blood from the heart, the rigid arterial vessels fail to stretch. What is the medical diagnosis to which this condition refers?

    a. Arteriosclerosis

    b. Coronary occlusion

    c. Ischemia

    d. Atherosclerosis

9. A client has chest pain and is admitted to the hospital. The procedure that the client undertakes is described as a balloon-tipped catheter inserted through the skin and threaded from a peripheral artery into the diseased coronary artery. The inflation of the balloon compresses the atherosclerotic plaque against the arterial wall, increasing the diameter of the artery. What is the procedure called?

    a. Coronary stent

    b. Atherectomy

    c. Percutaneous transluminal coronary angioplasty (PTCA)

    d. Coronary artery bypass grafting (CABG)

10. Which of the following is the gold standard laboratory test in identifying heart damage from an acute myocardial infarction?

    a. Myoglobin

    b. Troponin

    c. Creatine kinase (CK)

    d. Aspartate aminotransferase (AST)

Caring for Clients with Cardiac Dysrhythmias

1. Name and describe common cardiac dysrhythmias.
2. Identify medications to control or eliminate dysrhythmias.
3. Explain the purpose and advantages of elective cardioversion.
4. Explain when defibrillation is used to treat dysrhythmias.
5. Discuss the purpose for implanting an automatic internal cardiac defibrillator.
6. Name various types of artificial pacemakers and the purpose for their use.
7. Describe nursing management of the client with a dysrhythmia treated by drug therapy, elective cardioversion, defibrillation, or pacemaker insertion.

SECTION I: ASSESSING YOUR UNDERSTANDING

Activity A *Fill in the blanks by choosing the correct word from the options given in parentheses.*

1. A _____ is a conduction disorder that results in an abnormally slow or rapid heart rate or one that does not proceed through the conduction system in the usual manner. _____ *(Dysrhythmia, Sinus bradycardia, Sinus tachycardia)*

2. In _____, several areas in the right atrium initiate impulses resulting in disorgan-ized, rapid activity. *(Atrial flutter, Atrial fibrillation, Heart block)*

3. In _____ the atrial impulse never gets through, and the ventricles develop their own rhythm independent of the atrial rhythm. *(First-degree heart block, Second-degree heart block, Complete heart block)*

4. _____ is a ventricular contraction that occurs early and independently in the cardiac cycle before the SA node initiates an electrical impulse. *(Premature ventricular contraction, Ventricular tachycardia, Ventricular fibrillation)*

5. _____ is the rhythm of a dying heart; the ventricles do not contract effectively and there is no cardiac output. *(Premature ventricular contraction, Ventricular tachycardia, Ventricular fibrillation)*

6. An_____ is commonly located in public places such as worksites and locations where large numbers of people gather. It is also carried on some airplanes and police cars. The machine analyzes the heart's rhythm to determine if defibrillation is needed. *(Automatic external defibrillator, Automatic implanted cardioverter defibrillator, Implanted pacemaker)*

7. A _____ provides an electrical stimulus to the heart muscle to treat an ineffective bra-dydysrhythmia. *(Defibrillator, Pacemaker, Cardioversion)*

8. _____ is a procedure in which a heated catheter tip destroys dysrhythmia producing

tissue. *(Automatic external defibrillator, Radiofrequency catheter ablation, Elective electrical cardioversion)*

Activity B *Mark each statement as either "T" (True) or "F" (False). Correct any false statements.*

1. T F   Cardiac dysrhythmias may originate in the atria, atrioventricular node, or ventricles.

2. T F   Sinus tachycardia occurs in clients with healthy hearts as a physiologic response to strenuous exercise, anxiety and fear, pain, fever, hyperthyroidism, hemorrhage, shock, or hypoxemia.

3. T F   In first- and second-degree heart block, the impulse arises outside the normal conduction pathway.

4. T F   Premature atrial contractions often cause a flip-flop sensation in the chest, sometimes described as "fluttering."

5. T F   Premature ventricular contractions are always harmless.

6. T F   Ventricular fibrillation is an indication for cardiopulmonary resuscitation (CPR) and immediate defibrillation.

7. T F   Because of the altered rate and rhythm, all dysrhythmias affect the heart's pumping action and cardiac output to some degree.

Activity C *Write the correct term for each description given below.*

1. The usual cardiac rhythm. _____

2. The most common cause of dysrhythmias. _____

3. The use of drugs to eliminate dysrhythmia. _____

4. Refers to disorders in the conduction pathway that interfere with the transmission of impulses from the SA node through the AV node to the ventricles. _____

5. If performed within the first 5 minutes of ventricular fibrillation or cardiac arrest, the potential for survival is 50%; after 10 minutes without treatment, the chance for resuscitation is unlikely. _____

6. A nonemergency procedure done by a physician to stop rapid, but not necessarily life-threatening, atrial dysrhythmias._____

7. The only treatment for a life-threatening ventricular dysrhythmia; used when there is no functional ventricular contraction._____

8. A totally implanted device used to manage a chronic bradydysrhythmia. _____

Activity D *Given in Column A are types of premature ventricular contractions. Match these with their descriptions given in Column B.*

Column A

____ 1. Bigeminy

____ 2. Couplets

____ 3. A run of PVCs

____ 4. Multifocal PVCs

____ 5. R-on-T-phenomenon

Column B

a. PVCs that originate from more than one location.

b. A PVC whose R wave falls on the T wave of the preceding complex.

c. Two PVCs in a row.

d. Every other beat is a PVC.

e. Three or more PVCs in a row.

Activity E *Using Table 26-1 on p. 130, compare the dysrhythmias based on the given criteria.*

Activity F *Consider the following figure.*

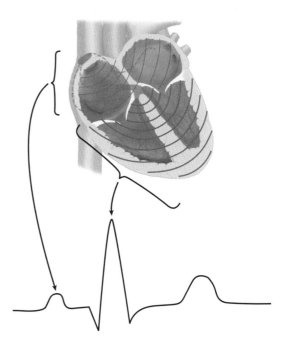

TABLE 26-1

	Rhythm	Atrial beats per minute	Ventricular beats per minute	Treatment
Normal sinus rhythm				
Sinus bradycardia				
Sinus tachycardia				
Premature atrial contraction				
Supraventricular tachycardia				
Atrial flutter				
Atrial fibrillation				
First-degree AV block Second-degree AV block				
Complete heart block				
Ventricular tachycardia				
Ventricular fibrillation				

1. Identify the first wave before the complex. What does this wave correlate with?

   _____

2. Identify the complex. What does the complex correlate with?

   _____

3. Identify the first wave following the complex. What does this wave correlate with?

   _____

Activity H *Briefly answer the following questions.*

1. Describe atrial flutter.

   _____

   _____

2. How can atrial fibrillation result in the formation of blood clots? What is the treatment?

   _____

   _____

   _____

3. What is the Maze procedure? What dysrhythmia is it used to treat?

   _____

   _____

   _____

4. Identify common causes of occasional premature ventricular contractions that are usually harmless. What are the associated symptoms?

   _____

   _____

   _____

5. What does electrical cardioversion do to the heart?

   _____

   _____

   _____

6. What is the purpose of an electrophysiology study?

   _____

   _____

   _____

SECTION II: APPLYING YOUR KNOWLEDGE

Activity I *Give rationale for the following questions.*

1. Why can sinus bradycardia be dangerous for the client?

   _____

   _____

2. Why is supraventricular tachycardia dangerous for the client?

_____

_____

_____

3. Why does atrial fibrillation result in an irregular ventricular heart rate?

_____

_____

_____

4. Why do clients with coronary artery disease and supraventricular tachycardia develop chest pain?

_____

_____

_____

5. Why do some clients with dysrhythmias not require antidysrhythmic drugs?

_____

_____

_____

6. Why are digitalis and diuretics withheld for 24 to 48 hours before cardioversion?

_____

_____

_____

Activity J _Answer the following questions related to caring for clients with cardiac dysrhythmias._

1. Describe the origin and appearance of a premature atrial contraction. What are common causes of the dysrhythmia?

_____

_____

2. Describe the characteristics of ventricular tachycardia.

_____

_____

_____

3. What are assessment findings for a client with a dysrhythmia?

_____

_____

_____

4. What is an automatic implanted cardioverter defibrillator?

_____

_____

5. What is the difference between demand (synchronous) mode pacemakers and fixed-rate (asynchronous) mode pacemakers?

_____

_____

_____

6. What is the difference between the following temporary pacemakers; transcutaneous, transvenous, and transthoracic?

_____

_____

_____

Activity K _Think over the following questions. Discuss them with your instructor or peers._

1. You are preparing a client for an elective electrical cardioversion. What are the nursing assessments and interventions indicated pre- and post-procedure?

_____

_____

_____

2. Your client is symptomatic with a heart rate of 42 and unresponsive to medication. What nursing assessments and interventions are indicated with the use of a transcutaneous pacemaker?

_____

_____

_____

3. Your client goes into ventricular fibrillation. What actions will you take?

_____

_____

_____

SECTION III: GETTING READY FOR NCLEX

Activity L *Answer the following questions.*

1. Which of the following dysrhythmias is frequent during the early post-implantation period of an internal pacemaker?
   a. Ventricular tachycardia
   b. Ventricular fibrillation
   c. Premature ventricular contractions
   d. Premature atrial contractions

2. Which of the following is an indication of an alarm sound when a client with transvenous pacemaker is on a cardiac monitor?
   a. Client's heart rate drops below the lowest level set on the alarm system.
   b. Client is confused or restless and physical movement disturbs external pacemaker.
   c. Client's heartbeat is greater than 60 beats/minute.
   d. Client's blood pressure drops below the lowest level set on the alarm system.

3. A client with dysrhythmia has decreased cardiac output. Which of the following nursing interventions is essential to maintain adequate cardiac output?
   a. Encourage mild exercises
   b. Place the client in supine position
   c. Ensure a client IV access
   d. Provide supplemental oxygen

4. Which of the following adverse effects should a nurse check for when administering lidocaine?
   a. Convulsions
   b. Amnesia
   c. Dyspnea
   d. Urinary retention

5. A nurse is required to monitor a client with dysrhythmia during the administration of isoproterenol. Which of the following nursing interventions will help to determine the drug response?

   a. Monitor vital signs.
   b. Closely monitor the pulse rate.
   c. Monitor blood pressure.
   d. Monitor fluid intake and output.

6. A client is admitted to the hospital with a dysrhythmia. Which of the following is the most common cause of dysrhythmias?
   a. Hypothermia
   b. Metabolic acidosis
   c. Drug therapy
   d. Ischemic heart disease

7. A nurse responds to a telemetry alarm and determines that the client is in which rhythm, where the rate is greater than 150, diastole is shortened, and the heart does not have sufficient time to fill?
   a. Sinus bradycardia
   b. Sinus tachycardia
   c. Supraventricular Tachycardia
   d. Atrial flutter

8. What is the best rationale for acting quickly to restore an elderly client's heart rate from a new onset of atrial fibrillation to normal sinus rhythm?
   a. Increased risk of stroke
   b. Increased risk of heart attack
   c. Increased risk of endocarditis
   d. Increased risk of bradycardia

9. A nurse is teaching a client with a history of dysrhythmias about changes in diet. Which of the following does the nurse suggest to the client to prevent catecholamine release, which may cause dangerous dysrhythmias?
   a. Eat a low salt, high fiber diet.
   b. Drink no more than 6 oz. of beer or wine per day.
   c. Drink at least 10 glasses of water per day.
   d. Eat a variety of foods according to the food pyramid.

CHAPTER 27

Caring for Clients with Hypertension

Learning Objectives

1. Identify the two physiologic components that create blood pressure.
2. List factors that influence blood pressure.
3. List three structures that physiologically control arterial pressure.
4. Explain systolic and diastolic arterial pressure.
5. Define hypertension and identify groups at risk for it.
6. Differentiate essential and secondary hypertension.
7. Identify causes of secondary hypertension.
8. List consequences of chronic hypertension.
9. Discuss the assessment findings in hypertension.
10. Discuss the medical and nursing management of the client with hypertension.
11. Differentiate between accelerated and malignant hypertension.
12. Identify potential complications of uncontrolled malignant hypertension.
13. Discuss the medical and nursing management of the client with malignant hypertension.

SECTION I: ASSESSING YOUR UNDERSTANDING

Activity A *Fill in the blanks by choosing the correct word from the options given in parentheses.*

1. _____ is the force produced by the volume of blood in arterial walls. *(Stroke volume, Cardiac output, Blood pressure)*

2. _____ is determined by the force and volume of blood that the left ventricle ejects and the ability of the arterial system to distend at the time of ventricular contraction. *(Systolic blood pressure, Diastolic blood pressure, Hypertensive disease)*

3. _____ is a systolic blood pressure of 120 to 139 mm Hg or a diastolic blood pressure between 80 and 89 mm Hg. *(Normal blood pressure, Prehypertension, Stage 1 hypertension)*

4. _____ may cause a persistent cough until the medication is discontinued. *(Thiazide diuretics, ACE inhibitors, Beta blockers)*

5. _____ describes markedly elevated BP, accompanied by hemorrhages and exudates in the eyes. *(Stage 1 hypertension, Stage 2 hypertension, Accelerated hypertension)*

Activity B *Mark each statement as either "T" (True) or "F" (False). Correct any false statement.*

1. T F Blood pressure is represented by the following formula: BP = CO (cardiac output) × SV (stroke volume).

2. T F Hypertension is a sustained elevation in systolic or diastole blood pressure that exceeds Stage 1 hypertension levels.

3. **T F** Stage 2 hypertension is defined as a systolic blood pressure of 140 to 159 or a diastolic blood pressure between 90 and 99.

4. **T F** Clients with hypertension may be asymptomatic. The onset of hypertension, considered "the silent killer," often is gradual.

5. **T F** Accelerated and malignant hypertension usually have gradual onset.

Activity C *Write the correct term for each description below.*

1. Reflects arterial pressure during ventricular relaxation. _____

2. The ethnic group at highest risk for development of hypertension. _____

3. Vascular changes in the eyes, retinal hemorrhages, or edema of the optic nerves associated with hypertension. _____

4. A possible adverse effect with all antihypertensive drugs. _____

5. Describes dangerously elevated BP accompanied by papilledema. _____

Activity D *Match the various terms given in Column A to their associated definitions or effects given in Column B*

Column A

_____ 1. Essential hypertension

_____ 2. Secondary hypertension

_____ 3. White-coat hypertension

Column B

a. A term describing elevated BP that develops during evaluation by medical personnel. This hypertension most likely results from anxiety that is accompanied by a surge of epinephrine and norepinephrine, powerful neurohormones that cause vasoconstriction.

b. Sustained elevated BP with no known cause.

c. Elevated BP that results from or is secondary to some other disorder.

Activity E *Identify the correlation of the electrolytes and body chemicals to essential hypertension based on the given criteria.*

	Effects on Blood Pressure
Sodium	
Potassium	
Calcium	
Renin-angiotensin-aldosterone mechanism	
Catecholamines	
Natriuretic factor	

Activity F *Briefly answer the following questions.*

1. What does the measured BP reflect?

_____

_____

_____

2. What factors affect blood pressure?

_____

_____

_____

3. What causes an in increase in peripheral vascular resistance, which in turn increases systolic blood pressure?

_____

_____

_____

4. Describe the difference between hypertensive heart disease, hypertensive vascular disease, and hypertensive cardiovascular disease.

_____

_____

_____

5. How is medication usually prescribed for the hypertensive client?

_____

_____

_____

6. What types of clients develop accelerated or malignant hypertension?

_____

_____

_____

7. How is accelerated and malignant hypertension medically managed?

_____

_____

_____

SECTION II: APPLYING YOUR KNOWLEDGE

Activity G *Provide rationale for the questions.*

1. Why does blood pressure tend to increase with age?

_____

_____

_____

2. How can hypertension lead to heart failure?

_____

_____

_____

3. How can hypertension lead to angina?

_____

_____

_____

4. Why is caffeine intake reduced or eliminated in clients with hypertension?

_____

_____

_____

5. Why is the client on antihypertensive medication advised to rise slowly from a sitting or lying position?

_____

_____

_____

6. Why is malignant hypertension fatal unless BP is quickly reduced?

_____

_____

_____

Activity H *Answer the following questions related to caring for clients with hypertension.*

1. What predisposing conditions may cause secondary hypertension?

_____

_____

_____

2. What changes to the arterial vascular system and serious complications may occur as a result of hypertension?

_____

_____

_____

3. What are risk factors for the development of hypertension?

_____

_____

_____

4. What are the signs and symptoms of hypertension?

_____

_____

_____

5. What nonpharmacologic interventions are used for clients with prehypertension?

_____

_____

_____

6. How is the client with hypertension assessed?

_____

_____

_____

7. Describe the signs and symptoms associated with accelerated and malignant hypertension.

_____

_____

_____

Activity I *Think over the following questions. Discuss them with your instructor or peers.*

1. Your client is admitted with malignant hypertension. What are the indicated nursing assessments and interventions to care for this client?

_____

_____

_____

2. Your client requires education on the DASH diet. What information would you provide?

_____

_____

_____

3. Your client is diagnosed with prehypertension. The client asks how he can reduce his blood pressure without the use of medications. What information will you provide?

_____

_____

_____

SECTION III: GETTING READY FOR NCLEX

Activity J *Answer the following questions.*

1. Which of the following is a nursing intervention when assessing clients with hypertension?
   a. The nurse takes the temperature when the client is in a standing, sitting, and then supine position.
   b. The nurse teaches the client about non-pharmacologic and pharmacologic methods for restoring BP.
   c. The nurse takes BP in both arms when the client is in a standing, sitting, and then supine position.
   d. The nurse weighs the client each morning.

2. Which of the following must the nurse consider when administering IV fluids to clients with hypertension?
   a. The nurse checks the client's BP every hour.
   b. The nurse checks the site and progress of the infusion every hour.
   c. The nurse checks the progress of the infusion once a day.
   d. The nurse checks the clients pulse rate every hour.

3. Why does the nurse instruct the client to avoid Valsalva maneuvers?
   a. Client's BP will decrease momentarily.
   b. Client may suffer from a myocardial infarction.
   c. Client may lose consciousness.
   d. Client's BP will increase momentarily.

4. Which of the following is a nursing intervention to ensure that the client is free from injury caused by falls?
   a. Nurse monitors for chest pain and elevated LDL levels.
   b. Nurse monitors for swelling and heaviness of legs.
   c. Nurse monitors postural changes in BP.
   d. Nurse monitors temperature for mild fever.

5. Which of the following diets does the nurse recommend for clients with hypertension under the physician's guidance?
   a. The food guide pyramid
   b. The step one diet
   c. The South Beach diet
   d. The DASH diet

6. A male client, age 78, complains of dizziness, especially when he stands up after sleeping or sitting. The client also informs the nurse that he periodically experiences nosebleeds and blurred vision. Which of the following conditions should the nurse assess for the client?
   a. Postural hypotension
   b. White-coat hypertension
   c. Postural hypertension
   d. White-coat hypotension

7. Why should the nurse monitor ACE inhibitors cautiously in clients with renal or hepatic impairment and older adults?

   a. A sudden raise in BP may occur during the first 1 to 3 hours after the initial dosage.

   b. A sudden drop in BP may occur during the first 1 to 3 hours after the initial dosage.

   c. A sudden drop in body temperature may occur during the first 1 to 3 hours after the initial dosage.

   d. A sudden raise in pulse rate may occur during the first 1 to 3 hours after the initial dosage.

8. A nurse takes a 40-year-old client's blood pressure in the doctor's office during a routine follow up for a blood pressure check. The client's systolic pressure is 160 and the diastolic is 90. What type of hypertension is the client exhibiting if this is the third result at this level?

   a. Stage 2 hypertension

   b. Prehypertension

   c. Stage 1 hypertension

   d. Hypertensive heart disease

9. Which of the following current conditions for a client might necessitate the doctor to prescribe an ACE inhibitor as the first line of antihypertensive therapy in a client with hypertension?

   a. Chronic kidney disease

   b. Heart failure

   c. Diabetes

   d. High CVD risk

10. How might the blood pressure be affected in a client whose body mass index (BMI) is 31 (obese)?

    a. increased

    b. decreased

    c. no change

    d. a change either way

Caring for Clients with Heart Failure

Learning Objectives

1. Discuss the pathophysiology and etiology of heart failure.
2. Distinguish between acute and chronic heart failure.
3. Identify differences between left-sided and right-sided heart failure.
4. Describe the symptoms, diagnosis, and treatment of left-sided and right-sided heart failure.
5. Discuss the nursing management of clients with heart failure.
6. Discuss the pathophysiology, etiology, symptoms, diagnosis, and treatment of pulmonary edema.
7. Discuss the nursing management of clients with pulmonary edema.

SECTION I: ASSESSING YOUR UNDERSTANDING

Activity A *Fill in the blanks by choosing the correct word from the options given in parentheses.*

1. An estimate of the heart's efficiency as a pump is its _____, the percentage of blood the left ventricle ejects when it contracts. *(ejection fraction, preload, afterload)*

2. _____ is a sudden change in the heart's ability to contract. It can cause life-threatening symptoms and pulmonary edema. *(Acute heart failure, Chronic heart failure, Intermittent heart failure)*

3. _____ is the force that the ventricle must overcome to empty its diastolic volume; it may increase as a result of arterial hypertension, aortic stenosis, pulmonary hypertension, or excessive blood volume from renal failure. *(Preload, Afterload, Interload)*

4. _____ restores synchrony in the contractions of the right and left ventricles which is achieved with a biventricular pacemaker. *(Intra-aortic balloon pump, Cardiac resynchronization therapy, Multiple gated acquisition scan)*

5. _____ may be used if cardiogenic shock accompanies acute left ventricular heart failure. *(An intra-aortic balloon pump, Cardiac resynchronization therapy, A multiple gated acquisition scan)*

Activity B *Mark each statement as either "T" (True) or "F" (False). Correct any false statements.*

1. T F Congestive heart failure (CHF) describes the accumulation of blood and fluid in organs and tissues from impaired circulation.

2. T F Left-sided heart failure occurs when the ventricle fails to eject its total diastolic filling volume into the pulmonary artery, causing congestion of blood in the venous vascular system.

3. T F A loss of muscle elasticity due to cardio-myopathy, or a reduced ventricular ejection volume because diastole is shortened due to a tachydysrhythmia, can cause a decreased preload.

4. T F Usually when a client has chronic heart failure, he or she develops signs and symptoms of both right-sided and left-sided heart failure.

5. T F When clients with acute pulmonary edema are oxygenated, a mask, rather than nasal cannula, is needed to deliver the maximum percentages of oxygen.

Activity C *Write the correct term for each description given below.*

1. The inability of the heart to pump sufficient blood to meet the body's metabolic needs.

   _____

2. Occurs when the heart's ability to pump effectively is gradually compromised and its impaired contractility remains prolonged.

   _____

3. A reduction in the ventricular ejection volume because diastole is shortened as a result of a tachydysrhythmia. _____

4. The major cause of right-sided heart failure.

   _____

5. The most accurate noninvasive test that measures the left ventricle's ejection fraction during rest and activity. _____

6. Some clients awaiting heart transplants are treated with an auxiliary heart pump that supplements the heart's ability to eject blood.

   _____

Activity D *Compare right sided heart failure and left sided heart failure based on the given criteria.*

Criteria	Left Ventricular Failure	Right Ventricular Failure
Function		
Pathophysiology		
Affects of congestion		
Signs and symptoms		

Activity E *Match the medication in Column A with their mechanisms of action in Column B.*

Column A

_____ 1. Cardiac glycosides

_____ 2. Diuretics

_____ 3. Vasodilators

_____ 4. Nonglycoside inotropic agents

_____ 5. ACE inhibitors

_____ 6. hBNP

Column B

a. Promote sodium and water excretion, thus reducing circulating blood volume and decreasing heart's workload.

b. Improve stroke volume by reducing afterload; reduce preload by dilating veins and arteries.

c. Block ACE from converting angiotensin I to angiotensin II (a potent vasoconstrictor); promote fluid and sodium loss and decrease peripheral vascular resistance.

d. Increase cardiac output by slowing heart rate and increasing force of contraction.

e. Peptide hormone that acts on the kidney to increase the excretions of sodium and water and reduce blood pressure.

f. Relieve cardiogenic shock by strengthening force of myocardial contraction.

Activity F *Briefly answer the following questions.*

1. What two mechanisms can cause heart failure?

   _____

   _____

   _____

2. How do chronic respiratory disorders affect the right side of the heart?

   _____

   _____

   _____

3. What is the compensatory response of the renal system to a decrease in cardiac output?

_____

_____

_____

4. What is the compensatory response of the adrenal gland to the presence of angiotensin in response to a decrease in cardiac output?

_____

_____

_____

5. Describe a cardiomyoplasty.

_____

_____

_____

6. What are the signs and symptoms of acute pulmonary edema?

_____

_____

_____

SECTION II: APPLYING YOUR KNOWLEDGE

Activity G *Give rationale for the following questions.*

1. How does β-type natriuretic peptide decrease blood pressure?

_____

_____

_____

2. Why are small, frequent meals offered to clients with heart failure?

_____

_____

_____

3. Why are clients with heart failure instructed to avoid activities that engage the Valsalva maneuver, such as straining with bowel elimi-

nation or using the arms to pull and reposition oneself?

_____

_____

_____

4. Why is pulmonary edema a serious complication of left sided heart failure?

_____

_____

_____

5. Why is morphine administered to clients with acute pulmonary edema?

_____

_____

_____

Activity H *Answer the following questions related to caring for clients with heart failure.*

1. Describe the compensatory response of the sympathetic nervous system to a decrease in cardiac output.

_____

_____

_____

2. What is the medical treatment for heart failure?

_____

_____

_____

3. What types of medications are used to manage heart failure?

_____

_____

_____

4. What is ventricular restoration?

_____

_____

_____

5. What is an artificial heart?

_____

_____

_____

6. What is the pathophysiology of acute pulmonary edema?

_____

_____

_____

Activity I *Think over the following questions. Discuss them with your instructor or peers.*

1. Your client has a new onset of heart failure and requires education. What information will you provide to assist the client in managing this disease process?

_____

_____

_____

2. What nursing assessments and interventions are indicated for the client with heart failure?

_____

_____

_____

3. Your client has signs and symptoms of acute pulmonary edema. What are the nursing assessments and interventions indicated?

_____

_____

_____

SECTION III: GETTING READY FOR NCLEX

Activity J *Answer the following questions.*

1. A client with a suspected left-sided heart failure is scheduled to undergo a multiple gated acquisition scan (MUGA). Which of the following actions are required before undergoing the test?

a. Diuretics are administered.

b. Client is medicated to relieve cough.

c. Client should avoid fluid intake six hours before the test.

d. Client is administered analgesics.

2. Clients with symptomatic heart failure should limit sodium intake to _____ mg of sodium daily.

3. Which of the following dietary recommendations should a nurse give a client taking diuretics?

a. Include potassium-rich foods.

b. Include protein-rich foods.

c. Avoid fruit and fruit juices.

d. Avoid dairy products.

4. Which of the following should the nurse identify as the earliest symptom of heart failure in many older clients?

a. Increased urine output

b. Swollen joints

c. Dyspnea on exertion

d. Nausea and vomiting

5. Which of the following nursing interventions should a nurse perform when caring for a client with congestive heart failure who has decreased cardiac output?

a. Encourage activities that engage the Valsalva maneuver.

b. Encourage the client to perform exercises.

c. Assess apical heart rate before administering digitalis.

d. Offer small, frequent feedings.

6. Which of the following symptoms is observed in the client with right-sided heart failure?

a. Dependent pitting edema

b. Exertional dyspnea

c. Orthopnea

d. Hemoptysis

7. Which of the following classifications of heart failure is defined as marked limitation of physical activity with the client being comfortable at rest, but less than ordinary activity causes fatigue, heart palpitation, or dyspnea?

a. Class II

b. Class I

c. Class IV

d. Class III

8. Which of the following predisposes a client to right-sided heart failure and is a condition in which the heart is affected secondarily by lung damage?
   a. Myocardial infarction
   b. Cor pulmonale
   c. Hypertension
   d. Cardiomyopathy

9. A client comes to the clinic with dyspnea on exertion and a MUGA scan is ordered. The client's ejection fraction should be within which of the following ranges?
   a. 45%–55%
   b. 55% and above
   c. 35%–45%
   d. Less than 35%

10. Which assessment is the most important in determining the amount of fluid that the client is retaining?
    a. Heart sounds
    b. Peripheral pulses
    c. Daily weights
    d. Peripheral edema

CHAPTER 29

Caring for Clients Undergoing Cardiovascular Surgery

Learning Objectives

1. Describe the purpose of cardiopulmonary bypass and its disadvantages.
2. Name indications for cardiac surgery.
3. Describe how coronary artery blood flow is surgically restored.
4. Name four surgical procedures for revascularizing the myocardium.
5. Identify techniques to correct valvular disorders.
6. Describe two methods for controlling bleeding from heart trauma.
7. List five problems associated with heart transplantation.
8. List three types of surgery performed on central or peripheral blood vessels.
9. Discuss the nursing management of clients undergoing cardiovascular surgery.

SECTION I: ASSESSING YOUR UNDERSTANDING

Activity A *Fill in the blanks by choosing the correct word from the options given in parentheses.*

1. _____ refers to surgical techniques that improve the delivery of oxygenated blood to the myocardium for clients who have coronary artery disease. *(Myocardial revasculariza-*

tion, Cardiopulmonary bypass, Extracorporeal circulation)

2. _____ uses a balloon catheter to stretch the stenosed valve. *(A commissurotomy, A balloon valvuloplasty, An annuloplasty)*

3. When a donor heart becomes available, it must be removed from the donor and transplanted within _____ hours of being harvested. *(3, 6, 10)*

4. _____ is the resection and removal of the lining of an artery. It is performed to remove obstructive atherosclerotic plaques from the carotid, femoral, or popliteal arteries. *(A thrombectomy, An embolectomy, An endarterectomy)*

Activity B *Mark each statement as either "T" (True) or "F" (False). Correct any false statements.*

1. T F The internal mammary artery in the chest is the relocated vessel most often used for grafting in coronary artery bypass.

2. T F A valvuloplasty and annuloplasty are procedures that surgically tighten an incompetent valve.

3. T F Surgical replacement of a heart valve with a mechanical valve or a

bioprosthetic valve does not require cardiopulmonary bypass.

4. **T F** The most common method of heart transplant is an orthotopic heart transplant, in which the recipient's failing heart is removed and the donor heart is sutured onto the native great vessels of the heart.

Activity C *Write the correct term for each description related to cardiovascular surgery given below.*

1. This type of surgery improves myocardial oxygenation by bypassing or detouring around the occluded portion of one or more coronary arteries with a relocated blood vessel._____

2. This procedure is performed by means of a thoracotomy. The surgeon places a purse-string suture in the wall of the heart, makes an incision, and inserts his or her finger or a metal dilator into the narrowed valve, stretching its opening. _____

3. To prevent tissue rejection following a heart transplant, recipients are given this type of medication. As a result of taking this medication clients are at risk for infection._____

4. Body surface area is obtained from a chart based on height and weight. _____

Activity D *Match the types of heart valves given in Column A with their corresponding disadvantages given in Column B*

Column A

_____ 1. Hemodynamic monitoring

_____ 2. Direct blood pressure monitoring

_____ 3. Central venous pressure

_____ 4. Pulmonary artery pressure monitoring

_____ 5. Pulmonary capillary wedge pressure

_____ 6. Cardiac index

Column B

a. Reflects the cardiac output in relation to the particular client's body size.

b. A monitor continuously displays the waveform and indicates the client's systolic, diastolic, and mean arterial pressures.

c. Methods include direct BP monitoring, central venous pressure (CVP) monitoring,

and pulmonary artery pressure monitoring.

d. By inserting a multi-lumen catheter into a peripheral vein with a distal tip in the pulmonary artery, pressures and cardiac output can be measured to assess left ventricular function.

e. The retrograde pressure from the fluid on the left side of the heart at the end of left ventricular diastole.

f. Measures the pressure produced by venous blood in the right atrium.

Activity E *Compare the types of surgical myocardial revascularization listed in the table based on the following criteria.*

Surgery	Description	Procedure
Conventional Coronary Artery Bypass Graft (CABG)		
Off-Pump Coronary Artery Bypass (OPCAB)		
Minimally Invasive Direct Coronary Artery Bypass (MIDCAB)		
Port Access Coronary Artery Bypass (PACAB)		

Activity F *Briefly answer the following questions.*

1. How are heart tumors surgically managed?

_____

_____

_____

2. When is a heart transplant indicated in adults, newborns, and infants?

_____

_____

_____

3. When is coronary artery bypass performed?

_____

_____

_____

4. Where are clients who have undergone cardiovascular surgery cared for postoperatively?

_____

_____

_____

5. What problems are associated with heart transplants?

_____

_____

_____

SECTION II: APPLYING YOUR KNOWLEDGE

Activity G _Give rationales for the following questions._

1. Why is antibiotic therapy given for 1 to 2 months following a prosthetic heart valve replacement?

_____

_____

_____

2. Why does a transplanted heart beat faster than the client's natural heart? Why do transplant recipients not experience angina?

_____

_____

_____

3. Why can a thrombectomy or embolectomy be an emergency surgical procedure? How is it performed?

_____

_____

_____

4. Why does the nurse hyperoxygenate with 100% oxygen before suctioning and suction for no longer than 10 to 15 seconds?

_____

_____

_____

5. Why does the nurse provide preoperative instruction for coughing, deep breathing, leg exercises and splinting?

_____

_____

_____

Activity H _Answer the following questions related to caring for clients undergoing cardiovascular surgery._

1. What is the most lethal complication among clients who survive the acute stage of a myocardial infarction? What is the treatment?

_____

_____

_____

2. How are penetrating and non-penetrating heart trauma injuries medically and surgically managed?

_____

_____

_____

3. How are central and peripheral graft procedures preformed?

_____

_____

_____

4. What nursing assessments and interventions will the nurse implement to monitor for postoperative hemorrhage?

_____

_____

_____

Activity I *Think over the following questions. Discuss them with your instructor or peers.*

1. Your client has undergone an aortic graft. What nursing assessments and interventions are indicated?

_____

_____

_____

2. You client has undergone a myocardial revascularization. What nursing assessments and interventions are indicated?

_____

_____

_____

3. You client has undergone a heart transplant. What signs and symptoms are indicative of organ rejection?

_____

_____

_____

SECTION III: GETTING READY FOR NCLEX

Activity J *Answer the following questions.*

1. What are the signs of organ rejection a nurse should closely monitor for when caring for a client after heart transplantation?
   a. Low white blood cell count
   b. ECG changes
   c. Amnesia
   d. Dyspnea

2. Which of the following vessels is often used for grafting?
   a. The basilic and cephalic veins in the arm
   b. The internal mammary and internal thoracic arteries in the chest
   c. The saphenous vein in the leg
   d. The radial artery in the arm

3. Which of the following nursing interventions are required when caring for a client who has had cardiac surgery and is at risk for ineffective tissue perfusion?
   a. Restrict fluid intake.
   b. Ensure client avoids prolonged sitting.

   c. Position lower extremities below level of heart.
   d. Instruct client to avoid leg exercises.

4. Which of the points should a nurse include in the discharge teaching plan for a client after cardiac surgery?
   a. Avoid shower bath and take tub bath until all incisions are healed.
   b. Notify the physician if a painless lump is felt at the top of the chest incision.
   c. Continue to wear support hose or elastic stockings during the night and remove them during the day.
   d. Sexual relations typically can be resumed in two to four weeks depending on tolerance for activity.

5. Why are heart biopsies performed throughout a client's lifetime after heart transplantation?
   a. To detect rejection
   b. To check the rate of the heart beat
   c. To check the heart functionality
   d. To check for heart tumor

6. The average heart beat of a transplanted heart is about _____ beats/minute.

7. Which of the following procedures for coronary artery bypass grafting highlights a shortened operative procedure from 3 to 6 hours to 2 hours and shows promise of decreased mortality from complications?
   a. Minimally invasive direct coronary artery bypass (MIDCAB)
   b. Off-pump coronary artery bypass (OPCAB)
   c. Conventional coronary artery bypass graft (CABG)
   d. Port access coronary artery bypass (PACAB)

8. A client is undergoing a minimally invasive valve approach for surgery by the heart surgeon. What is the main advantage of this type of approach?
   a. Increased surgical trauma
   b. Decreased blood loss
   c. Slower mobility
   d. Less anxiety

9. What short term pharmacological approach is used after a client has a prosthetic heart valve replacement for 1 to 2 months postoperatively?

   a. Anticoagulant therapy

   b. Antibiotic therapy

   c. Ace Inhibitor therapy

   d. Beta Blocker therapy

10. In penetrating heart injuries such as a stab wound, which of the following tears in the heart continues to bleed and does not seal with a clot?

   a. Pericardial tear

   b. Endocardial tear

   c. Epicardial tear

   d. Myocardial tear

CHAPTER 30

Introduction to the Hematopoietic and Lymphatic Systems

Learning Objectives

1. Define hematopoiesis.
2. Name the major structures in the hematopoietic system.
3. Name three types of blood cells produced by bone marrow, and discuss the function of each.
4. List at least five components of plasma.
5. Name three plasma proteins and explain the function of each.
6. Identify the four blood groups and discuss the importance of transfusing compatible types.
7. Explain the components and function of the lymphatic system and its role in hematopoiesis.
8. Describe the pertinent assessments of the hematopoietic and lymphatic systems when obtaining a health history and conducting a physical examination.
9. Name laboratory and diagnostic tests for disorders of the hematopoietic and lymphatic systems.
10. Discuss the nursing management of clients with hematopoietic or lymphatic disorders.

SECTION I: ASSESSING YOUR UNDERSTANDING

Activity A *Fill in the blanks by choosing the correct word from the options given in parentheses.*

1. The _____ manufactures blood cells and hemoglobin. *(Red marrow, Yellow marrow, White marrow)*

2. _____ require iron, B_{12}, B_6, and folate to mature properly. *(Leukocytes, Thrombocytes, Erythrocytes)*

3. The red color of blood is caused by _____ an iron-containing pigment attached to erythrocytes. *(Hemoglobin, Red marrow, Yellow marrow)*

4. Approximately _____ of the thrombocytes remain in the spleen unless needed in cases of significant bleeding. *(1/3, 1/2, 2/3)*

5. Blood cells are suspended in a fluid called plasma, which consists of 90% water and 10% _____ *(Marrow, Lymphokine, Protein)*

Activity B *Mark each statement as either "T" (True) or "F" (False). Correct any false statements.*

1. **T F** The lymphatic system, which includes the thymus gland and spleen, assists in the maturation of certain lymphocytes.

2. **T F** The yellow marrow can not form blood cells.

3. **T F** All blood cells are produced from undifferentiated precursors called pluripotential stem cells in the bone marrow.

4. **T F** Leukocytes only circulate in the blood.

5. **T F** Thrombocytes release a substance known as glycoprotein IIb/IIIa, which causes the platelets to adhere and form a plug, or clot, that occludes the injured vessel.

6. **T F** Globulins plays a key role in forming blood clots. They can be transformed from a liquid to fibrin, a solid that controls bleeding.

Activity C *Write the correct term for each description given below.*

1. The manufacture and development of blood cells. _____

2. The soft tissue that fills spaces in the interior of the long bones and spongy bones of the skeleton. _____

3. The type of marrow that consists primarily of fat cells and connective tissue. _____

4. This hormone, released by the kidneys, regulates the rate of erythrocyte production. _____

5. The most abundant protein in the plasma, formed in the liver. _____

Activity D *Match the cell type in Column A with the normal range Column B.*

Column A

_____ **1.** Normal amount of hemoglobin in an adult.

_____ **2.** Normal leukocyte count

_____ **3.** Normal thrombocyte count

_____ **4.** Normal erythrocyte count

Column B

a. 3.6 to 5.4 million/mm^3

b. 150,000 to 350,000/mm^3

c. 12 to 17.4 g/dL

d. 5000 to 10,000/mm^3

Activity E *Compare the types of blood cells based on the given criteria.*

Type of Blood Cell	Function
Leukocytes	
Neutrophils	
Basophils	
Eosinophils	
B Lymphocytes	
T Lymphocytes	
Monocytes	
Erythrocytes	
Thrombocytes	

Activity F *Briefly answer the following questions.*

1. Where is red marrow primarily found?

   _____

   _____

   _____

2. How do red blood cells deliver oxygen to the cells of the body?

   _____

   _____

   _____

3. What happens to red blood cells when they are removed from circulation by the body?

   _____

   _____

   _____

4. What is a Schilling test? How is it performed?

   _____

   _____

   _____

SECTION II: APPLYING YOUR KNOWLEDGE

Activity G *Give rationale for the following questions.*

1. Why are leukocytes in constant demand by the body?

   _____

   _____

   _____

2. Why is a bone marrow aspiration performed?

   _____

   _____

   _____

3. Why is vitamin C important in hematopoiesis?

   _____

   _____

   _____

4. Why are older adults susceptible to infections and malignancies?

   _____

   _____

   _____

Activity H *Answer the following questions related to caring for clients with hematopoietic and lymphatic disorders.*

1. What is the role of proteins in the hematopoietic and lymphatic systems?

   _____

   _____

   _____

2. Explain the relationship between blood type and antigen/antibodies.

   _____

   _____

   _____

3. Describe the lymphatic system and its function.

   _____

   _____

   _____

4. What assessment data is significant to the hematopoietic and lymphatic systems?

   _____

   _____

   _____

5. Some medications affect the hematopoietic system, causing a decrease in various blood components. What signs and symptoms should be monitored for?

   _____

   _____

   _____

6. When obtaining a history, the nurse asks about foreign travel. How is this related to the hematopoietic and lymphatic systems?

   _____

   _____

   _____

Activity I *Think over the following questions. Discuss them with your instructor or peers.*

1. Your client is advised they need to change their dietary habits to improve red blood cell formation. How will you instruct them?

   _____

   _____

   _____

2. Your client is scheduled for a bone marrow aspiration. What is your role in this procedure?

   _____

   _____

   _____

SECTION III: GETTING READY FOR NCLEX

Activity J *Answer the following questions.*

1. Which of the following is the effect of a decrease in the number of lymphocytes with age?

   a. Decreased resistance to infection

   b. Cognitive problems

   c. Urinary incontinence

   d. Decrease in various blood components

2. When can a donor and recipient of blood be considered compatible?

    a. If there is no change in the blood color when both samples are mixed in the laboratory.

    b. If there are blood clots when both samples are mixed in the laboratory.

    c. If there is no clumping or hemolysis when both samples are mixed in the laboratory.

    d. If a blood drop does not sink when dropped in water after both samples are mixed in the laboratory.

3. When assessing a client with a disorder of the hematopoietic or the lymphatic system, why is it important for the nurse to obtain a dietary history?

    a. Compromised nutrition interferes with the production of blood cells and hemoglobin.

    b. Diet consisting of excessive fat interferes with the production of blood cells and hemoglobin.

    c. Inconsistent dieting interferes with the production of blood cells and hemoglobin.

    d. Diet consisting of excessive iron and protein elements interferes with the production of blood cells and hemoglobin.

4. A client is prescribed medications that depress thrombocytes. The nurse should monitor for which of the following signs and symptoms in the client?

    a. Sore throat

    b. Bleeding gums and dark, tarry stools

    c. Pernicious anemia

    d. Thickening of blood

5. Which of the following nursing interventions is essential for a client during the Schilling test?

    a. Collecting urine 24 to 48 hours after the client has received nonradioactive B12.

    b. Collecting blood samples of 50ml for 24 to 48 hours after the client has received the nonradioactive B12.

    c. Not allowing any oral fluid consumption for 24 to 48 hours after the client has received nonradioactive B12.

    d. Making the client lie down in supine position for 24 to 48 hours after the client has received nonradioactive B12.

6. Which of the following organs releases erythropoietin, a hormone determining the rate of the production of red blood cells?

    a. Pancreas

    b. Spleen

    c. Liver

    d. Kidneys

7. How long do erythrocytes circulate in the blood?

    a. 25 days

    b. 80 days

    c. 120 days

    d. 60 days

8. Which component of blood has proteins that function primarily as immunologic agents that prevent or modify some types of infectious diseases?

    a. Plasma

    b. Erythrocytes

    c. Leukocytes

    d. Platelets

9. What is the definition of the Rh factor and where is it located?

    a. Specific antigen on the RBC nucleus

    b. Specific protein on the RBC membrane

    c. Specific antibody on the RBC membrane

    d. Specific protein on the RBC nucleus

10. A client comes to the clinic and the nurse inspects the client's mouth and throat. The nurse documents that the tonsil size is 2+. What does this mean?

    a. Tonsils touch the uvula

    b. Tonsils extend medially toward the uvula

    c. Tonsils touch each other

    d. Tonsils are visible

Caring for Clients with Disorders of the Hematopoietic System

1. List seven types of anemia, including examples of inherited types.
2. Identify nutritional deficiencies that can lead to anemia.
3. Discuss clinical problems that clients with any type of anemia experience.
4. Discuss factors that cause sickling of erythrocytes and related adverse effects.
5. List activities a person with sickle cell disease can do to reduce the potential for a sickle cell crisis.
6. Explain the term *erythrocytosis*, give one example of a characteristic disease, and list possible complications.
7. Explain how forms of leukemia are classified.
8. List clinical problems or nursing diagnoses common among clients with leukemia.
9. Explain how the bone marrow dysfunction of multiple myeloma has an effect on the skeletal system.
10. Differentiate agranulocytosis from leucopenia.
11. Explain the term *pancytopenia* and give an example of a disorder that represents this condition.
12. Discuss the meaning of *coagulopathy* and name two coagulopathies.
13. Discuss nursing responsibilities when managing the care of clients with coagulopathies.

SECTION I: ASSESSING YOUR UNDERSTANDING

Activity A *Fill in the blanks by choosing the correct word from the options given in parentheses.*

1. _____ are abnormalities in the numbers and types of blood cells. (*Blood dyscrasias, coagulopathies, thalassemia*)

2. _____ are found in people from Southeast Asia and Africa. (*Alpha-thalassemias, Beta-thalassemias, Gamma-thalassemias*)

3. _____ is an increase in circulating erythrocytes. (*Erythrocytosis, Leukocytosis, Leukemia*)

4. _____ refers to any malignant blood disorder in which proliferation of leukocytes, usually in an immature form, is unregulated. There often is an accompanying decrease in production of erythrocytes and platelets. (*Erythrocytosis, Leukocytosis, Leukemia*)

5. _____ is a malignancy involving plasma cells, which are B-lymphocyte cells in bone marrow. (*Leukemia, Multiple myeloma, Agranulocytosis*)

6. _____ is a decreased production of granulocytes which places the client at risk

for infection. *(Aplastic anemia, Agranulocytosis, Multiple Myeloma)*

7. _____ is a consequence of inadequate stem cell production in the bone marrow. *(Aplastic anemia, Multiple myeloma, Coagulopathy)*

8. _____ refers to conditions in which a component that is necessary to control bleeding is missing or inadequate. *(Aplastic anemia, Agranulocytosis, Coagulopathy)*

Activity B *Mark each statement as either "T" (True) or "F" (False). Correct any false statements.*

1. T F Anemia is a term that refers to a deficiency of erythrocytes.

2. T F The need for iron increases during periods of rapid growth, pregnancy, and the female reproductive years when intermittent blood loss accompanies menses.

3. T F Beta-thalassemias are found in people from Mediterranean islands and the Po Valley in Italy.

4. T F For people who live at high altitudes, erythrocytosis is a normal phenomenon and usually requires no treatment.

5. T F Leukemia is a genetic disorder.

6. T F The most common cause of agranulocytosis is a disease process.

7. T F Aplastic anemia may be autoimmune in nature, or in many cases, the bone marrow becomes dysfunctional from exposure to toxic chemicals, radiation, or drug therapy with anticancer drugs and some antibiotics.

8. T F Purpura is small hemorrhages in the skin, mucous membranes, or subcutaneous tissues.

9. T F Hemophilia is inherited from mother to daughter as a sex-linked recessive characteristic. Sons can inherit the trait but seldom develop the disease.

Activity C *Write the correct term for each description given below.*

1. Bleeding disorders that involve platelets or clotting factors. _____

2. Hereditary hemolytic anemias. _____

3. A severe form of beta-thalassemia. Clients exhibit symptoms of severe anemia and a bronzing of the skin caused by hemolysis of erythrocytes. _____

4. Characterized by a greater-than-normal number of erythrocytes, leukocytes, and platelets. _____

5. An increased number of leukocytes above normal limits. _____

6. A general reduction in all WBCs. _____

7. Insufficient numbers of erythrocytes, leukocytes, and platelets. _____

8. A lower-than-normal number of thrombocytes. _____

9. A disorder involving an absence or reduction of a clotting factor. _____

Activity D *Given in Column A are different types of anemia. Match these with their associated signs and symptoms given in Column B.*

Column A

_____ 1. Hypovolemic anemia

_____ 2. Iron deficiency anemia

_____ 3. Sickle cell anemia

_____ 4. Hemolytic anemia

_____ 5. Thalassemias

_____ 6. Pernicious anemia

_____ 7. Folic acid deficiency anemia

Column B

a. Symptoms are similar to those associated with hypovolemic anemia. In more severe forms the client is jaundiced and the spleen is enlarged.

b. The reduced blood flow during sickle cell crisis leads to localized ischemia, severe pain, and possible tissue infarction if the oxygen supply is inadequate. Fever, pain, and swelling of one or more joints are common.

c. Severe fatigue, a sore and beefy-red tongue, dyspnea, nausea, anorexia, headaches, weakness, and lightheadedness occur.

d. Pallor, fatigue, chills, postural hypotension, and rapid heart and respiratory rates occur.

e. Some clients develop stomatitis and glossitis, digestive disturbances, and diarrhea.

f. Clients with this disorder, also known as Cooley's anemia, exhibit symptoms of severe anemia and a bronzing of the skin caused by hemolysis of erythrocytes.

g. Clients have reduced energy, feel cold all the time, and experience fatigue and dyspnea with minor physical exertion. The heart rate usually is rapid even at rest.

Activity E *Compare the types of anemia based on the following criteria.*

Type of Anemia	Cause	Treatment
Hypovolemic anemia		
Iron deficiency anemia		
Sickle cell anemia		
Hemolytic anemia		
Thalassemias		
Pernicious anemia		
Folic acid deficiency anemia		

Activity F *Briefly answer the following questions.*

1. What are possible reasons a client may develop iron deficiency anemia?

_____

_____

_____

2. What ethnic groups are affected by sickle cell anemia? How does sickle cell anemia differ from carrying the sickle cell trait?

_____

_____

_____

3. What clients are at risk for developing pernicious anemia?

_____

_____

_____

4. What types of clients are at risk for developing folic acid anemia?

_____

_____

_____

5. What are the symptoms of polycythemia vera?

_____

_____

_____

6. How are leukemias classified? What are the 4 types?

_____

_____

_____

7. What are the signs and symptoms of agranulocytosis?

_____

_____

_____

8. What is the medical management of aplastic anemia?

_____

_____

_____

9. Describe the pathophysiology of thrombocytopenia.

_____

_____

_____

10. What is the medical treatment for hemophilia?

_____

_____

_____

SECTION II: APPLYING YOUR KNOWLEDGE

Activity G *Give rationale for the following questions.*

1. Why is iron deficiency anemia unusual in older adults?

_____

_____

2. Why are older adults more susceptible to hemolytic anemia?

_____

_____

3. There are many leukocytes present with leukemia, so why is the client at risk for infection? Why are clients at risk for anemia and bleeding?

_____

_____

4. Why do clients with multiple myeloma experience hypercalcemia, pathologic fractures and significant pain?

_____

_____

_____

5. How does multiple myeloma interfere with the immune response and cause renal failure?

_____

_____

_____

Activity H *Answer the following questions related to caring for clients with disorders of the hematopoietic system.*

1. What problems do clients with sickle cell anemia have?

_____

_____

_____

2. What is the pathophysiology of polycythemia vera?

_____

_____

_____

3. What is the treatment for polycythemia vera?

_____

_____

_____

4. How is leukemia medically managed?

_____

_____

_____

5. What are the signs and symptoms of multiple myeloma?

_____

_____

_____

6. What is the medical treatment for multiple myeloma?

_____

_____

_____

7. What are the signs and symptoms of aplastic anemia?

_____

_____

_____

8. What is the medical treatment for thrombocytopenia?

_____

_____

_____

Activity I *Think over the following questions. Discuss them with your instructor or peers.*

1. Your client is diagnosed with sickle cell anemia. What educational information will you provide to this client?

_____

_____

_____

2. Your client is diagnosed with acute lymphocytic leukemia. Their absolute neutrophil count indicates they are at high risk for infection. You place the client in neutropenic precautions. What guidelines will you follow?

_____

_____

_____

3. What general nursing assessments and interventions will you provide to all clients diagnosed with anemia?

_____

_____

_____

4. What nursing assessments and interventions will you provide to clients that are specific to each type of the 7 anemias?

_____

_____

_____

SECTION III: GETTING READY FOR NCLEX

Activity J *Answer the following questions.*

1. For a client with low blood volume, what is the major implication of decreasing blood pressure, and a rapid heart rate?

a. Compression of blood vessels due to blood loss
b. Increase in the circulating blood volume
c. Inadequate renal perfusion
d. Hypovolemia and shock

2. What is the period in life when the need for iron increases?

a. Pregnancy
b. Infancy
c. Old age
d. Male reproductive years

3. For a client with sickle cell anemia, how does the nurse assess for jaundice?

a. The nurse assesses the mental status, verbal ability, and motor strength.
b. The nurse observes the joints for signs of swelling.
c. The nurse inspects the skin and sclera for jaundice.
d. The nurse collects a urine specimen.

4. Severe and extensive hemolysis causes:

a. Leg ulcers
b. Shock
c. Priapism
d. Compromised growth

5. What are the nursing interventions for a client with thalassemia?

a. Maintain the client on bed rest and protect him or her from infections.
b. Ambulate the client frequently.
c. Advise drinking 3 quarts (L) of fluid per day.
d. Instruct the client to elevate the lower extremities as much as possible.

6. For a client with polycythemia vera, how can the nurse help decrease the risk for thrombus formation?

a. Teach the client how to perform isometric exercises.
b. Help the client don thromboembolic stockings or support hose during waking hours.
c. Advise drinking 3 quarts (L) of fluid per day.
d. Instruct the client to rest immediately if chest pain develops.

7. Which of the following decreases the absorption of iron in clients who are taking an iron supplement due to iron deficiency anemia?
   a. Coffee
   b. Butter
   c. Flour
   d. Bread

8. Which of the following types of hemoglobin is responsible for the sickle cell crescent shape in hemoglobin under hypoxic conditions?
   a. Hemoglobin A1C
   b. Hemoglobin S
   c. Hemoglobin A
   d. Hemoglobin F

9. What is the major symptom in sickle cell crisis for clients with sickle cell anemia?
   a. Fever
   b. Lethargy
   c. Atelectasis
   d. Pain

10. What is the major nursing intervention in educating clients who have leukemia?
   a. Monitor temperature at least once per shift
   b. Implement contact isolation precautions
   c. Explain the need to limit exposure to those who are ill
   d. Keep the client warm as they chill easily

Caring for Clients with Disorders of the Lymphatic System

Learning Objectives

1. Explain the cause and characteristics of lymphedema.
2. Discuss the role of the nurse when managing the care of clients with lymphedema.
3. Describe nursing interventions that promote the resolution of lymphangitis and lymphadenitis.
4. Explain the nature and transmission of infectious mononucleosis.
5. List suggestions the nurse can offer to individuals who acquire infectious mononucleosis.
6. Define the term *lymphoma* and name two types.
7. Name the type of malignant cell diagnostic of Hodgkin's disease.
8. List three forms of treatment used to cure or promote remission of lymphomas.
9. Name at least four problems that nurses address when caring for clients with Hodgkin's disease and non-Hodgkin's lymphoma.

SECTION I: ASSESSING YOUR UNDERSTANDING

Activity A *Fill in the blanks by choosing the correct word from the options given in parentheses.*

1. The tonsils, thymus gland, and spleen are _____ lymphatic structures. *(Specialized, Accessory, Primary)*

2. _____ is a condition that results from impaired lymph circulation. *(Lymphedema, Lymphangitis, Lymphadenitis)*

3. _____ refers to a group of cancers that affect the lymphatic system. *(Infectious mononucleosis, Lymphangitis, Lymphoma)*

4. Symptoms of _____ include fatigue, fever, sore throat, headache, and cervical lymph node enlargement. The tonsils ooze white or greenish-gray exudates. *(Infectious mononucleosis, Lymphoma, Lymphedema)*

5. Monoclonal antibody therapy is a form of _____. *(Radiation, Chemotherapy, Immunotherapy)*

Activity B *Mark each statement as either "T" (True) or "F" (False). Correct any false statements.*

1. T F The lymph nodes contain lymphocytes and macrophages, specialized immune defensive cells that trap, destroy, and remove infectious microorganisms, cellular debris, and cancer cells.

2. T F When inflammation of the lymphatic vessels affects nearby lymph nodes, the condition is called lymphadenitis.

3. T F Lymphedema affects more than one fourth of women who have received treatment for breast cancer.

4. T F Lymphangitis and lymphadenitis are usually caused by a congenital disorder.

5. T F Non-Hodgkin's lymphoma is treated with radiation, chemotherapy, or both.

6. T F Symptoms of non-Hodgkin's lymphoma include lymph node enlargement, which usually is localized.

Activity C *Write the correct term for each description given below.*

1. Clusters of bean-sized structures located primarily in the neck, axilla, chest, abdomen, pelvis, and groin. _____

2. Worldwide, the most common cause of lymphedema is a parasitic worm; mosquitoes transmit the parasite. _____

3. Inflammation of lymphatic vessels. _____

4. A viral disease that affects lymphoid tissues such as the tonsils and spleen, caused by the Epstein-Barr virus. _____

5. This form of treatment for lymphoma requires marrow from a human donor. _____

Activity D *Match the type of complex decongestive physiotherapy treatment for lymphedema given in Column A with the description given in Column B.*

Column A

____ **1.** Distal-to-proximal massage

____ **2.** Compression dressings

____ **3.** Active exercise

____ **4.** Mechanical pulsating compression device

Column B

a. Relieves edema by reducing the excess volume of fluid in the interstitial space.

b. The alternating filling and emptying "milk" the lymph toward the duct, leading to venous drainage.

c. Facilitates lymphatic drainage into collateral vessels.

d. Promotes lymphatic circulation and maintains functional use of the limb.

Activity E *Compare the two types of lymphomas based on the given criteria.*

Type of Lymphoma	Description	Cause
Hodgkin's disease		
Non-Hodgkin's lymphomas		

Activity F *Briefly answer the following questions.*

1. How is lymphatic fluid circulated?

_____
_____
_____

2. What are the assessment findings with lymphangitis and lymphadenitis?

_____
_____
_____

3. How is infectious mononucleosis spread? Whom does it most commonly affect?

_____
_____
_____

4. What is monoclonal antibody therapy? How is it performed?

_____
_____
_____

5. How is an autologous bone marrow transplant performed?

_____
_____
_____

6. What are the advantages of an allogenic bone marrow transplant?

_____
_____
_____

SECTION II: APPLYING YOUR KNOWLEDGE

Activity G *Give rationale for the following questions.*

1. Why are antibiotics not prescribed for uncomplicated infectious mononucleosis?

_____

_____

_____

2. Why is the risk of lymphoma increased in older adults?

_____

_____

_____

3. Why do clients with Hodgkin's disease develop pain, fever, and itching?

_____

_____

_____

4. Why is staging and subclassification an important part of medical care for Hodgkin's disease?

_____

_____

_____

5. Why would an endotracheal tube, laryngoscope, and bag-valve mask be placed at the bedside for a client with Hodgkin's disease?

_____

_____

_____

Activity H *Answer the following questions related to caring for clients with disorders of the lymphatic system.*

1. Describe the pathophysiology of lymphedema

_____

_____

_____

2. What are Reed-Sternberg cells? How are the cells identified?

_____

3. What are the signs and symptoms of Hodgkin's disease?

_____

_____

4. What is the medical treatment for Hodgkin's disease?

_____

_____

5. A client with Hodgkin's disease is at risk for infection related to immunosuppression secondary to impaired lymphocytes and drug or radiation therapy. What precautions would be taken?

_____

_____

6. What is the pathophysiology of non-Hodgkin's lymphoma? How is the disease classified?

_____

_____

Activity I *Think over the following questions. Discuss them with your instructor or peers.*

1. Your client is diagnosed with lymphedema. What nursing assessments and interventions are indicated?

_____

_____

2. You client is diagnosed with Hodgkin's disease. What are your priority nursing diagnoses? What is your rationale for these diagnoses? What nursing assessments and interventions are indicated?

_____

_____

SECTION III: GETTING READY FOR NCLEX

Activity J *Answer the following questions.*

1. A female client with lymphedema expresses her anxiety about the abnormal enlargement of an arm. Which of the following suggestions should a nurse give to support the client's self-image?

   a. Place the arm in a sling

   b. Introduce variations in styles of clothing

   c. Apply cold soaks to the affected arm

   d. Tie a tight bandage to the arm

2. Under which of the following situations should a nurse notify the physician when caring for a client with lymphangitis?

   a. Affected area appears to enlarge

   b. Lymph nodes remain the same

   c. Red streaks appear

   d. Liver and spleen become enlarged

3. Which of the following are the most significant symptoms of the B subclassification of Hodgkin's disease?

   a. Fever and weight loss

   b. Night sweats and fever

   c. Weight loss and anemia

   d. Anemia and fever

4. Which of the following nursing interventions ensures that a client with Hodgkin's disease remains free of infection?

   a. Apply ice to the skin for brief periods.

   b. Practice conscientious hand washing.

   c. Provide cool sponge baths.

   d. Use cotton gloves.

5. Which of the following instructions should a nurse give a client with non-Hodgkin's lymphoma who is being treated with radiation and chemotherapy?

   a. Increase fluid intake

   b. Intake soft, bland foods

   c. Intake low-fat meals

   d. Intake food rich in folic acid

6. Which of the following instructions should a nurse give a client with Hodgkin's disease who is at risk of impaired skin integrity?

   a. Do not trim nails

   b. Use mild soap

   c. Rub skin dry

   d. Keep the neck in midline

7. A client comes to the clinic complaining of sore throat, fatigue, and headache. The client lives in a dormitory and has been feeling ill for several weeks. Upon assessment of the client the nurse notes the cervical lymph nodes are enlarged. What does the nurse suspect the client has?

   a. Lymphomas

   b. Lymphedema

   c. Lymphangitis

   d. Infectious Mononucleosis

8. A nurse is assisting a client with Hodgkin's lymphoma and has assessed shallow respirations associated with enlarged cervical lymph nodes. What would be the best nursing intervention to assist the client to avoid unnecessary pressure on the trachea and provide for increased lung expansion and improved air exchange?

   a. Encourage the use of incentive spirometry.

   b. Monitor the pulse oximetry and keep at 90% or greater.

   c. Place the client in high Fowler's position.

   d. Keep the environment quiet and free of distraction.

9. A client has just received an allogenic bone marrow transplant as treatment for non-Hodgkin's lymphoma. The client is showing signs of rejection. What is this term called?

   a. Lymphoma relapse

   b. Short remission

   c. Bone marrow transplant rejection

   d. Graft versus host disease

10. Which of the following is responsible for infections of mononucleosis?

    a. Elephantiasis

    b. Reed-Sternberg cells

    c. Lymphogranulomatosis

    d. Epstein-Barr virus

CHAPTER 33

Introduction to the Immune System

Learning Objectives

1. Explain the meaning of an immune response.
2. List two general components of the immune system.
3. Discuss the role of T-cell and B-cell lymphocytes.
4. Differentiate between an antigen and an antibody.
5. Name examples of lymphoid tissue.
6. List some cells and chemicals that enhance the function of the immune system.
7. Name three types of immunity, describing how each develops.
8. Discuss techniques for detecting immune disorders.
9. Describe the role of the nurse when caring for a client with an immune disorder.

SECTION I: ASSESSING YOUR UNDERSTANDING

Activity A *Fill in the blanks by choosing the correct word from the options given in parentheses.*

1. Primary targets of the _____ are infectious, foreign, or cancerous cells. *(Immune system, Colony-stimulating factor, Tumor necrosis factor)*

2. Formation of antibodies is called a _____ response. *(Cell-mediated, Humoral, Cytotoxic)*

3. _____ are chemical messengers released by lymphocytes, monocytes, and macrophages. There are many subgroups including interleukins, interferons, tumor necrosis factor, and colony-stimulating factors *(Immunoglobulins, Nonantibody Proteins, Cytokines)*

4. _____ results from the administration of a killed or weakened microorganism or toxoid. *(Naturally acquired active immunity, Artificially acquired active immunity, Passive immunity)*

5. _____ is the inability to mount an immune response. *(Anergy, Inergy, Energy)*

Activity B *Mark each statement as either "T" (True) or "F" (False). Correct any false statements.*

1. T F When tissue cell markers detects a non-self substance, the immune system protects, defends, and destroys what it perceives as atypical or abnormal.

2. T F The B-cell lymphocytes are manufactured in the bone marrow and travel to the thymus gland, where they mature.

3. T F Natural killer cells require the assistance of T and B lymphocytes to target non-self substances.

4. T F Naturally acquired active immunity occurs as a direct result of infection by a specific microorganism.

5. T F All invading microorganisms produce a response that gives lifelong immunity.

6. T F A genetically engineered form of human interleukin-2 is being used to stimulate the immune system's ability to target tumor cells as biologic therapy for clients who have not responded to conventional cancer treatment.

Activity C *Write the correct term for each description given below.*

1. Markers act as "fingerprints" that enable the immune system to differentiate self from non-self. _____

2. Occurs when T cells survey proteins in the body, actively analyze the surface features, and respond to those that differ from the host by directly attacking the invading antigen. _____

3. The process of engulfing and digesting bacteria and foreign material. _____

4. These tissues filter bacteria from tissue fluid. Because they are exposed to pathogens in the oral and nasal passages, they can become infected and locally inflamed. _____

5. Lymphocyte-like cells that circulate throughout the body looking for virus-infected cells and cancer cells. _____

Activity D *Match the cytokines in Column A with their function in Column B.*

Column A

_____ **1.** Interleukins

_____ **2.** Interferons

_____ **3.** Tumor necrosis factor

_____ **4.** Colony-stimulating factors

Column B

a. Chemicals that primarily protect cells from viral invasion. They enable cells to resist viral infection and slow viral replication.

b. Helps in cellular repair when administered in small doses. Excess amounts destroy healthy tissue.

c. Carry messages between leukocytes and tissues that form blood cells. Some enhance the immune response, whereas others suppress it

d. Regulate the production, maturation, and function of blood cells.

Activity E *Compare the specialized white blood cells based on the given criteria.*

Type of Cells	Function
Neutrophils (microphages)	
Monocytes (macrophages)	
Regulator T cells:	
Helper T cells (also called T4 or CD4 cells)	
Suppressor T cells	
Effector T cells:	
Cytotoxic T cells (also called T8 or CD8 cells)	
B-cell lymphocytes:	
Plasma cells	
Memory cells	

Activity F *Briefly answer the following questions.*

1. What are the types of lymphocytes? What is their function?

   _____

   _____

   _____

2. What are the functions of the thymus gland?

   _____

   _____

   _____

3. What is the function of the spleen?

   _____

   _____

   _____

4. Explain the process of artificially acquired active immunity.

   _____

   _____

   _____

5. How does the complement system assist in the immune response?

   _____

   _____

   _____

SECTION II: APPLYING YOUR KNOWLEDGE

Activity G *Give rationale for the following questions.*

1. Why are immunosuppressive drugs prescribed following an organ transplant?

_____

_____

_____

2. Why are viral vaccines less effective in older adults?

_____

_____

_____

3. Why are natural killer cells unable to destroy cancer cells?

_____

_____

_____

4. Why is the older client at increased risk for problems related to immunity?

_____

_____

_____

Activity H *Answer the following questions related to the immune system.*

1. Where is lymphoid tissue found?

_____

_____

_____

2. What is the function of the lymph nodes?

_____

_____

_____

3. How do antibodies destroy invading cells? What is another name for antibodies?

_____

_____

_____

4. What information will the nurse explain and what interventions will the nurse take when preparing a client for laboratory testing.

_____

_____

_____

5. What are examples of interleukin activity?

_____

_____

_____

Activity I *Think over the following questions. Discuss them with your instructor or peers.*

1. What dietary modifications can clients make to boost their immune system?

_____

_____

_____

2. A client states that he has heard that high levels of vitamins and minerals can provide assistance to the immune system. What would you tell him?

_____

_____

_____

3. A mother states she does not want her child immunized. Her rationale is that her child was born with natural immunities and immunizations are not required. What information would you provide?

_____

_____

_____

SECTION III: GETTING READY FOR NCLEX

Activity J *Answer the following NCLEX-style questions.*

1. Which of the following causes memory cells to convert to plasma cells?

    a. An organ transplant

    b. Release of lymphokines

    c. Re-exposure to a specific antigen

    d. Initial exposure to an antigen

2. A male client is suspected of an immune system disorder. Which of the following important factors will the nurse document while assessing the client?

    a. The client's diet

    b. The client's drug history

    c. The client's ability to produce antibodies

    d. The client's family members' history of chronic diseases

3. Which of the following factors makes it important for the nurse to provide special care to older clients with immune system disorders?

    a. Age-related changes

    b. Poor diet

    c. Use of multiple drugs (polypharmacy)

    d. Reduced activity levels

4. A pregnant client requires immediate but temporary protection from chickenpox. Which type of immunization would be required?

    a. Naturally acquired active immunization

    b. Artificially acquired active immunization

    c. Passive immunization

    d. Artificially acquired passive immunization

5. What are the essential nursing actions that should be taken for a client with an immune system disorder?

    a. Monitor client for depression.

    b. Monitor client for infusion reactions.

    c. Review drug references.

    d. Advise the client on modifying the home environment.

6. Which of the following is the best dietary advice to maximize the immune function in healthy people?

    a. To include immune-enhancing formulas.

    b. To avoid polyunsaturated fatty acids.

    c. To increase intake of essential fatty acids and omega-3 fatty acids.

    d. To follow a balanced and varied diet.

7. A nurse attends a seminar on the immune system and learns about the different lymphocytes in the body. Where do the T lymphocytes originate from and where do they travel to?

    a. Bone marrow and the lymph nodes

    b. Bone marrow and plasma

    c. Bone marrow and spleen

    d. Bone marrow and thymus

8. Which of the following white blood cells is small, present in blood and migrates to tissue as necessary?

    a. Neutrophils

    b. Leukocytes

    c. Monocytes

    d. Lymphocytes

9. Which of the following lymphoid tissues has both hematopoietic and immune functions and acts as an emergency reservoir of blood and filters the blood as well?

    a. Tonsils and adenoids

    b. Thymus gland

    c. Spleen

    d. Lymph nodes

10. A nurse is taking care of a client with cancer and is teaching about the types of drugs that promote the natural production of blood cells in people whose own hematopoietic functions have become compromised. What class of drugs are these?

    a. Tumor necrosis factors

    b. Colony-stimulating factors

    c. Interferons

    d. Interleukins

Caring for Clients with Immune-Mediated Disorders

Learning Objectives

1. Describe an allergic disorder.
2. List five examples of allergic signs and symptoms.
3. Name four categories of allergens, and give an example of each.
4. Give four examples of allergic reactions, including two that are potentially life-threatening.
5. Describe diagnostic skin testing.
6. Name three methods for treating allergies.
7. Discuss the nursing management of a client with an allergic disorder.
8. Explain the meaning of autoimmune disorder, and give at least three examples of related diseases.
9. Discuss theories that explain the development of an autoimmune disorder.
10. Name three categories of drugs used in the treatment of autoimmune disorders.
11. Discuss the nursing management of a client with an autoimmune disorder.
12. Give two explanations for how chronic fatigue syndrome develops.
13. List common symptoms experienced by people with chronic fatigue syndrome.
14. Name common nursing diagnoses, desired outcomes, and related nursing interventions for clients who have chronic fatigue syndrome.

SECTION I: ASSESSING YOUR UNDERSTANDING

Activity A *Fill in the blanks by choosing the correct word from the options given in parentheses:*

1. An _____ is characterized by a hyper-immune response to weak antigens that usually are harmless. *(Allergic disorder, Allergen, Anaphylaxis response)*

2. _____ is the process by which cellular and chemical events occur after a second or subsequent exposure to an allergen. *(Anaphylaxis, Chemotaxis, Sensitization)*

3. Immediate hypersensitivity response: type _____ is mediated by immunoglobulin E (IgE) antibodies. IgE antibodies attach to basophils or mast cells; the response occurs within minutes. *(I, II, III)*

4. In an _____, killer T cells and autoantibodies attack or destroy natural cells—those cells that are "self." *(Allergic disorder, Autoimmune disorder, Anaphylaxis response)*

5. Autoimmune disorders have inflammatory symptoms that are episodic. Periods of acute flare-ups are called _____ *(Exacerbations, Remissions, Alloimmunity)*

6. _____ is a complex of symptoms primarily characterized by profound fatigue with no identifiable cause. *(An autoimmune disorder, Chronic fatigue syndrome, An allergic disorder)*

7. A _____ is a test in which the client lays horizontally on a table whose incline is elevated to approximately 70 degrees for 45 minutes. *(Tilt-table test, Flat-table test, Elevated-table test)*

Activity B *Mark each statement as either "T" (True) or "F" (False). Correct any false statement.*

1. T F Allergens have a protein component and gain entry to the host from the environment.

2. T F An immediate hypersensitivity response: Type II is mediated by immunoglobulin M or G (IgM or IgG) antibodies and occurs within minutes.

3. T F The radioallergosorbent blood test (RAST) can indicate what is causing an allergic response.

4. T F An intradermal injection test is usually performed prior to a scratch test.

5. T F The treatment used to relieve allergic symptoms depends on the type of allergy. Besides avoiding the allergen if possible, many clients experience symptomatic relief with drug therapy.

6. T F Autoantibodies are antibodies against self-antigens; they are immunoglobulins.

7. T F Some believe that chronic fatigue syndrome is associated with fibromyalgia because both conditions share many symptoms.

Activity C *Write the correct term for each description below.*

1. The antigens that can cause an allergic response. _____

2. This type of immediate hypersensitivity response is mediated by IgG antibodies and responses reach a peak within 6 hours after exposure. _____

3. A process of attracting migratory cells to a particular area in the body. _____

4. Acute swelling of the face, neck, lips, larynx, hands, feet, genitals, and internal organs. _____

5. Autoantibodies target cells whose antigens match the individual's own genetic code. _____

6. These autoimmune disorders have inflammatory symptoms that are episodic; during some periods, clients are asymptomatic. _____

7. Pain in fibrous tissues of the body such as muscles, ligaments, and tendons. _____

Activity D *Match the medications in Column A with their mechanisms of action in Column B.*

Column A	Column B
____ 1. Antihistamines	a. Block receptors for leukotrienes
____ 2. Oral corticosteroids	b. Block histamine (H$_1$) receptors
____ 3. Oral decongestant agents	c. Act on alpha or beta receptors
____ 4. Bronchodilators	d. Dilate airways by stimulating the B2-adrenergic receptors located throughout the lungs.
____ 5. Oral or parenteral sympathomimetic agents	e. Regulate immune response, control inflammatory response
____ 6. Leukotriene antagonists	f. Vasoconstrict nasal membranes

Activity E *Compare the theories for autoimmune disorders based on the given criteria.*

Theory	Description of Theory
Triggering event	
Genetically predisposed	
Sequestered antigen theory	

Activity F *Briefly answer the following questions.*

1. Describe the pattern of allergies.

_____

_____

_____

2. Which organs and structures are primarily involved in allergic reactions?

_____

_____

_____

3. Describe a delayed hypersensitivity response: Type IV.

_____

_____

_____

4. What happens to the client during anaphylaxis?

_____

_____

_____

5. What is a patch test?

_____

_____

_____

6. What are complications of inhalant allergies?

_____

_____

_____

7. What types of tests are used to detect autoimmune disorders?

_____

_____

_____

SECTION II: APPLYING YOUR KNOWLEDGE

Activity G   *Give rationale for the following questions.*

1. When testing for food allergies with an elimination diet, why may clients experience symptoms based on their expectations, not from a true allergy?

_____

_____

_____

2. Why does the nurse instruct clients who are scheduled for diagnostic skin testing to avoid taking prescribed or over-the-counter antihistamine or cold preparations for at least 48 to 72 hours before testing?

_____

_____

_____

3. Why are older adults more susceptible to autoimmune disorders?

_____

_____

_____

4. Why does drug therapy for autoimmune disorders cause the client to be at increased risk for infection?

_____

_____

_____

5. Why do some believe that chronic fatigue syndrome should be called "chronic viral reactivation syndrome"?

_____

_____

_____

Activity H   *Answer the following questions.*

1. How does the body suppress the allergic response via the eosinophil chemotactic factor?

_____

_____

_____

2. What signs and symptoms can occur with anaphylaxis?

_____

_____

_____

3. What is a scratch (prick) test?

_____

_____

_____

4. What is desensitization?

_____

_____

_____

5. How is an autoimmune disorder medically managed?

_____

_____

_____

6. What is included in the nursing assessment of a client with an autoimmune disorder?

_____

_____

_____

7. Explain the theory of the HPA axis as it relates to chronic fatigue syndrome.

_____

_____

_____

8. What are signs and symptoms of chronic fatigue syndrome?

_____

_____

_____

Activity I *Think over the following questions. Discuss them with your instructor or peers.*

1. What educational informational would you provide to a client diagnosed with an autoimmune disorder?

_____

_____

_____

2. What educational information would you provide to a client diagnosed with an allergic disorder?

_____

_____

_____

3. What would be your priority nursing diagnoses for a client with chronic fatigue syndrome? Why? What nursing assessments and interventions are indicated?

_____

_____

_____

SECTION III: GETTING READY FOR NCLEX

Activity J *Answer the following questions.*

1. What is the role of a nurse during the scratch test to detect allergies?

  a. Applying the liquid test antigen

  b. Measuring the length and width of the raised wheal

  c. Determining the type of allergy

  d. Documenting the findings

2. Which of the following is the most severe complication among clients with allergies, regardless of type?

  a. Bronchitis

  b. Cardiac arrest

  c. Anaphylactic shock and angioneurotic edema

  d. Asthma and nasal polyps

3. Why must clients, who will undergo diagnostic skin tests, avoid taking antihistamine or cold preparations for at least 48 to 72 hours before testing?

  a. Antihistamines may increase the potential for excessive bleeding.

  b. Antihistamines may aggravate the allergic reaction.

  c. Antihistamines may increase the potential for false-negative test results.

  d. Antihistamines may cause wheezing.

4. Which of the following would help a client with allergic skin reaction reduce itching and maintain intact skin?

    a. Humidifying the environment

    b. Avoiding a skin lubricant

    c. Bathing with a bar soap that contains lye

    d. Bathing with hot water

5. Which of the following should a client with autoimmune disorder be advised to avoid?

    a. Rest during the periods of severe exacerbation

    b. Regular exercise during the periods of remission

    c. Being in crowds during the periods of immunosuppression

    d. Humid environment during the periods of remission

6. When assessing a client with autoimmune disorder, what signs should the nurse look for in the client?

    a. Hypotension

    b. Localized inflammation

    c. Hives or rashes

    d. Cramping and vomiting

7. Many clients with chronic fatigue syndrome (CFS) report severe, ongoing fatigue without any explanation that has lasted for at least __ months.

8. Which of the following is the most important factor in the nursing management of a client with CFS?

    a. Teaching the client how to avoid aggravating the disease

    b. Informing the client about the drug therapy that will provide significant improvement

    c. Advising the client to alter the diet and environment

    d. Educating the client about the disease process and its limitations

9. Antihistamines are used cautiously in older men with prostatic hypertrophy for which of the following reasons?

    a. Because these clients may experience increased drowsiness

    b. Because these clients may experience difficulty voiding

    c. Because these clients face a greater risk of cardiac arrest

    d. Because these clients have a lower autoimmune response

10. What percent of clients with chronic fatigue syndrome (CFS) will experience hypotension during a tilt table test, which can eventually be diagnostic for these clients?

    a. 60%

    b. 96%

    c. 80%

    d. 20%

Caring for Clients with HIV/AIDS

Learning Objectives

1. Explain the term *acquired immunodeficiency syndrome (AIDS)*.
2. Identify the virus that causes AIDS.
3. Discuss the characteristics of a retrovirus.
4. Explain how human immunodeficiency virus (HIV) is transmitted.
5. Name at least four methods for preventing transmission of HIV.
6. List three criteria for diagnosing AIDS.
7. Discuss the pathophysiologic process of AIDS.
8. List at least five manifestations characteristic of acute retroviral syndrome.
9. Name two laboratory tests used to screen for HIV antibodies and one that confirms a diagnosis of AIDS.
10. Name two laboratory tests used to measure viral load, and give two purposes for their use.
11. Identify categories of drugs that are used to treat individuals infected with HIV, and give an example of a specific drug in each category.
12. Give the criterion for successful drug therapy for HIV/AIDS.
13. Discuss the nursing management of a client with AIDS, including client teaching.
14. Describe techniques for preventing HIV infection among healthcare workers who care for infected clients.
15. Discuss two ethical issues that affect healthcare workers in relation to clients with HIV infection.

SECTION I: ASSESSING YOUR UNDERSTANDING

Activity A *Fill in the blanks by choosing the correct word from the options given in parentheses.*

1. _____ is an infectious and eventually fatal disorder that profoundly weakens the immune system. *(Acquired immunodeficiency syndrome, Opportunistic infection, Human immunodeficiency virus)*

2. At the time of primary HIV infection, one third to more than one half of those infected develop _____, which often is mistaken for "flu" or some other common illness. *(Acute retroviral syndrome, Kaposi's sarcoma, Pneumocystis pneumonia)*

3. _____ is ineffective response to a prescribed drug because of the survival and duplication of exceptionally virulent mutations and noncompliance with drug therapy regimens. *(Drug resistance, Drug dominance, Drug cross-resistance)*

4. When _____ is done, the blood is examined for genetic changes in circulating HIV particles. *(Genotype testing, ELISA testing, Phenotype testing)*

5. _____ inhibits an enzyme that functions in DNA synthesis. When combined with antiretrovirals, this drug interferes with viral replication, increasing anti-HIV effects. *(Interferon, Interleukin-2, Hydroxyurea)*

6. _____ is an opportunistic infection that affects immunosuppressed people such as clients with AIDS. The infection can infect the choroid and retinal layers of the eye, leading to blindness. *(Cryptosporidium, Cytomegalovirus, Candidiasis)*

7. Immunosuppressed clients may develop serious diarrhea as a result of infection with a protozoan called _____.
(Cryptosporidium, Cytomegalovirus, Candidiasis)

Activity B *Mark each statement as either "T" (True) or "F" (False). Correct any false statements.*

1. **T F**   Opportunistic infections cause acquired immunodeficiency syndrome.

2. **T F**   People infected with HIV who are asymptomatic cannot infect others with the virus.

3. **T F**   Physicians are the largest group of healthcare workers to have occupationally acquired HIV infection.

4. **T F**   Although viral replication is rapid during acute retroviral syndrome, antibody tests cannot detect the infection.

5. **T F**   When drug therapy is begun, clients are started on a combination of generally three antiretroviral drugs: two reverse transcriptase inhibitors and one protease inhibitor.

6. **T F**   Interleukin-2 is used to increase the numbers of T4 helper and natural killer lymphocytes.

7. **T F**   Pneumocystis pneumonia is a form of pneumonia that is rare among individuals with an intact immune system.

Activity C *Write the correct names for the following conditions and treatment of clients with AIDS.*

1. A disease infecting large numbers of people throughout the world; HIV/AIDS is an example. _____

2. A double layer of lipid material surrounding the incomplete HIV. _____

3. A type of connective tissue cancer common among those with AIDS. _____

4. Diminished drug response to similar HIV drugs. _____

5. Scientists are able to look for these points on HIV genes where mutations occur. _____

6. A measured amount of this antiviral drug is mixed with the virus until there is a quantity that prevents the virus from reproducing. The higher the dose of drug that eventually inhibits viral growth, the greater the viral drug resistance. _____

7. Activates the cell's own defenses against viruses and is believed to increase blood levels of antiretroviral drugs. _____

8. This yeast infection may develop in the oral, pharyngeal, esophageal, or vaginal cavities or in folds of the skin. _____

Activity D *Match diagnostic tests in Column A with the descriptions given in Column B.*

Column A	Column B
____ 1. Enzyme-linked immunosorbent assay (ELISA) test	a. If results of a second ELISA test are positive, this test is performed. A positive result confirms the diagnosis; however, false-positive and false-negative results on both tests are possible.
____ 2. Western blot	
____ 3. A total T-cell count	
____ 4. p24 antigen test and polymerase chain reaction test	b. This type of cancer screening is recommended for women infected with HIV.
____ 5. Papanicolaou cervical test	c. An initial HIV screening test; results are positive when there are sufficient HIV antibodies; it also is positive when there are antibodies from other infectious diseases. The test is repeated if results are positive.
	d. Measures viral loads. Used as a guide for drug therapy and to follow the progression of the disease.
	e. Determines the status of T lymphocytes.

Activity E *Compare the following antiretroviral medications based on the given criteria.*

Classification	Mechanism of Action
Reverse Transcriptase Inhibitors	
Nucleoside Reverse Transcriptase Inhibitors (NRTIs)	
Non-Nucleoside Reverse Transcriptase Inhibitors (NNRTIs)	
Nucleotide Analogues	
Protease Inhibitors	
Entry Inhibitors (Fusion Inhibitors)	
Integrase Inhibitors	

Activity F *Briefly answer the following questions.*

1. What factors have contributed to the decline in the mortality from AIDS?

2. How did HIV originate?

3. How does the capsid insert its contents into the helper T cell?

4. How is HIV transmitted?

5. What events mark the conversion from HIV to AIDS?

6. What determines the rate of progression from HIV to AIDS?

7. What are the benefits of highly active antiretroviral therapy (HAART)?

SECTION II: APPLYING YOUR KNOWLEDGE

Activity G *Give rationale for the following questions.*

1. Why is AIDS a major public health problem in the United States, especially among African Americans?

2. How can a person with HIV donate blood and the virus not be detected?

3. Why must nurses immediately report any needlestick or sharp injury to a supervisor?

4. Why should client take antiretroviral medications exactly as prescribed?

5. Most people infected with HIV die of their disease; a few are long-term survivors. Why do some individuals have long term survival?

_____

_____

_____

6. Why do some physicians feel that delaying drug therapy is justified?

_____

_____

_____

7. Why is it difficult to diagnose distal sensory polyneuropathy?

_____

_____

_____

8. What is AIDS dementia complex? What are the symptoms?

_____

_____

_____

Activity H   *Answer the following questions related to caring for the client with HIV/AIDS.*

1. What are the characteristics of HIV-1 and HIV-2?

_____

_____

_____

2. How does HIV replicate?

_____

_____

_____

3. What prevention strategies can reduce or eliminate the transmission of HIV?

_____

_____

_____

4. How does immunodeficiency develop?

_____

_____

_____

5. What are symptoms of acute retroviral syndrome?

_____

_____

_____

6. What are current guidelines for initiation of drug therapy?

_____

_____

_____

7. What is the approximate cost of drug therapy? What are options for funding?

_____

_____

_____

Activity I   *Think over the following questions. Discuss them with your instructor or peers.*

1. When providing education to the client with HIV/AIDS what information would you provide related to diet?

_____

_____

_____

2. When caring for the HIV/AIDS client on an outpatient basis what educational information would you provide?

_____

_____

_____

3. What steps will you take to ensure safe handling of needles and sharp instruments as a health care provider?

_____

_____

_____

SECTION III: GETTING READY FOR NCLEX

Activity J *Answer the following questions.*

1. A client is being taught about the transmission of HIV and is taught that body fluids such as blood, semen, and vaginal secretions can transmit the virus. What is the other body fluid that the HIV virus can be transmitted through?
   a. Saliva
   b. Tears
   c. Sweat
   d. Breast milk

2. Which of the following symptoms is associated with AIDS-related distal sensory polyneuropathy (DSP)?
   a. Staggering gait and muscle incoordination
   b. Abnormal sensations such as burning and numbness
   c. Delusional thinking
   d. Incontinence

3. Which of the following precautions must a nurse take while caring for clients with HIV/AIDS to reduce occupational risks?
   a. Transport specimens of body fluids in leak proof containers.
   b. Seek prescription for a fusion inhibitor to reduce risk of infection.
   c. Avoid administering IV drugs.
   d. Avoid cleaning the client's room, especially cleaning urine, stool, or vomit.

4. Which of the following is an important nursing intervention for HIV-positive clients?
   a. Suggesting the use of herbal medications and alternate therapies.
   b. Suggesting the use of psychostimulants such as methamphetamine.
   c. Advising client to avoid clinical drug trials.
   d. Providing referral to support groups and resources for information.

5. A client with HIV has been prescribed antiviral medications. What instructions related to administration of medications should the nurse give such a client?
   a. Comply with the timing of antiviral medications around meals.
   b. Avoid exposure to harsh sunlight for about two hours after taking the medication.
   c. Have the medications with plenty of fruit juice.
   d. Have an increased dose of the medications if the symptoms worsen.

6. In a client with AIDS, a CD4 cell count above _____ mm^3 would indicate that antiretroviral therapy is being effective.

7. What dietary advice should the nurse give to clients with HIV/AIDS?
   a. Encourage intake of fat-soluble vitamins in amounts two to five times the RDA
   b. Encourage intake of water-soluble vitamins in amounts two to five times the RDA
   c. Increase the intake of iron and zinc
   d. Decrease the intake of trace element and antioxidant supplements

8. Which of the following is the main reason why older clients with AIDS need more care than their younger counterparts?
   a. Because older clients lack in balanced diet and activity
   b. Because older clients lack knowledge about disorders
   c. Because older clients have a faster progression of disease
   d. Because older clients do not generally adhere to a therapy

9. A client with AIDS is terminally ill and wants to name a person as a beneficiary to his life insurance in exchange for immediate cash. What is the term that best describes this arrangement?
   a. Power of attorney
   b. Beneficiary settlement
   c. Viatical settlement
   d. Life insurance guardianship

10. A client with AIDS is experiencing bouts of diarrhea, anorexia, nausea, and vomiting. Cryptosporidiosis is diagnosed and the nurse goes to hang the first antibiotic. Which type of macrolide antibiotic is the nurse going to hang?
    a. Humatin
    b. Azithromycin
    c. Penicillin
    d. Ancef

Introduction to the Nervous System

Learning Objectives

1. Name the two anatomic divisions of the nervous system.
2. Name the three parts of the brain.
3. List the four lobes of the cerebrum.
4. Give two functions of the spinal cord.
5. Name and describe the function of the two parts of the autonomic nervous system.
6. Describe methods used to assess motor and sensory function.
7. List six diagnostic procedures performed to detect neurologic disorders.
8. Discuss the nursing management of the client undergoing neurologic diagnostic testing.

SECTION I: ASSESSING YOUR UNDERSTANDING

Activity A *Fill in the blanks by choosing the correct word from the options given in parentheses.*

1. The basic structure of the nervous system is the _____. *(Neuron, Dendrite, Axon)*

2. _____ transmit impulses from the CNS. *(Sensory neurons, Myelin, Motor neurons)*

3. The _____ is the surface of the cerebrum. It contains motor neurons, which are responsible for movement, and sensory neurons, which receive impulses from peripheral sensory neurons located throughout the body. *(Corpus callosum, Cerebral cortex, Midbrain)*

4. The two main functions of the _____ are to provide centers for reflex action and to serve as a pathway for impulses to and from the brain. *(Spinal cord, Meninges, Vertebrae)*

5. _____ allergies suggest an allergy to iodine. *(Dairy, Peanut, Seafood)*

Activity B *Mark each statement as either "T" (True) or "F" (False). Correct any false statements.*

1. T F The central nervous system (CNS) consists of the brain and spinal cord.

2. T F The nervous system is divided into two anatomical divisions: the central nervous system and the peripheral nervous system

3. T F Dendrites are nerve fibers that conduct impulses away from the cell body.

4. T F Neurons are directly connected to one another.

5. T F The medulla contains vital centers concerned with respiration, heartbeat, and vasomotor activity.

Activity C *Write the correct term for each description given below.*

1. The part of the nervous system that consists of all the sensory and motor nerves outside the CNS. It includes the cranial, spinal, and sympathetic and parasympathetic nerves of the autonomic nervous system. _____

2. The type of neurons that transmit impulses to the CNS. _____

3. These substances accomplish the transmission of an impulse from one neuron to the next; they can either excite or inhibit neurons. _____

4. The cerebrum consists of two hemispheres: each hemisphere has four lobes. _____, _____, _____, and _____

5. The part of the brain, located behind and below the cerebrum, which controls and coordinates muscle movement. _____

6. Within the brain are four hollow structures called the ventricles, which manufacture and absorb this fluid. _____.

Activity D *Match the levels of consciousness (LOC) given in Column A with their corresponding characteristics given in Column B.*

Column A

____ **1.** Conscious

____ **2.** Somnolent or lethargic

____ **3.** Stuporous

____ **4.** Semicomatose

____ **5.** Comatose

Column B

a. The client is aroused only by vigorous and continuous stimulation, usually by manipulation or strong auditory or visual stimuli.

b. Spontaneous motion is uncommon, but the client may groan or mutter.

c. There is no spontaneous movement, and the respiratory rate is irregular.

d. The client responds immediately, fully, and appropriately to visual, auditory, and other stimulation.

e. The client is drowsy or sleepy at inappropriate times but can be aroused, only to fall asleep again.

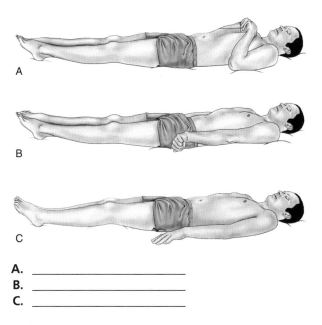

A. _____
B. _____
C. _____

Activity F *Match the cranial nerve in Column A to its corresponding function in Column B.*

Column A

____ **1.** Olfactory nerve

____ **2.** Optic nerve

____ **3.** Oculomotor nerve

____ **4.** Trochlear nerve

____ **5.** Trigeminal nerve

____ **6.** Abducens nerve

____ **7.** Facial nerve

____ **8.** Vestibulocochlear (or auditory) nerve

____ **9.** Glossopharyngeal nerve

____ **10.** Vagus nerve

____ **11.** Accessory (or spinal accessory) nerve

Column B

a. Facial expression, taste, secretions of salivary and lacrimal glands

b. Head and shoulder movement

c. Eye movement

d. Taste, sensory fibers of pharynx and tongue, swallowing, secretions of parotid gland

e. Eye movement

f. Contraction of iris and eye muscles

g. Sense of smell

h. Movement of the tongue

i. Sensory nerve to face, chewing

j. Hearing, balance

k. Sight

l. Motor fibers to glands producing digestive enzymes, heart rate, muscles of speech,

TABLE 36-1

Test	Method	Purpose	Precautions
Computed Tomography			
Magnetic Resonance Imaging			
Positron Emission Tomography			
Single-photon Emission Computed Tomography			
Lumbar Puncture			
Contrast Studies			
Electroencephalogram			
Brain Scan			
Electromyography			
Nerve Conduction Studies			
Echoencephalogram			

_____ **12.** Hypoglossal nerve — gastrointestinal motility, respiration, swallowing, coughing, vomiting reflex

Activity G *Identify the method, purpose, and precautions for the diagnostic tests related to the nervous system that are listed in Table 36-1.*

Activity H *Briefly answer the following questions.*

1. What pharmacological considerations should be noted when performing a neurologic assessment?

_____

_____

_____

2. How are intellectual and speech patterns assessed?

_____

_____

_____

3. What assessments will the nurse make if the client has sustained trauma?

_____

_____

_____

4. How is motor response evaluated in the comatose or unconscious client?

_____

_____

_____

5. What are the three parts to the Glasgow Coma Scale?

_____

_____

_____

SECTION II: APPLYING YOUR KNOWLEDGE

Activity I *Give rationale for the following questions.*

1. Why does the nurse stand close to the client when performing the Romberg test?

_____

_____

_____

2. Why can assessment of the older adult be difficult?

_____

_____

_____

3. Why do some rehabilitation centers prefer the Rancho Los Amigos Scale to the Glasgow Coma Scale?

_____

_____

_____

4. Why is it important to monitor temperature with a CNS disorder?

_____

_____

_____

Activity J *Answer the following questions related to the nervous system.*

1. Describe the function of the spinal nerves.

_____

_____

_____

2. What information is essential to gather when obtaining a history?

_____

_____

_____

3. Describe the assessment of motor function during a neurologic examination.

_____

_____

_____

4. Describe the assessment of sensory function during a neurological examination.

_____

_____

_____

5. When assessing client pupils what information should be reported to the physician immediately?

_____

_____

_____

Activity K *Think over the following questions. Discuss them with your instructor or peers.*

1. Calculate the client's Glasgow Coma Scale: Eye opening response – to pain, Best verbal response – incomprehensible sounds, Best motor response – withdraws (pain). What is the client's total score? What high-priority nursing diagnoses would be pertinent? What nursing interventions would you provide?

_____

_____

_____

2. You are assessing an older client's pupillary response and note pupil response is sluggish. What further information will you need to obtain?

_____

_____

_____

3. You are preparing a client for a lumbar puncture. The client is fearful about the procedure. How will you explain the procedure? What educational information will you provide? What nursing interventions will you utilize to reduce the client's fears?

_____

_____

_____

SECTION III: GETTING READY FOR NCLEX

Activity L *Answer the following questions.*

1. A client, age 45, undergoes a lumbar puncture in which CSF is extracted for a particular neurological diagnostic procedure. After the procedure, he complains of dizziness and a slight headache. Which of the following steps must the nurse take to provide comfort to the client?

   a. Position the client flat for at least three hours or as directed by the physician.

   b. Keep the room well lighted and play some soothing music in the background.

   c. Help the client ambulate and perform a few light leg exercises.

   d. Provide some easy reading material to the client.

2. Why should the nurse wake up a client, who is to undergo an EEG, at midnight?

   a. Because excess sleep may make the client lazy and nervous for the EEG

   b. Because optimum sleep helps regulate the breathing patterns during the EEG

   c. Because it helps the client to fall asleep naturally during the EEG

   d. Because it reduces the chances of getting a headache when electrodes are fixed to the client's scalp

3. During the physical examination of a client for a possible neurological disorder, how can the nurse examine the client for stiffness and rigidity of the neck?

   a. By positioning the client flat on the bed for at least three hours

   b. By moving the head and chin of the client towards the chest

   c. By asking the client to bend and pick up small and large objects on the floor

   d. By introducing a painful stimulus on the neck

4. A nurse has been examining the vital signs of a client for the past two days. On a particular day, she observes a sudden change in the vital signs of the client. Which of the following steps should the nurse take immediately?

   a. Inform the physician

   b. Change the environmental settings of the client

   c. Alter the diet intake of the client

   d. Decrease the physical activity of the client, if any

5. The nurse assesses the motor functions during a neurologic examination of a client. Which of the following steps will help the nurse perform the examination effectively?

   a. Check the client's sensitivity to heat, cold, touch, and pain.

   b. Ask the client to pick up small and large objects between the thumb and forefinger.

   c. Ask questions that require cognition and logic.

   d. Evaluate the client's level of consciousness (LOC).

6. In which of the following clients will an MRI scan be contraindicated?

   a. Overweight clients

   b. Clients over the age of 60

   c. Clients with metal implants in their body

   d. Clients with brain tumor

7. A client is undergoing neurological testing for a brain tumor. Which anatomic division of the nervous system is affected in this individual?

   a. Peripheral nervous system

   b. Autonomic nervous system

   c. Sympathetic nervous system

   d. Central nervous system

8. A nurse is caring for a client with a problem with the cerebrum. Which of the following four lobes of the cerebrum is located just above the ear?

   a. Parietal lobe

   b. Temporal lobe

   c. Frontal lobe

   d. Occipital lobe

9. A client is on the neurological floor and the nurse performs an assessment on the client's level of consciousness. What would the nurse document after her assessment if the client is unresponsive except to superficial, relatively mild painful stimuli to which the client makes some purposeful motor response (movement) to evade stimulation?

   a. Client is somnolent or lethargic.

   b. Client is in a stuporous state.

   c. Client is semicomatose.

   d. Client is comatose.

CHAPTER 37

Caring for Clients with Central and Peripheral Nervous System Disorders

Learning Objectives

1. Discuss at least four signs and symptoms and nursing care of the client with increased intracranial pressure.
2. Name four infectious or inflammatory diseases that affect the central or peripheral nervous system.
3. Discuss three neuromuscular disorders, common related problems, and nursing management.
4. Discuss the nursing management of clients with a cranial nerve disorder.
5. List the signs and symptoms of Parkinson's disease.
6. Discuss the purpose of drug therapy and drugs commonly prescribed for Parkinson's disease.
7. Describe signs and symptoms of Huntington's disease and related nursing management.
8. Discuss the pathophysiology of seizure disorders and different types of seizures.
9. Discuss the nursing management of clients with seizure disorders.
10. Discuss the nursing management of clients with brain tumors.

SECTION I: ASSESSING YOUR UNDERSTANDING

Activity A *Fill in the blanks by choosing the correct word from the options given in parentheses.*

1. Shallow, rapid breathing followed by periods of apnea is known as _____. *(Cushing's triad, Cheynes-Stokes respirations, Papilledema)*

2. Normal intracranial pressure (ICP) in the ventricles is _____ mm Hg. *(0 to 5, 1 to 15, 5 to 20)*

3. Although the ICP varies, a rise of _____ mm Hg from a previous measurement is cause for concern. *(2, 4, 6)*

4. A viral link is suspected as the cause for _____. Inflammation occurs around the nerve, blocking motor impulses to facial muscles. Inflammation or ischemia resulting from nerve compression leads to impaired nerve function. *(Bell's palsy, Trigeminal neuralgia, Parkinson's disease)*

5. _____ is an extrapyramidal disorder that is transmitted genetically and inherited by people of both genders. *(Parkinson's disease, Trigeminal neuralgia, Huntington's chorea)*

6. A _____ is a growth of abnormal cells within the cranium. *(Brain abscess, Brain tumor, Brain lesion)*

Activity B *Mark each statement as either "T" (True) or "F" (False). Correct any false statements.*

1. T F Inside the cranium, there is (1) brain tissue, (2) blood, and (3) cerebrospinal fluid (CSF). If one or more of these increases significantly without a decrease in either of the other two, ICP becomes elevated.

2. **T F**   Temperature regulation is not a concern for the client with IICP.

3. **T F**   Encephalitis is medically managed with antibiotic therapy.

4. **T F**   Parkinson's disease and parkinsonism result from a deficiency of the neurotransmitter acetylcholine.

5. **T F**   A seizure is a brief episode of abnormal electrical activity in the brain.

6. **T F**   An akinetic seizure affects the muscles. The person loses consciousness briefly and falls to the ground. Recovery is rapid.

Activity C *Write the correct term for each of the following descriptions that relate to nervous system disorders or conditions.*

1. An increase in systolic BP and decrease in diastolic BP (widened pulse pressure), bradycardia, and irregular respirations. _____

2. The client's head is maintained in this position to promote venous drainage of blood and CSF. _____

3. An inflammation of the meninges caused by various infectious microorganisms such as bacteria, viruses, fungi, or parasites. _____

4. This treatment for Guillain-Barré may include removal of plasma from the blood and reinfusion of the cellular components with saline. This treatment has been shown to shorten the course of the disease if performed within the first 2 weeks. _____

5. A collection of purulent material in the brain. If untreated, it can be fatal. _____

6. A surgical procedure that destroys a part of the globus pallidus to eliminate or reduce tremor, stooped posture, shuffling gait, and stiff movement. _____

Activity D *Match the neurological disorders in Column A with their signs and symptoms in Column B.*

Column A

_____ Bell's palsy

_____ Huntington's disease

_____ Trigeminal neuralgia

_____ Parkinson's disease

Column B

a. Early signs include stiffness, referred to as rigidity, and tremors of one or both hands, described as pill-rolling. Bradykinesia develops; clients have a masklike expression, stooped posture, hypophonia, and difficulty swallowing saliva. Weight loss occurs, a shuffling gait is apparent, and the client has difficulty turning or redirecting forward motion.

b. The client describes the pain as sudden, severe, and burning. The pain ends as quickly as it begins, usually lasting a few seconds to several minutes. The cycle repeats many times each day. During a spasm, the face twitches and the eyes tear.

c. Symptoms develop slowly and include mental apathy and emotional disturbances, choreiform movements, grimacing, difficulty chewing and swallowing, speech difficulty, intellectual decline, and loss of bowel and bladder control. Severe depression is common and can lead to suicide.

d. Involves the seventh cranial nerve, which is responsible for movement of the facial muscles. Symptoms develop in a few hours or over 1 to 2 days. Facial pain, pain behind the ear, numbness, diminished blink reflex, ptosis of the eyelid, and tearing on the affected side occur. Speaking and chewing become difficult.

TABLE 37-1

Neuromuscular Disorder	Cause	Signs and Symptoms	Treatment
Multiple Sclerosis			
Myasthenia Gravis			
Amyotrophic Lateral Sclerosis			

Activity E *Compare and contrast the early and late signs of increased ICP.*

1. Early signs: _____

2. Late signs: _____

Activity F *Compare the neuromuscular disorders in Table 37-1 with regard to cause, signs and symptoms, and treatment.*

Activity G *Briefly answer the following questions.*

1. Why are isotonic intravenous solutions and supplemental oxygen or mechanical ventilation significant to the medical care of the client with increased ICP?

_____

_____

2. The physician may order medications such as anticonvulsants and benzodiazepines. Why would these medications be used in the treatment of increased ICP?

_____

_____

3. Describe the treatment for meningitis.

_____

_____

4. What is encephalitis? What are common causes?

_____

_____

5. Surgical division of the sensory root of the trigeminal nerve may be performed as treatment for trigeminal neuralgia. What problems may result from this procedure?

_____

_____

_____

6. What are signs and symptoms of a brain tumor?

_____

_____

_____

SECTION II: APPLYING YOUR KNOWLEDGE

Activity H *Give rationale for the following questions.*

1. Why are hypotonic intravenous solutions and solutions containing dextrose not administered to clients with increased ICP?

_____

_____

2. Why are narcotics withheld from clients with increased ICP unless absolutely necessary?

_____

_____

3. Why are respiratory status, nutrition and immobility priority concern for the caring for the client with Guillain-Barré?

_____

_____

4. Why are CT scans, MRIs, and skull radio-graphs safer techniques for diagnosing and locating a brain abscess than a lumbar puncture?

_____

_____

_____

5. Why may an absence seizure go unnoticed?

_____

_____

_____

6. Why should anticonvulsant medications be withdrawn slowly?

_____

_____

_____

Activity I *Answer the following questions related to central and peripheral nervous system disorders.*

1. Describe the signs and symptoms of meningitis.

_____

_____

_____

2. What are signs and symptoms of encephalitis?

_____

_____

_____

3. Describe the pathophysiology of Guillain-Barré syndrome and the usual course of the disorder.

_____

_____

_____

4. Describe the mechanism of action for dopa-minergics, antiparkinson agents, dopamine agonists, and anticholinergics.

_____

_____

_____

5. Describe the difference between a partial elementary seizure with motor symptoms, a partial elementary seizure with sensory symptoms, and a partial seizure with complex symptoms.

_____

_____

_____

6. Describe the difference between generalized seizures: a myoclonic seizure and a tonic-clonic seizure.

_____

_____

_____

Activity J *Think over the following questions. Discuss them with your instructor or peers.*

1. What priority nursing diagnoses and interventions would you identify for clients with increased ICP?

_____

_____

2. What priority nursing diagnoses and interventions would you identify for clients with neurologic infectious or inflammatory disorders?

_____

_____

3. What priority nursing diagnoses and interventions would you identify for clients with neuromuscular disorders?

_____

_____

4. What educational information would you provide to the family of a client diagnosed with an extrapyramidal disorder?

_____

_____

5. What educational information would you provide to a client diagnosed with a seizure disorder?

_____

_____

_____

SECTION III: GETTING READY FOR NCLEX

Activity K *Answer the following questions.*

1. A female client recovers from a serious phase of insect bites. What skin-related advice must the nurse give to the client and all her family members to prevent the recurrence of the ailment?
   a. Ensure minimum crowd interactions when outdoors
   b. Apply insect repellant to clothing and exposed skin
   c. Wear thick woolen clothing to cover the skin while outdoors
   d. Apply a good sunscreen lotion while going outdoors

2. The nurse observes the temperature record of a client and relates the fever to the brain infection the client currently has. The nurse knows that a high temperature may lead to an increased cerebral irritation. Which of the following measures can help the nurse control the client's body temperature?
   a. Administering prescribed antipyretics
   b. Reducing body hydration
   c. Applying ice packs
   d. Keeping the room temperature warm

3. Which of the following is the characteristic of a cacogenic diet that is suggested for children with seizures?
   a. High-carbohydrate diet
   b. High-protein diet
   c. High-fat diet
   d. Low-fat diet

4. A 34-year-old male client is diagnosed with encephalitis. Medication has been started for him and he is receiving nursing care. Which of the following nursing interventions are the most critical for such a client?
   a. Evaluating the client's ventilation capacity and lung sounds frequently
   b. Observing closely for signs of respiratory distress
   c. Administering an indwelling urethral catheter
   d. Monitoring vital signs and LOC frequently

5. A client with neuromuscular disorder is receiving intensive nursing care. The client is likely to face the risk for impaired skin integrity. Which of the following must the nurse ensure to prevent skin breakdown in the client?
   a. Prevent strenuous exercises by the client
   b. Use pressure-relieving devices when the client is in bed
   c. Place the client in a Fowler's position
   d. Avoid giving daily baths to the client with soaps

6. Why do emotional counseling and helping the client perform common daily activities become important nursing care interventions in clients with Parkinson's or Huntington's diseases, or even epilepsy?
   a. Because clients suffer from depression, anxiety, and inability to perform basic self-care
   b. Because clients become paralytic throughout the body
   c. Because the clients' bones become weak, brittle, and painful to even move
   d. Because clients generally become very aggressive and violent with other people

7. A client comes to the Emergency Room following a fall at her home and is diagnosed with increased intracranial pressure. What is the first sign or symptom that occurs with this diagnosis?
   a. Decrease in LOC (level of consciousness)
   b. Headache
   c. Vomiting
   d. Papilledema

8. A graduate nurse is taking a test on neurological conditions. Which of the following nursing interventions is used as a gastrointestinal preventative measure for the client with intracranial pressure?

   a. Insertion of an NG tube

   b. Administration of a histamine antagonist (Pepcid)

   c. Sips of clear fluid

   d. Insertion of a rectal tube

9. Which of the following signs is present in a client with meningitis and is described as the inability to extend the leg when the thigh is flexed on the abdomen?

   a. Opisthotonos

   b. Positive Brudzinski's sign

   c. Positive Kernig's sign

   d. Nuchal rigidity

10. The nursing management of a client with Guillain-Barré syndrome who is immobile should concentrate on what aspects of care once the respiratory system has been managed?

    a. Turn the client every 2 hours to prevent skin breakdown

    b. Range-of-motion (ROM) exercises every 8 hours

    c. Encourage the client to participate in self-care

    d. Consult with a physical or occupational therapist on independence activities

11. A nurse is taking care of a client with ptosis (drooping) of the eyelids, difficulty chewing and swallowing, diplopia, voice weakness, masklike facial expression, and weakness of the extremities. Which of the following conditions does the nurse suspect?

    a. Parkinson's disease

    b. Extrapyramidal disorder

    c. Multiple sclerosis

    d. Myasthenia gravis

Caring for Clients with Cerebrovascular Disorders

Learning Objectives

1. Identify three common types of headaches and their characteristics.
2. List nursing techniques that supplement drug therapy in reducing or relieving headaches.
3. Explain the cause and significance of a transient ischemic attack.
4. Discuss medical and surgical techniques used to reduce the potential for a cerebrovascular accident.
5. Differentiate between ischemic and hemorrhagic strokes.
6. Identify five manifestations of a cerebrovascular accident; discuss those that are unique to right-sided and left-sided infarctions.
7. Identify at least five nursing diagnoses common to the care of a client with a cerebrovascular accident and interventions for them.
8. Describe a cerebral aneurysm and the danger it presents.
9. Discuss appropriate nursing interventions when caring for a client with a cerebral aneurysm.

SECTION I: ASSESSING YOUR UNDERSTANDING

Activity A *Fill in the blanks by choosing the correct word from the options given in parentheses.*

1. _____, the most common of the three types of headaches, occur when a person contracts the neck and facial muscles

for a prolonged period of time. *(Tension headaches, Migraine headaches, Cluster headaches)*

2. Prophylactic drug therapy may be necessary if _____ occur several times a month and produce severe impairment or if acute attacks are not adequately relieved. *(Tension headaches, Migraine headaches, Cluster headaches)*

3. A _____ is a sudden, brief attack of neurologic impairment caused by a temporary interruption in cerebral blood flow. *(Cerebrovascular accident (CVA), Cerebral aneurysms, Transient ischemic attack (TIA))*

4. _____ is the antidote for oral anticoagulants. *(Vitamin A, Vitamin E, Vitamin K)*

5. _____ develop at a weakened area in the blood vessel wall. The defect is congenital or secondary to hypertension and atherosclerosis. *(TIAs, CVAs, Aneurysms)*

Activity B *Mark each statement as either "T" (True) or "F" (False). Correct any false statements.*

1. T F Migraine headaches, which are recurrent and severe and last for a day or more, have a vascular origin.

2. T F A person with a cluster headache has pain on one side of the head, usually behind the eye, accompanied by nasal congestion, rhinorrhea, and tearing and redness of the eye.

3. T F A CVA is a prolonged interruption in the flow of blood through one of the arteries supplying the brain.

4. T F An ischemic stroke occurs when a cerebral blood vessel ruptures and blood is released in brain tissue.

5. T F Confusion and emotional liability are characteristic symptoms of a CVA.

6. T F Tissue plasminogen activator (TPA) and anticoagulant therapy are the treatments of choice for a hemorrhagic CVA.

Activity C *Write the correct term for each description given below.*

1. These types of headaches may be a variant of migraine headaches; they are episodic, reoccurring over 6 to 8 weeks, with only brief periods of recovery between multiple daily attacks. _____

2. These types of headaches are usually relieved by rest, a mild analgesic, and stress management techniques such as relaxation or imaging. _____

3. A warning that a cerebrovascular accident can occur in the near future; one third of people who experience this develop stroke.

   _____

4. An abnormal sound caused by blood flowing over the rough surface of one or both carotid arteries. _____

5. This type of medication has been found to limit neurologic deficits when given within 3 hours after the onset of an ischemic CVA.

   _____

Activity D *Match the nursing intervention listed in Column A with the rationale in Column B.*

Column A

_____ 1. Eliminate environmental factors that intensify pain, such as bright light and noise.

_____ 2. Administer prescribed medications as early as possible and note their effects.

_____ 3. Offer a back massage to promote muscle relaxation.

_____ 4. Apply warm (or cool) cloths to the forehead or back of the neck.

_____ 5. Provide distraction with soft, soothing music, or suggest using a relaxation tape or one that provides guided imagery.

Column B

a. Relaxes tense muscles, causes local dilation of blood vessels, and relieves headache. This approach is not likely to help a client with migraine or cluster headache.

b. Reduced anxiety can relieve a tension headache; clients with migraine or cluster headaches are not receptive to this approach.

c. Sensory stimuli decrease pain tolerance.

d. There are many different categories with various mechanisms of action. If treatment is ineffective collaborate with the physician to modify.

e. Warmth promotes vasodilation; cool stimuli reduce blood flow.

Activity E *Compare and contrast the symptoms of right-sided hemiplegia (stroke on left side of brain) and left-sided hemiplegia (stroke on right side of brain).*

_____

_____

_____

Activity F *Briefly answer the following.*

1. A client who has "classic" migraines may experience an "aura." What is an "aura"? What other symptoms do clients often experience with a "common" migraine?

   _____

   _____

   _____

2. What are the symptoms of a TIA?

   _____

   _____

   _____

3. What procedures may be performed on the carotid arteries to increase blood flow to the brain?

   _____

   _____

   _____

4. Define hemiplegia, expressive aphasia, receptive aphasia, and hemianopia.

_____

_____

_____

5. What are the clinical manifestations following a cerebral hemorrhage?

_____

_____

_____

6. What are the symptoms of a cerebral aneurysm?

_____

_____

_____

SECTION II: APPLYING YOUR KNOWLEDGE

Activity G _Give rationale for the following questions._

1. Why may an older adult ignore symptoms of a TIA?

_____

_____

_____

2. Why are clients at risk for a TIA given aspirin prophylactically?

_____

_____

_____

3. Why may an older adult diagnosed with hypertension receiving medication to treat the disorder still be at risk for a CVA?

_____

_____

_____

4. Why is it essential to monitor a client's cardiac rhythm following carotid artery surgery?

_____

_____

_____

5. Why is surgery not always an option for treatment of an aneurysm?

_____

_____

_____

Activity H _Answer the following questions related to caring for clients with cerebrovascular disorders._

1. Describe the pathophysiology of a TIA.

_____

_____

_____

2. Describe the basic events and effects that occur as a result of a CVA.

_____

_____

_____

3. What are the signs of an impending CVA?

_____

_____

_____

4. How are clients at risk for a TIA or CVA medically managed?

_____

_____

_____

5. What assessment data should the nurse obtain when caring for a client with a cerebrovascular disorder?

_____

_____

_____

6. How are clients with an aneurysm medically managed?

_____

_____

_____

Activity I *Think over the following questions. Discuss them with your instructor or peers.*

1. What educational information will you provide to clients about controllable risk factors to prevent a TIA or CVA?

   _____

   _____

   _____

2. What do you identify as high priority nursing diagnoses and nursing interventions for the client experiencing a CVA? What educational information will you provide?

   _____

   _____

   _____

3. What appropriate nursing interventions will you implement when caring for the client with an aneurysm?

   _____

   _____

   _____

SECTION III: GETTING READY FOR NCLEX

Activity J *Answer the following questions.*

1. Which of the following would describe the discomfort experienced by a client with a tension headache?

   a. A heavy feeling over the frontal region, and sensitivity to light

   b. Pressure or steady constriction on both sides of the head

   c. Headache and temporary unilateral paralysis

   d. Vague headache, especially periorbital

2. What should the nurse teach an older client with TIA?

   a. Not to worry about the symptoms that are part of the normal aging process

   b. Admit oneself in a rehabilitation center or a nursing home for rehabilitation

   c. Comply with the medication regimen

   d. Observe any changes in the nails and skin

3. Why should clients who take warfarin (Coumadin®) refrain from food items such as green, leafy vegetables and soybeans?

   a. Because the foods contain vitamin K, which reduces the anticoagulant effect of the medication

   b. Because the foods contain vitamin K, which increases the anticoagulant effect of the medication

   c. Because the foods help stimulate salivation

   d. Because the foods minimize the volume of food consumption

4. The nurse in the postoperative unit prepares to receive a client after a balloon angioplasty of the carotid artery. Which of the following items should the nurse keep at the bedside for such a client in the case of an emergency situation based on the procedure that was done?

   a. BP apparatus

   b. Call bell

   c. IV infusion stand

   d. Endotracheal intubation

5. A young male client visits a nurse with a complaint of chronic tension headaches. Which of the following is the most appropriate nursing instruction to manage the client?

   a. Instructing the client to monitor for signs of bruising or bleeding

   b. Suggesting eating and swallowing techniques that reduce the potential for aspiration

   c. Counseling on alternate therapies

   d. Advising the client to change sleeping positions frequently

6. Why would a Heimlich maneuver be performed on a client?

   a. To increase the absorption of the prescribed medication

   b. To clear the airway if the client cannot speak or breathe after swallowing food

   c. To reduce the potential for injuries as a result of falls

   d. To maintain extremities in proper anatomic position

7. Which of the following conditions is the result of a ruptured cerebral blood vessel and the release of blood into the brain tissue?

   a. Ischemic stroke

   b. Transient ischemic attack

   c. Cerebral aneurysm

   d. Hemorrhagic stroke

8. Which of the following are controllable risk factors for CVAs?

   a. Race

   b. Sex

   c. HTN

   d. Age

9. A client enters the emergency room due to a left sided CVA. Tissue plasminogen activator (TPA) is ordered for the client, who has had an ischemic stroke. Within how many hours does the drug need to be given to be most successful?

   a. 6 hours

   b. 3 hours

   c. 8 hours

   d. 10 hours

10. In performing discharge teaching to a client with a cerebral aneurysm, the nurse instructs the client to do which of the following?

    a. Lift heavy objects if you are able

    b. Limit emotional upsets to no more than 3 per day

    c. Do not bend over for long periods of time

    d. Do not strain during a bowel movement

Caring for Clients with Head and Spinal Cord Trauma

1. Differentiate a concussion from a contusion.
2. Explain the differences between epidural, sub-dural, and intracerebral hematomas.
3. Discuss the nursing management of a client with a head injury.
4. Discuss the nursing management of a client undergoing intracranial surgery.
5. Explain spinal shock, listing four symptoms.
6. Discuss autonomic dysreflexia and at least five manifestations.
7. List possible long-term complications of spinal cord injury.
8. Describe the nursing management of a client with a spinal cord injury.
9. Identify the anatomic difference between intramedullary and extramedullary spinal nerve root compression.

SECTION I: ASSESSING YOUR UNDERSTANDING

Activity A *Fill in the blanks by choosing the correct word from the options given in parentheses.*

1. When the head is struck, dual bruising can result if the force is strong enough to send the brain ricocheting to the opposite side of the skull. This is called a _____. *(Coup injury, Contrecoup injury, Skull fracture)*

2. A _____ is a surgical opening in the skull. *(Craniotomy, Craniectomy, Cranioplasty)*

3. To detect any CSF drainage the nurse looks for a _____, which is a blood stain surrounded by a clear or yellowish stain. *(Battle sign, Periorbital ecchymosis, Halo sign)*

4. _____ results in weakness, paralysis and sensory impairment of all extremities and the trunk when there is a spinal injury at or above the first thoracic (T1) vertebrae. *(Tetraplegia, Paraplegia, Hemiplegia)*

5. _____ is a neuroprotective drug that blocks the neurotoxic effects of glutamate. *(Rilutek, Cetherin, A corticosteroid)*

6. An _____ lesion is a type of spinal nerve root compression that involves the spinal cord. *(Extramedullary, Laminectomy, Intramedullary)*

Activity B *Mark each statement as either "T" (True) or "F" (False). Correct any false statements.*

1. T F A contusion results in diffuse and microscopic injury to the brain. The force of the blow causes temporary neurologic impairment but no serious damage to cerebral tissue.

2. T F People at high risk for cerebral hematomas are those receiving anticoagulant

therapy or those with an underlying bleeding disorder.

3. **T F** All clients with cerebral hematomas require surgical intervention.

4. **T F** A cranioplasty is the repair of a defect in a cranial bone.

5. **T F** A head injury is always considered an emergency.

6. **T F** After the initial period of therapeutic care for a spinal cord injury, the focus of treatment turns to rehabilitative and restorative measures.

Activity C *Write the correct term for each description given below.*

1. A contusion caused when the head is struck directly. _____

2. Removal of part of the cranial bone. _____

3. A break in the continuity of the cranium. _____

4. Weakness or paralysis and compromised sensory functions of both legs and lower pelvis, occurs with spinal injuries below the T1 level. _____

5. May be used to activate paralyzed muscles and prevent muscle atrophy. _____

6. A type of spinal nerve root compression that involves the tissues surrounding the spinal cord. _____

Activity D *Match the type of cerebral hematoma given in column A with the corresponding description given in Column B.*

Column A

____ 1. Epidural hematoma

____ 2. Subdural hematoma

____ 3. Acute subdural hematoma

____ 4. Subacute and chronic subdural hematomas

____ 5. Intracerebral hematoma

____ 6. Uncal herniation

Column B

a. Results from venous bleeding, with blood gradually accumulating in the space below the dura.

b. Symptoms progressively worsen within the first 24 hours of the head injury.

c. Bleeding within the brain that results from an open or closed head injury or from a cerebrovascular

condition such as a ruptured cerebral aneurysm.

d. Stems from arterial bleeding, usually from the middle meningeal artery, and blood accumulation above the dura. It is characterized by rapidly progressive neurologic deterioration.

e. Unrelieved increased ICP can cause the brain to shift to the lateral side or herniate downward through the foramen magnum.

f. Clients become symptomatic after 24 hours and up to 1 week later.

Activity E *Provide the description and manifestations/causes of complications associated with spinal cord injury.*

Complication	Description	Manifestations/ Causes
Respiratory failure		
Spinal shock		
Autonomic dysreflexia		
Pressure ulcers		
Respiratory infections		
Urinary impairment		
Fecal impairment		
Spasticity and contractures		
Weight change		
Calcium depletion		
Urinary calculi		
Sexual dysfunction: male		
Sexual dysfunction: female		
Pain		

Activity F *Briefly answer the following questions.*

1. When a client is discharged following a concussion, what changes would the family be instructed to watch for as common signs of increased ICP?

_____

_____

_____

2. The rapidity and severity of neurological changes caused by a cerebral hematoma depend on which factors?

_____

_____

_____

3. What is the purpose of Burr holes?

_____

_____

_____

4. What are common sites and causes of spinal cord injuries?

_____

_____

_____

5. What is the purpose of treadmill training? Is it appropriate for all clients with spinal cord injuries?

_____

_____

_____

6. What types of clients may benefit from tendon transfer surgery?

_____

_____

_____

7. Describe the usual symptoms of a spinal nerve root compression.

_____

_____

_____

SECTION II: APPLYING YOUR KNOWLEDGE

Activity G *Give rationale for the following questions.*

1. Why do epidural hematomas require prompt intervention?

_____

_____

_____

2. Why would mannitol be used following intracranial surgery?

_____

_____

_____

3. Why are fluids restricted before intracranial surgery?

_____

_____

_____

4. Why is it important to monitor temperature following intracranial surgery?

_____

_____

_____

5. Why are open head injuries more likely to create a risk for infection but less likely to result in increased ICP?

_____

_____

_____

6. Why are basilar skull fractures especially dangerous?

_____

_____

_____

Activity H *Answer the following questions related to caring for the client with head and spinal cord trauma.*

1. To reduce the potential for both minor and life-threatening head injuries, the nurse will stress the importance of which activities?

   _____

   _____

   _____

2. What types of signs and symptoms can a basilar skull fracture produce?

   _____

   _____

   _____

3. Describe the medical and surgical treatment for a skull fracture.

   _____

   _____

   _____

4. Describe how trauma, edema, and bleeding can cause damage to the spinal cord.

   _____

   _____

   _____

5. Describe how immobilization and traction are used with a spinal cord injury.

   _____

   _____

   _____

6. Describe the benefits of functional electrical stimulation.

   _____

   _____

   _____

7. What is the medical and surgical treatment involved with a spinal nerve root compression?

   _____

   _____

   _____

Activity I *Think over the following questions. Discuss them with your instructor or peers.*

1. What nursing care would you provide for a client returning to your unit after intracranial surgery?

   _____

   _____

2. A client who has suffered a traumatic spinal cord injury is being transferred to your unit following the acute care phase. What will be your priority nursing diagnoses and interventions for the physiological needs of the client? What will be your priority nursing diagnoses and interventions for the psychosocial needs of the client? What educational information will you need to provide to the client and family?

   _____

   _____

   _____

3. What are the ethical considerations related to spinal cord injuries and embryonic stem cell transplantation?

   _____

   _____

   _____

SECTION III: GETTING READY FOR NCLEX

Activity J *Answer the following questions.*

1. Which of the following is a symptom of basilar skull fracture?

   a. Raccoon eyes

   b. Halo sign

   c. Amnesia

   d. Paresthesia

2. Which of the following statements justifies the administration of the prescribed anticonvulsant phenytoin to a client before the intracranial surgery?

   a. To reduce the risk of seizures before and after surgery

   b. To avoid intraoperative complications

   c. To reduce cerebral edema

   d. To prevent postoperative vomiting

3. Which of the following dietary interventions prevents the precipitation of calcium renal stones?
   a. High-fiber diet
   b. Increase protein intake
   c. High fluid intake
   d. Intake of zinc

4. A client with spinal cord injury at the level of T3 complains of a sudden severe headache and nasal congestion. The nurse observes that the client has a flushed skin with goosebumps. Which of the following actions should the nurse first take?
   a. Raise the client's head
   b. Place the client on a firm mattress
   c. Call the physician
   d. Administer an analgesic to relieve the pain

5. Which of the following nursing interventions is taken as a precautionary measure if shock develops when a client with spinal cord injury is hospitalized?
   a. An IV line is inserted to provide access to a vein.
   b. Head and back are immobilized mechanically with a cervical collar and back support.
   c. Traction with weights and pulleys is applied.
   d. A turning frame is used.

6. Which of the following clients are more likely to suffer from a cerebral hematoma?
   a. A client with a family history of hemophilia; no symptoms
   b. A client receiving platelets for a low platelet count
   c. A client with anemia taking iron
   d. A client with atrial fibrillation on Coumadin

7. Which of the following intracranial surgeries involves the repair of a defect in a cranial bone?
   a. Craniectomy
   b. Craniotomy
   c. Cranioplasty
   d. Cranial lysis

8. Which of the following drugs is used to decrease intracranial pressure following intracranial surgery?
   a. Benadryl
   b. Mannitol
   c. Prednisone
   d. Corticosteroids

9. Which of the following nursing interventions should be done in the case of a client who has a head injury obtained from being thrown off of a motorcycle?
   a. Assess LOC every hour or more often if needed
   b. Put the code cart outside the client's room
   c. Keep the client quiet in bed
   d. Allow one visitor at a time

Caring for Clients with Neurologic Deficits

1. Define neurologic deficit.
2. Describe the three phases of a neurologic deficit.
3. Give the primary aims of medical treatment of a neurologic deficit.
4. Name six members of the healthcare team involved with the management of a client with a neurologic deficit.
5. Describe nursing management of a client with a neurologic deficit.

SECTION I: ASSESSING YOUR UNDERSTANDING

Activity A *Fill in the blanks by choosing the correct word from the options given in parentheses.*

1. A _____ position facilitates functional use of the limbs. *(Flexed, Neutral, Hyperextended)*

2. The urge to void occurs when the bladder contain between _____ of urine. *(50mL to 100mL, 150mL to 300mL, 350mL to 500mL)*

3. _____ is a normal response to loss. *(Grief, Despair, Hopelessness)*

Activity B *Mark each statement as either "T" (True) or "F" (False). Correct any false statements.*

1. T F All clients with neurologic deficit eventually accept their disability.

2. T F Massage bony prominences when areas remain reddened with relief of pressure.

3. T F A behavioral or cognitive change such as irritability may be the only sign of urinary retention in older adults with a neurologic deficit.

Activity C *Write the correct term for each description given below.*

1. A condition in which one or more functions of the central and peripheral nervous systems are decreased, impaired, or absent. _____

2. Increases fecal bulk and pulls water in to the feces to promote regular bowel elimination. _____

3. Exercises that should be performed slowly and smoothly, with momentary pause when spasticity causes resistance. _____

Activity D *Given in Column A are some measures used in the treatment of clients with neurologic deficit. Match these with the corresponding benefits given in Column B.*

Column A	Column B
____ 1. Flotation mattress	a. Positions the foot and ankle in such a way as to prevent plantar flexion.
____ 2. Footboard	
____ 3. Disposable porous pads	b. Used for safe transfer of the client.
____ 4. Mechanical lift	

c. Keeps urine away from skin and bedding dry.

d. Relieves pressure when the client is lying and sitting.

Activity E *There are three phases of neurologic deficit; compare and contrast these phases based on the given criteria.*

Phase	Time Frame	Client's Condition	Focus of Treatment
Acute Phase			
Recovery Phase			
Chronic Phase			

Activity F *Briefly answer the following questions.*

1. What are examples of a neurological deficit?

_____

_____

_____

2. What is the purpose of occupational and recreational therapy?

_____

_____

_____

3. Who are the members of the healthcare team involved in the care of the client with a neurological deficit?

_____

_____

_____

SECTION II: APPLYING YOUR KNOWLEDGE

Activity G *Give rationale for the following questions.*

1. Why are social services and other agencies involved in client care following discharge?

_____

_____

_____

2. Why is it important for the family to discuss medication administration with the physician when the client has impaired swallowing?

_____

_____

_____

3. Why should the client with paraplegia or tetraplegia be regularly position in an upright posture?

_____

_____

_____

4. Why should caution be used when moving and lifting clients who have been immobile?

_____

_____

_____

Activity H *Answer the following questions related to caring for clients with neurological deficits.*

1. What types of psychosocial issues may the client and family have as a result of the change in the client's condition?

_____

_____

_____

2. How can the nurse assist the client in coping with their disability?

_____

_____

_____

3. How can the nurse facilitate positive family processes in coping with altered lifestyles, strained financial resources, conflicts, and the new responsibilities people must accept?

_____

_____

_____

4. What elements are included in the assessment for a client with a neurological deficit?

_____

_____

_____

Activity I *Think over the following questions. Discuss them with your instructor or peers.*

1. A client you are caring for is in the chronic phase after recovering from an accident which left the client a paraplegic. What will be your priority nursing diagnoses and interventions for the physiological needs of the client? What will be your priority nursing diagnoses and interventions for the psychosocial needs of the client?

_____

_____

_____

2. What information about sexuality and reproduction will you need to provide if the client is male? If the client is female?

_____

_____

_____

SECTION III: GETTING READY FOR NCLEX

Activity J *Answer the following questions.*

1. Which of the following actions should the nurse perform to monitor for electrolyte imbalances and dehydration in a client with neurologic deficit?
   a. Measure intake and output
   b. Use the Glasgow Coma Scale
   c. Mini-Mental Status Examination
   d. Assess vital signs

2. Which of the following is a sign of urinary retention in older adults with neurologic deficit?
   a. Amnesia
   b. Hypotension
   c. Hypertension
   d. A behavior change

3. Which of the following conditions are more likely to develop in a client who is relatively immobile for the rest of his or her life?
   a. Bladder infection
   b. Diarrhea
   c. Paralysis
   d. Bladder inflammation

4. Which of the following instructions should be given to the client's family if a client with impaired swallowing has to take solid medication?
   a. Mix the medication with food
   b. Use the liquid form of the medication
   c. Check with the physician or pharmacist before crushing or breaking tablets, or opening capsules
   d. Perform ROM exercises after the medication is administered

5. Which of the following actions should the nurse perform before a client with impaired physical mobility gets up?
   a. Use parallel bars or walker
   b. Apply an abdominal binder
   c. Use incontinence pads
   d. Use footboard

6. Which of the following nursing interventions may reduce hemostasis and decrease the potential for thrombophlebitis for a client with neurologic disorder?
   a. Remove and reapply elastic stockings
   b. Change the client's position
   c. Keep extremities at neutral position
   d. Use a flotation mattress

7. Which of the following nursing diagnoses pertain to a client with a neurological deficit in relation to his marriage?
   a. Risk for Disuse Syndrome related to musculoskeletal inactivity and neuromuscular impairment
   b. Total Urinary Incontinence or Urinary Retention related to effects of disease or injury to the nervous system or spinal cord nerves, loss of bladder tone
   c. Impaired Physical Mobility related to muscle weakness and paralysis
   d. Risk for Sexual Dysfunction related to disturbance or loss of nerve function to genitalia

8. A client who has been immobile from a neurological deficit is moved to another bed in the nursing home and, following the move, complains of pain in his leg. Which complication is possible?

   a. TIA's

   b. Paralysis

   c. Fractures

   d. Bruising

9. Which of the following activity-related strategies would a nurse teach a client who is going home?

   a. Avoid fatigue and take frequent rest periods if needed

   b. Take deep breaths every 4 hours while awake

   c. Make your daily routine rigid so that you can remember what to do

   d. Avoid exposure to the outdoors

10. The nurse instructs a client who has a neurological deficit in which of the following regarding nutrition and diet?

    a. Eat two large meals instead of frequent small meals.

    b. Consume a diet low in fiber.

    c. Chew foods quickly.

    d. Be sure to take fluids frequently.

Introduction to the Sensory System

Learning Objectives

1. Describe the anatomy and physiology of the eyes.
2. Discuss tests that are used for visual screening.
3. Identify questions to ask during an eye assessment.
4. Describe diagnostic studies for eye function.
5. Explain the anatomy and physiology of the ears.
6. Describe methods for assessing the ear and hearing acuity.
7. Describe specific diagnostic tests for ear function.

SECTION I: ASSESSING YOUR UNDERSTANDING

Activity A *Fill in the blanks by choosing the correct word from the options given in parentheses.*

1. The superior and inferior rectus muscles permit eye movement _____. *(Up and down, Toward the nose and the temple, Left and right)*

2. The eyelids, eyelashes, and tears _____ the anterior or exposed surface of the eye. *(Maintain placement of, Protect, Nourish)*

3. The process of _____ occurs when the ciliary muscles contract or relax, changing the shape of the lens, which allows the person to clearly see distant or near objects. *(Refraction, Near point, Accommodation)*

4. The _____ is used to evaluate near vision. *(Snellen eye chart, Rosenbaum Pocket Vision Screener, Ishihara polychromatic plates)*

5. The _____ equalizes pressure in the middle ear. *(Eustachian tube, Labyrinth, External acoustic meatus)*

6. A _____ is used to measure gross auditory acuity. *(Weber test, Romberg test, Whisper test)*

Activity B *Mark each statement as either "T" (True) or "F" (False). Correct any false statements.*

1. T F The medial and lateral rectus muscles move the eye to the left and right.

2. T F Lysozyme is an antibacterial enzyme found in tears.

3. T F The Ishihara polychromatic plates assess extraocular muscle function.

4. T F Sound is perceived because of a chain reaction involving the middle and inner ear.

5. T F The American Speech-Language-Hearing Association recommends that adults be screened at least every decade through the age of 50 and every 3 years after that.

6. T F Hearing acuity is determined by measuring the intensity at which a person first perceives sound using a caloric stimulation test.

Activity C *Write the correct term for each description given below.*

1. These innervate the eye, ocular muscles, and lacrimal apparatus. They include the optic, oculomotor, trochlear, trigeminal, abducens, and facial nerves. _____

2. The closest point at which a person can clearly focus on an object. _____

3. A simple screening tool for determining visual acuity, the ability to see far images clearly. _____

4. This part of the ear helps maintain balance. _____

5. An examination which involves inspecting the external acoustic canal and tympanic membrane. _____

6. A more precise method for evaluating vestibular function, the mechanisms that facilitate maintaining balance. It is performed in conjunction with caloric stimulation. _____

Activity D *Match the structures of the eye given in Column A with their related descriptions given in Column B.*

Column A

____ 1. Sclera

____ 2. Uvea

____ 3. Iris

____ 4. Pupil

____ 5. Ciliary process

____ 6. Ciliary muscle

____ 7. Aqueous humor

____ 8. Vitreous humor

____ 9. Retina

____ 10. Macula

____ 11. Cornea

Column B

a. An opening that dilates and constricts in response to light.

b. A nutrient-rich liquid that nourishes eye structures.

c. Commonly referred to as the "white of the eye." It is composed of tough connective tissue which protects structures in the eye.

d. Produce aqueous humor.

e. The vascular coat of the eye. This structure includes the choroid which prevents light from scattering inside the eye.

f. Helps change the shape of the lens when adjusting to near or far vision.

g. Contains nerve cells called rods and cones.

Rods function in night or dim light and assist in distinguishing black and white. Cones function in bright light and are sensitive to color.

h. The highly vascular, pigmented portion of the eye.

i. Provides central vision, the ability to discriminate letters, words, and the details of any image.

j. A thick, gelatinous material that maintains the spherical shape of the eyeball and maintains the placement of the retina.

k. The transparent domelike structure that covers most of the anterior portion of the eyeball.

Activity E *Differentiate among the following eye tests based on the given criteria.*

Test	Purpose
Ophthalmoscopy	
Retinoscopy	
Tonometry	
Visual Field Examination	
Color Vision Testing	
Amsler Grid	
Slit-Lamp Examination	
Retinal Angiography	
Ultrasonography	
Retinal Imaging	

Activity F *Briefly answer the following questions.*

1. Name the bones that form the walls of the orbit. What protects the posterior, superior, inferior, and lateral aspects of each eyeball?

_____

_____

_____

2. What conditions minimize glare for the older adult experiencing age-associated lens changes?

_____

_____

_____

3. What is the purpose of the corneal light reflex test? How is it performed?

_____

_____

_____

4. Identify common medications which are potentially ototoxic.

_____

_____

_____

5. Identify the structures and function of the outer ear.

_____

_____

_____

6. What is the difference between conductive and sensorineural hearing loss?

_____

_____

_____

SECTION II: APPLYING YOUR KNOWLEDGE

Activity G _Give rationale for the following questions._

1. Why does aging often result in the need for reading glasses for near vision?

_____

_____

_____

2. Why is a position test performed?

_____

_____

_____

3. Why should the examiner remain close to the client when performing the Romberg test?

_____

_____

_____

4. Why is it important to carefully document conduction times assessed using the Rinne and Weber tests?

_____

_____

_____

Activity H _Answer the following questions related to the sensory system._

1. Describe how the eyes convert light energy into nerve signals that are transmitted and interpreted in the cerebral cortex.

_____

_____

_____

2. What information is obtained in the nursing assessment of ocular health?

_____

_____

_____

3. What questions would the nurse ask during an eye examination?

_____

_____

_____

4. Describe the sequence of events that makes sound perception possible.

_____

_____

_____

5. What is the purpose of the Rinne and Weber test? How are they performed?

_____

_____

_____

Activity I *Think over the following questions. Discuss them with your instructor or peers.*

1. What high-priority nursing diagnoses and interventions would you implement for the client with diminished vision in the acute care setting? In the home care setting?

   _____

   _____

   _____

2. What high-priority nursing diagnoses and interventions would you implement for the client with diminished hearing?

   _____

   _____

   _____

SECTION III: GETTING READY FOR NCLEX

Activity J *Answer the following questions.*

1. During an ophthalmic assessment, which of the following is the nurse expected to observe carefully?
   a. Level of central vision
   b. Internal eye condition
   c. Pupil responses
   d. Rate of blinking

2. The following are the monometer measurements of four clients. Which of them has normal intraocular pressure (IOP)?
   a. 8 mm Hg
   b. 11 mm Hg
   c. 25 mm Hg
   d. 28 mm Hg

3. A client has undergone the Snellen eye chart and has 20/40 vision. Which of the following is true for this client?
   a. The client sees letters at 20 feet that others can read at 40 feet
   b. The client sees letters at 40 feet that others can read at 20 feet
   c. The client sees colors at 20 feet that others can see at 40 feet
   d. The client sees colors at 40 feet that others can see at 20 feet

4. When determining hearing acuity, if the client reports first perceiving sound at _____ dB, then his or her hearing is normal.

5. Which of the following should qualify as an abnormal result in a Romberg test?
   a. Hypotension
   b. Sneezing and wheezing
   c. Swaying, losing balance or arm drifting
   d. Excessive cerumen in the outer ear

6. Which of the following nursing actions is helpful for older clients who are experiencing lens changes associated with aging?
   a. Offering teaching aids with large-sized letters
   b. Suggesting reduced visual activity such as reading or watching television
   c. Suggesting the use of eye drops for comfort
   d. Suggesting the use of glasses or contact lenses

7. A 24 year old client asks a nurse at what point they should have an eye exam and states there is no history of any eye disease in their family. If the client has no eye problems, what would the nurse recommend?
   a. Annually after the age of 30
   b. Initially, a thorough exam at the age of 40
   c. Initially, a thorough exam at the age of 50
   d. Annually after the age of 50

8. A nurse is performing a health history on a client and determines that the client has lost some of his hearing. What drugs might this client have taken in the past that would have affected his hearing?
   a. Salicylates
   b. Penicillin
   c. Spironolactone
   d. Ceclor

9. The nurse is checking a client's color vision. Which of the following charts does the nurse use to check this?

   a. Ishihara polychromatic plates

   b. Rosenbaum Pocket Vision Screener

   c. Snellen eye chart

   d. Jaeger chart

10. A nurse assists a client with a test to determine if the client has hearing loss. Which of the following tests would a nurse use to test whether air conduction or bone conduction is greater in the client?

    a. Romberg test

    b. Rinne Test

    c. Weber test

    d. Otoscopic examination

CHAPTER 42

Caring for Clients with Eye Disorders

Learning Objectives

1. Explain the different types of refractive errors.
2. Differentiate the terms *blindness* and *visually impaired*.
3. Identify appropriate nursing interventions for a blind client.
4. Discuss the nursing management of clients with eye trauma.
5. Describe the technique for instilling ophthalmic medications.
6. Explain how different infectious and inflammatory eye disorders are acquired.
7. Specify the visual changes that result from delayed or unsuccessful treatment of macular degeneration.
8. Differentiate between open-angle and angle-closure glaucoma.
9. Distinguish categories and mechanisms of action of medications used to control intraocular pressure.
10. Identify a category of drugs contraindicated in clients with glaucoma.
11. Name activities clients with glaucoma should avoid because they elevate intraocular pressure.
12. Describe methods for improving vision after a cataract is removed.
13. Discuss postoperative measures that help prevent complications after a cataract extraction.
14. Give classic symptoms associated with a retinal detachment.
15. Discuss the care and cleaning of an eye prosthesis.

SECTION I: ASSESSING YOUR UNDERSTANDING

Activity A *Fill in the blanks by choosing the correct word from the options given in parentheses.*

1. In _____, vision is impaired because light rays are not sharply focused on the retina. *(Refractive errors, Infectious eye disorders, Eye trauma)*

2. Untreated _____, especially when caused by *Neisseria gonorrhoeae* and *Chlamydia trachomatis*, can lead to blindness. *(Conjunctivitis, Uveitis, Blepharitis)*

3. _____ seals the serous leak and destroys the encroachment of blood vessels in the area. It must be performed early to prevent progression of macular degeneration. *(Photodynamic therapy, Macular translocation, Laser photocoagulation)*

4. Carbonic anhydrase inhibitors used to treat glaucoma _____. *(Constrict the pupil, Decrease the flow rate of aqueous humor into the eye, Slow the production of aqueous fluid)*

5. A diet with cold-water fish, green leafy vegetables, and supplements including zinc, lutein, and zeaxanthin may be effective for slowing the progression of _____. *(Glaucoma, Age-related macular degeneration, Cataracts)*

6. A _____ occurs when the sensory layer becomes separated from the pigmented layer of the retina. *(Cataract, Retinal detachment, Age-related macular degeneration)*

Activity B *Mark each statement as either "T" (True) or "F" (False). Correct any false statements.*

1. **T F** When caring for a client with a visual impairment, one of the nurse's most important roles is to help the client with all ADLs so the client does not become frustrated.

2. **T F** For a chemical splash, take the client to the nearest sink or water fountain, instruct him or her to hold the eyes open, and flush the eyes with running water for 10 to 15 minutes.

3. **T F** Conjunctivitis is always treated with antibiotics or antiviral drops or ointment.

4. **T F** Common treatment of a chalazion includes surgical excision.

5. **T F** Miotics decrease the flow rate of aqueous humor into the eye.

6. **T F** Cataracts cannot be treated medically and are surgically removed.

Activity C *Write the correct term for each description given below.*

1. Treatment includes oral and topical corticosteroids, mydriatic (dilating) eyedrops such as atropine, and antibiotic eyedrops. Analgesics are prescribed for pain. Sunglasses reduce the discomfort of photophobia. _____

2. An inflammation of the cornea in which treatment is begun promptly to avoid permanent loss of vision. _____

3. This procedure uses an intravenous injection of a photosensitizing drug and a nonthermal laser application to reduce proliferation of abnormal blood vessels and eliminate the risk to the retina for clients with macular degeneration. _____

4. The purpose of eye drops used to treat glaucoma. _____

5. Signs and symptoms include gaps in vision or blind spots, a sensation that a curtain is being drawn over the field of vision, flashes of light, and seeing spots or moving particles, called floaters. Complete loss of vision may occur in the affected eye. This condition is not painful. _____

6. An alternative method of medication administration for clients with glaucoma that eliminates the need for frequent eyedrop instillation. _____

7. The surgical removal of an eye. _____

Activity D *Match the inflammatory and infectious eye disorders in column A with their description and symptoms in column B.*

Column A

___ 1. Keratitis
___ 2. Chalazion
___ 3. Uveitis
___ 4. Corneal Ulcer
___ 5. Hordeolum
___ 6. Conjunctivitis
___ 7. Blepharitis

Column B

a. Results from a bacterial, viral, or rickettsial infection; some forms are highly contagious. Symptoms include redness, excessive tearing, swelling, pain, burning or itching, and, possibly, purulent drainage from one or both eyes.

b. The cause is unknown; but it definitely produces inflammatory changes. Pathogens seldom are identified. Although the disorder occurs randomly, it is detected with some frequency among clients with autoimmune disorders; it may be an atypical antigen–antibody phenomenon.

c. Causes include trauma to the cornea and infectious agents. Symptoms include localized pain or the sensation that a foreign body is present; blinking increases the discomfort.

d. An erosion of the corneal tissue. Once corneal scar tissue has formed, the only treatment is corneal transplantation.

e. One form is associated with hypersecretion from sebaceous glands, which causes greasy scales to form. Infectious agents such as staphylococci cause other cases. Some cases are combinations of both. The lid margins appear inflamed. Patchy flakes cling to the eyelashes and are readily visible about the lids. Eyelashes may be missing. Purulent drainage may be present.

f. An inflammation and infection of the Zeis or Moll gland, a type of oil gland at the edge of the eyelid. *Staphylococcus aureus* is the most common causative pathogen. A sty appears as a tender, swollen, red pustule in the internal or external tissue of the eyelid.

g. A cyst of one or more meibomian glands, a type of sebaceous gland in the inner surface of the eyelid at the junction of the conjunctiva and lid margin. The swelling in the upper or lower eyelid is not tender and as it matures, it feels hard.

Activity E *Compare and contrast the pathophysiology and signs and symptoms of macular degeneration, glaucoma, and cataracts.*

Disorder	Pathophysiology	Signs and Symptoms
Dry macular degeneration		
Wet macular degeneration		
Open-angle glaucoma		
Angle-closure glaucoma		
Cataracts		

Activity F *Briefly answer the following questions.*

1. Define the following refractive errors: Emmetropia, Myopia, Hyperopia, Presbyopia, and Astigmatism.

   ———————————————————

   ———————————————————

   ———————————————————

2. Differentiate between blindness and visual impairment.

   ———————————————————

   ———————————————————

   ———————————————————

3. Identify potential causes of eye injuries.

   ———————————————————

   ———————————————————

   ———————————————————

4. How are minute foreign objects detected in the eye?

   ———————————————————

   ———————————————————

   ———————————————————

5. Describe why mydriatics (drugs that dilate the pupil) must never be administered to clients with glaucoma.

_____

_____

_____

6. Differentiate between intracapsular extraction, extracapsular extraction, and phacoemulsification.

_____

_____

_____

SECTION II: APPLYING YOUR KNOWLEDGE

Activity G *Give rationale for the following questions.*

1. Why should the nurse introduce himself or herself each time they enter the room when the client is visually impaired?

_____

_____

2. Why should the nurse call the client by name during group conversations when the client is visually impaired?

_____

_____

3. Why should a nightlight be used for older adults?

_____

_____

4. Why do clients with blepharitis become discouraged?

_____

_____

_____

5. Why are sties common in clients with diabetes mellitus?

_____

_____

_____

6. Why is acute angle-closure glaucoma an emergency?

_____

_____

_____

Activity H *Answer the following questions related to caring for clients with eye disorders.*

1. What are common signs of a refractive error? How are refractive errors commonly detected? What treatments are available to correct vision?

_____

_____

_____

2. Many types of conjunctivitis are contagious. What instructions would be provided to the client to reduce the risk of infection to others?

_____

_____

_____

3. What general instructions should be provided to the client with glaucoma?

_____

_____

_____

4. What post operative instructions will the nurse provide to the client who has undergone cataract surgery?

_____

_____

_____

5. Describe the nursing management for the client with a detached retina.

_____

_____

_____

6. Describe the procedure for teaching a client to clean a prosthetic eye.

_____

_____

_____

Activity I *Think over the following questions. Discuss them with your instructor or peers.*

1. Following cataract surgery vision may be corrected using one of three methods: corrective eyeglasses, a contact lens, or an intraocular lens (IOL) implant. Identify the benefits and disadvantages of each method.

_____

_____

_____

2. What are high priority nursing diagnoses and interventions would you identify for a client who is losing their vision?

_____

_____

_____

3. A neighbor seeks assistance from you because their child has a foreign object in their eye. What instructions would you provide?

_____

_____

_____

4. You are a friend's house when they suddenly announce bleach has splashed in their eye. What actions would you take?

_____

_____

_____

SECTION III: GETTING READY FOR NCLEX

Activity J *Answer the following questions.*

1. Which of the following actions should the nurse carry out first in a client with a chemical splash in the eye?
   a. Flush the eyes with running water
   b. Instill an antibiotic
   c. Apply an eye pad
   d. Rub the eyes vigorously

2. In addition to assessing the degree of the client's impairment, which of the following information should a nurse obtain from a client who has recently turned blind?
   a. About the client's diet
   b. About the client's allergy history
   c. About the client's family's medical history
   d. About how the client is coping with the visual problems

3. Which of the following are the treatments of a non-severe sty?
   a. Cold compresses
   b. Warm soaks
   c. Limited sensory stimulation
   d. Incision and drainage

4. Which of the following is the first symptom a client with dry macular degeneration may report?
   a. Blurred vision
   b. Loss of eyelashes
   c. Affected peripheral field
   d. Distortion of direct vision

5. Which of the following instructions should the nurse give a client with glaucoma?
   a. Avoid going outdoors in the daylight
   b. Avoid getting up too quickly
   c. Avoid heavy lifting
   d. Use cough syrups containing atropine

6. Which of the following symptoms should the nurse closely monitor for and report immediately in a client who has just undergone cataract surgery?
   a. Hypotension
   b. Nausea and vomiting

   c. Intense pain in the eye or near the brow

   d. Increased urine output

7. A nurse is working with an eye physician and the client is diagnosed with emmetropia. Which of the following statements best describes emmetropia?

   a. Difficulty with near vision

   b. Difficulty with far vision

   c. Visual distortion caused by an irregularly shaped cornea

   d. Normal vision

8. Which of the following eye procedures is used to remove the epithelial layer (top surface) of the cornea while a laser sculpts the cornea to correct refractive errors?

   a. Photorefractive keratectomy (PRK)

   b. Intrastromal corneal ring segments (ICRS)

   c. Laser-assisted in situ keratomileusis (LASIK)

   d. Conductive keratoplasty (CK)

9. A nurse is giving a lecture to a group of nursing students on blindness. What is the definition of blindness in terms of the best corrected visual acuity (BCVA)?

   a. Less than 20/200 even with correction

   b. Between 20/70 and 20/200 in the better eye with glasses

   c. 20/400 or greater with no light perception

   d. 20/40 in at least one eye with correction

10. A client is visually impaired and is admitted to the hospital. Which of the following interventions can help the client with a visual impairment achieve independence?

   a. Keep personal care items in a different location each day

   b. Ask client's preference for where to store hygiene articles and other objects needed for self-care.

   c. At mealtimes, ask the client to feel where food is on the plate

   d. Place meal tray on overbed tray and leave the room

Caring for Clients with Ear Disorders

1. List types of hearing impairment and the acuity levels for each.
2. Name techniques that clients with impaired hearing use to communicate with others.
3. Give examples of support services available for the hearing impaired.
4. Discuss the role of the nurse in caring for clients with a hearing loss.
5. Name conditions that involve the external ear.
6. Explain the technique for straightening the ear canal of adults to facilitate inspection and the administration of medication.
7. Discuss methods for preventing or treating disorders of the external ear.
8. Name conditions that affect the middle ear.
9. Describe nursing interventions appropriate for managing the care of a client with ear surgery.
10. Explain the pathophysiology of Ménière's disease, and name some consequences of this inner-ear disorder.
11. Discuss the nursing management of clients with Ménière's disease.

SECTION I: ASSESSING YOUR UNDERSTANDING

Activity A *Fill in the blanks by choosing the correct word from the options given in parentheses.*

1. Hearing impairment is described as mild, moderate, severe, or profound, depending on the _____ of sound required for a person to hear it. *(Quality, Intensity, Vibration)*

2. Diminished _____ results from a conductive loss, sensorineural loss, or both. *(Hearing, Ototoxicity, Otosclerosis)*

3. Clients with a _____ hearing loss benefit more from the use of a hearing aid because the structures that convert sound into energy and facilitate perception of sound in the brain continue to function. *(Sensorineural, Dual, Conductive)*

4. _____ is an acute inflammation or infection in the middle ear. *(Otitis externa, Ototoxicity, Otitis media)*

5. _____ is the result of a bony overgrowth of the stapes and a common cause of hearing impairment among adults. Fixation of the stapes occurs gradually over many years. *(Mastoiditis, Labyrinthitis, Otosclerosis)*

6. The best outcomes are achieved with the use of hearing aids with otosclerosis when the hearing loss is _____. *(Conductive, Sensorineural, Both)*

7. Generally, physicians attribute _____ to viral infections of the inner ear, a head injury, hereditary factors, or allergic reactions. More recent theories center on autoimmune factors. *(Ménière's disease, Ototoxicity, Acoustic neuromas)*

Activity B *Mark each statement as either "T" (True) or "F" (False). Correct any false statements.*

1. T F Hearing loss seriously impairs the ability to protect oneself and communicate with others.

2. T F The age at which hearing loss occurs plus the severity of the impairment have extensive consequences.

3. T F A cochlear implant restores normal hearing.

4. T F Purulent otitis media is a collection of pathogen-free fluid behind the tympanic membrane resulting from irritation associated with respiratory allergies and enlarged adenoids.

5. T F In some cases, the fluid is aspirated by needle in the treatment of otitis media.

6. T F Following a stapedectomy the client experiences an immediate, dramatic improvement in hearing but hearing diminishes over the next several days. This indicates the surgery was not successful.

7. T F Medications used to treat Ménière's disease often include antiemetics, antihistamines, tranquilizers, and diuretics.

Activity C *Write the correct term for each description given below.*

1. The client hears buzzing, whistling, or ringing noises in one or both ears. _____

2. A battery-operated device that fits behind the ear, in the ear, or in the ear canal and amplifies sound. _____

3. A method for communication that uses a hand-spelled alphabet and word symbols. _____

4. To reduce the consequences of spontaneous rupture of the eardrum, subsequent scarring, and hearing loss a physician may perform this procedure. The incised opening facilitates drainage of purulent material, eases pressure, and relieves throbbing pain. The incision heals readily, with little scarring. _____

5. A progressive, bilateral loss of hearing is the most characteristic symptom. Tinnitus appears as the loss of hearing progresses. The eardrum appears pinkish-orange from structural changes in the middle ear. _____

6. Episodic symptoms occur as a result of fluctuations in the production or reabsorption of fluid in the inner ear. _____

7. The detrimental effect of certain medications on the eighth cranial nerve or hearing structures. _____

Activity D *Match the item in column A with the alternate form of use for the hearing impaired in column B.*

Column A

____ 1. Telephones

____ 2. Television broadcasts

____ 3. Light-activated equipment

____ 4. Hearing dogs

____ 5. Theaters

Column B

a. Use closed-caption inserts in which the dialogue is printed on the bottom of the screen or a person who simultaneously signs is displayed in a corner of the screen.

b. Provide headsets that amplify actors' voices for individual patrons.

c. Text-based telecommunications equipment.

d. These products allow the hearing impaired to perceive rather than hear sound

e. Are specially trained to warn their owners when certain sounds occur.

Activity E *Identify the signs and symptoms and treatments for disorders of the external ear.*

Disorder	Signs and Symptoms	Treatment
Impacted Cerumen		
Foreign Objects		
Otitis Externa		

Activity F *Briefly answer the following questions.*

1. Describe how sound is transmitted with a cochlear implant.

   _____

   _____

   _____

2. What signs would the nurse look for to identify a hearing impairment?

   _____

   _____

   _____

3. What will influence the selection of a hearing aid?

   _____

   _____

   _____

4. Describe the pathophysiology of otitis media.

   _____

   _____

   _____

5. Describe the pathophysiology of otosclerosis.

   _____

   _____

   _____

6. What are the symptoms of Ménière's disease?

   _____

   _____

   _____

7. What are the symptoms of ototoxicity?

   _____

   _____

   _____

SECTION II: APPLYING YOUR KNOWLEDGE

Activity G *Give rationale for the following questions.*

1. Why might a client deny hearing loss and refuse to wear a hearing aid?

   _____

   _____

   _____

2. Why has the overuse of antibiotics created a problem?

   _____

   _____

   _____

3. Why can nystagmus occur with Ménière's disease?

   _____

   _____

   _____

4. Why is smoking contraindicated with Ménière's disease? Why are clients placed on a low sodium or sodium free diet?

   _____

   _____

   _____

5. Why does hearing loss occur with an acoustic neuroma?

   _____

   _____

   _____

6. Why is surgical removal of an acoustic neuroma the preferred treatment?

   _____

   _____

   _____

Activity H *Answer the following questions related to caring for clients with ear disorders.*

1. What considerations and interventions should be used when caring for a client with a hearing impairment?

_____

_____

_____

2. What complications can occur with otitis media?

_____

_____

_____

3. What is the etiology of otosclerosis?

_____

_____

_____

4. Describe the nursing management for the client undergoing ear surgery.

_____

_____

_____

5. Describe the pathophysiology of Ménière's disease.

_____

_____

_____

6. What are the signs and symptoms of an acoustic neuroma?

_____

_____

_____

Activity I *Think over the following questions. Discuss them with your instructor or peers.*

1. A client smiles and nods yes to everything you say while you are explaining instructions related to their care. How would you confirm the client has heard the instructions?

_____

_____

_____

2. A client you are caring for has a severe hearing impairment. The client is from a foreign country and is unable to read or write in English. What methods could you use to communicate with the client? It is determined the client requires surgery. What actions would you take to ensure the client can provide informed consent?

_____

_____

_____

3. A client you are caring for has a hearing impaired sibling who would like to visit. The sibling has a hearing dog. What would you tell your client about the hospital's policy on service dogs?

_____

_____

_____

SECTION III: GETTING READY FOR NCLEX

Activity J *Answer the following questions.*

1. Which of the following instructions should a nurse give a client who has been prescribed hearing aids and fears that wearing a hearing aid is a stigma?
   a. Purchase a hearing aid from a mail order catalogue
   b. Purchase a hearing aid from a company salesman
   c. Use a hearing aid that fits almost unnoticeably in the ear
   d. Avoid telling others about the use of a hearing aid

2. Which of the following findings should be observed when assessing a client for otitis externa?
   a. Swelling and pus
   b. Dried cerumen
   c. Client hears buzzing, whistling, or ringing noises
   d. Client has recently suffered from an upper respiratory infection

3. Which of the following should the nurse closely monitor for in a client who has undergone surgery for otosclerosis?

   a. Hypotension

   b. Nausea and vomiting

   c. Decreased urine output

   d. Abnormal facial nerve function

4. Which of the following is contraindicated for a client being treated for Ménière's disease?

   a. Alcohol

   b. Smoking

   c. A high-protein diet

   d. Cough syrups and other CNS depressants

5. What does tenderness behind the ear indicate in a client with otitis media?

   a. Mastoiditis

   b. Tinnitus

   c. Labyrinthitis

   d. Septicemia

6. Which of the following should prevent disorientation in older clients with hearing impairments?

   a. Use of written notes and a walking cane for proper balance

   b. Refer to a local support or self-help group

   c. Frequent contact and reorientation

   d. Avoid frequent outdoor activities

7. A client is sitting in the waiting room and another client begins to talk with them. Which of the following questions would encourage a client to respond to hearing deficits if the client denies having a hearing impairment?

   a. "Do you always ask people to repeat questions? If so, do you think that you have a hearing problem?"

   b. "Are you cupping your ear for a reason? Do you have trouble hearing?"

   c. "You did not answer several people who were talking with you in the waiting room. Did you not hear them?"

   d. "I saw you leaning over in the waiting room when Sylvia was talking to you. Can you describe any issues that you are having with your hearing?"

8. A nurse needs to irrigate a client's ear to remove wax. In which direction does the nurse hold the syringe when irrigating the ear?

   a. Toward the roof of the canal

   b. Toward the eardrum

   c. Toward the nasal cavity

   d. Toward the helix

9. Which of the following symptoms would a nurse suspect a client to have with a medical diagnosis of acoustic neuroma?

   a. Altered facial sensation

   b. Vertigo only when standing

   c. Tinnitus in the unaffected ear

   d. Impaired facial movement when smiling

10. What is a common cause of sensorineural hearing loss?

    a. Otitis media

    b. Temporal bone fractures

    c. Otitis externa

    d. Vascular conditions

CHAPTER 44

Introduction to the Gastrointestinal System and Accessory Structures

Learning Objectives

1. Identify major organs and structures of the gastrointestinal system.
2. Discuss important information to ascertain about gastrointestinal health.
3. Identify facts in the client's history that provide pertinent data about the present illness.
4. Discuss physical assessments that provide information about the functioning of the gastrointestinal tract and accessory organs.
5. Describe common diagnostic tests performed on clients with gastrointestinal disorders.
6. Describe nursing measures after liver biopsy.
7. Explain nursing management of clients undergoing diagnostic testing for a gastrointestinal disorder.

SECTION I: ASSESSING YOUR UNDERSTANDING

Activity A *Fill in the blanks by choosing the correct word from the options given in parentheses.*

1. The _____ GI tract begins at the mouth and ends at the jejunum. *(Upper, Middle, Lower)*

2. The client may receive up to three cleansing enemas prior to a _____ unless contra-

indicated in preparation for this test. *(Radionuclide imaging, Lower gastrointestinal series, Cholangiography)*

3. A client must have _____ prior to a percutaneous liver biopsy as bleeding is a major complication. *(Coagulation studies, An ultrasound, CT scanning)*

4. _____ allows for the direct visual examination of the lumen of the GI tract. *(Gastrointestinal endoscopy, Radionuclide imaging, Lower gastrointestinal series)*

5. _____, a bacterium, is believed to be responsible for the majority of peptic ulcers. *(Salmonella, Shigella, Helicobacter pylori)*

Activity B *Mark each statement as either "T" (True) or "F" (False). Correct any false statements.*

1. T F Accessory structures include the peritoneum, liver, gallbladder, and pancreas.

2. T F The client with a GI disorder may experience a wide variety of health problems that involve disturbances of ingestion, digestion, absorption, and elimination.

3. T F Instructions prior to an oral cholecystography include asking the client to eat a protein-free meal the night before the test.

4. T F If a contrast agent is going to be used with a cholangiography, the nurse must ask the client if he or she is allergic to iodine or peanut butter.

5. T F Polyethylene glycol/electrolyte solution produces watery stools, and is associated with increased risk of fluid and electrolyte imbalance.

Activity C *Write the correct term for each description given below.*

1. This portion of the GI tract begins at the ileum and ends at the anus. _____

2. In this test, to facilitate observation of the rectum, sigmoid colon, and descending colon fluoroscopically during filling, the examiner directs the client to make multiple position changes. _____

3. This test, contraindicated in pregnant women, requires that breast milk be pumped and discarded so that the nursing child remains safe from radioactivity. _____

4. Clients who are claustrophobic may need sedation before undergoing this test because it is imperative that they lie still and not panic during the test. _____

5. The physician obtains a small core of liver tissue by placing a needle through the client's lateral abdominal wall directly into the liver.

_____

Activity D *Match the diagnostic tests in Column A to their corresponding purpose in column B.*

Column A

____ **1.** Cholangiography

____ **2.** Upper Gastrointestinal Series

____ **3.** Magnetic Resonance Imaging

____ **4.** Radionuclide Imaging

____ **5.** Small Bowel Series

____ **6.** Lower Gastrointestinal Series (Barium Enema)

____ **7.** Computed Tomography

____ **8.** Magnetic Resonance Elastography

____ **9.** Oral Cholecystography (Gallbladder Series)

____ **10.** Ultrasonography

____ **11.** Enteroclysis

Column B

a. Used to visualize soft tissue structures. It is used to examine GI structures when CT scanning is inadequate.

b. Requires nasal or oral placement of a flexible feeding tube, the tip of which is positioned in the proximal jejunum. Contrast media fill in and pass through the intestinal loops. The examiner observes the intestine continuously by fluoroscopy and takes periodic radiographs of the various sections of the small intestine.

c. Detects lesions of the liver or pancreas and assists in evaluating gastric emptying.

d. Used to identify polyps, tumors, inflammation, strictures, and other abnormalities of the colon. 1000 to 1500 mL of barium solution is instilled rectally. The rectum, sigmoid colon, and descending colon are observed fluoroscopically during filling.

e. Shows the size and location of organs and outlines structures and abnormalities, helps detect cholecystitis, cholelithiasis, pyloric stenosis, and some disorders of the biliary system.

f. Facilitates the identification of structural abnormalities of the esophagus as well as swallowing dysfunction and oral aspiration. This procedure includes radiographic observation of the barium moving into the stomach and the first part of the small intestine.

g. May be performed to detect structural abnormalities of the GI tract. These tests help detect metastatic lesions that might not be apparent on regular GI radiographs.

h. Identifies stones in the gallbladder or common bile duct and tumors or other obstructions. The test also determines the ability of the gallbladder to concentrate and store a dyelike, iodine-based, radiopaque contrast medium.

i. Determines the patency of the ducts from the liver and gallbladder.

j. Fluoroscopy of the small intestine after the ingestion of a contrast medium. It is used to identify tumors, inflammation, or obstruction in the jejunum or ileum.

k. The resulting images enable physicians to ascertain the firmness of the liver, thus allowing them to better predict clients who are at risk for developing fibrosis and eventually cirrhosis.

Activity E *Identify the following functions of the gastrointestinal system and accessory structures.*

Structure	Function
Mouth	
Esophagus	
Stomach	
Small Intestine	
Large Intestine	
Peritoneum	
Liver	
Gallbladder	
Pancreas	

Activity F *Briefly answer the following questions:*

1. What is the objective of gathering the client history related to the gastrointestinal system? What information is gathered?

   _____

   _____

   _____

2. How is family and work history significant to the gastrointestinal system and accessory structure assessment?

   _____

   _____

   _____

3. What precautions are taken when a client undergoes an enteroclysis?

   _____

   _____

   _____

4. What are the therapeutic uses of a gastrointestinal endoscopy?

   _____

   _____

   _____

5. Following an endoscopy the nurse monitors for signs of perforation. Which signs and symptoms indicate a perforation?

   _____

   _____

   _____

SECTION II: APPLYING YOUR KNOWLEDGE

Activity G *Give rationale for the following questions.*

1. Why does disease of the large intestine or surgical removal of any portion of the large intestine place a client at risk for malabsorption,

fluid and electrolyte imbalances, and skin breakdown?

_____

_____

_____

2. Why may older adults have less control of the rectal sphincter?

_____

_____

_____

3. Why does the nurse have the client lie supine, with the knees flexed, for the abdominal examination?

_____

_____

_____

4. Why is abdominal auscultation completed to abdominal palpation during an examination?

_____

_____

_____

5. Why does the nurse examine client's anus and stool?

_____

_____

_____

6. Why does the nurse discourage drinking through a straw, smoking, or chewing gum prior to ultrasonography?

_____

_____

_____

Activity H _Answer the following questions related to the gastrointestinal system and accessory structures._

1. What is the significance of a skin assessment in relationship to the gastrointestinal system and accessory structures?

_____

_____

_____

2. Describe the process and purpose of the nursing examination of the mouth.

_____

_____

_____

3. Describe the process of the nursing examination of the abdomen.

_____

_____

_____

4. Describe the pre and post procedure care for an upper gastrointestinal series or small bowel series.

_____

_____

_____

5. What is the purpose of stool analysis?

_____

_____

_____

Activity I _Think over the following questions. Discuss them with your instructor or peers._

1. Your client is at risk for fluid volume deficit following a gastrointestinal procedure. What actions will you take to ensure adequate intake and output?

_____

_____

_____

2. Which clients are at higher risk for fluid volume deficit when undergoing gastrointestinal procedures?

_____

_____

_____

3. What interventions would you implement to prevent constipation following a gastrointestinal procedure?

_____

_____

_____

4. What action will you take to decrease a client's anxiety related to a gastrointestinal procedure?

_____

_____

_____

SECTION III: GETTING READY FOR NCLEX

Activity J *Answer the following questions:*

1. A client with a GI disorder has to undergo a barium swallow test. Which of the following diet restrictions are required prior to the test?

a. NPO for 8 to 12 hours before the test

b. NPO for 6 to 8 hours before the test

c. Maintain normal fluid intake 1 or 2 hours before the test

d. Avoidance of red meat 3 days prior to testing

2. A client has to undergo a barium enema for a suspected GI disorder. During the test, he experiences a strong urge to defecate and seeks the nurse's advice. Which of the following should the nurse do?

a. Advise him to clear his bowel immediately

b. Assure him that most people can retain the urge

c. Give him analgesics to relieve him of the urge

d. Instruct him to drink plenty of fluids

3. What instruction should be given to a client scheduled for a gallbladder series test?

a. To remain on a low-residue diet 1 to 2 days before the test

b. To take a laxative the evening before the test

c. Not to eat or drink until the test is complete

d. To take cleansing enemas the morning of the test

4. Which of the following diagnostic tests can be given to a client who cannot retain dye tablets given to test his gallbladder?

a. Oral cholecystography

b. Cholangiography

c. Barium enema

d. Barium swallow

5. Which of the following routes is used to instill a dye for a radionuclide imaging test?

a. Infusion through oral or IV route

b. Infusion through a T-tube

c. Infusion through a small nasogastric tube

d. Infusion through an endoscope

6. Which of the following tests is contraindicated for pregnant women?

a. Barium enema

b. Barium swallow

c. Radionuclide imaging

d. Gallbladder series test

7. Which of the following pretest evaluation measures should the nurse ensure before a client undergoes the gallbladder series test?

a. Determining the work environment of the client

b. Determining whether the client has a family history of GI disorders

c. Determining whether the client is pregnant

d. Determining whether the client is allergic to sea food or iodine

8. Which of the following will have the greatest implication on a client scheduled for a percutaneous liver biopsy?

a. History of coagulation studies

b. Allergy to iodine

c. Family history of GI disorders

d. Presence of radioactive material in the work environment

9. A client complained of sore throat after the procedure of EGD. The nurse observed that the client's gag reflex has returned. What measure can the nurse take to relieve the client's discomfort?

   a. Provide him with lots of fluids

   b. Provide him with ice chips

   c. Provide him with nourishments

   d. Provide him with medications

10. For which condition is magnetic resonance elastography showing great promise?

    a. Gallstones

    b. Liver cancer

    c. Cholecystitis

    d. Cirrhosis of the liver

Caring for Clients with Disorders of the Upper Gastrointestinal Tract

Learning Objectives

1. Discuss assessment findings and treatment of eating disorders, esophageal disorders, and gastric disorders.
2. Describe the nursing management of a client with a nasogastric or gastrointestinal tube or gastrostomy.
3. Identify strategies for relieving upper gastrointestinal discomfort.
4. Discuss the nursing management of clients undergoing gastric surgery.

SECTION I: ASSESSING YOUR UNDERSTANDING

Activity A *Fill in the blanks by choosing the correct word from the options given in parentheses.*

1. Gastric feedings are administered by bolus, intermittent, cyclic, or continuous methods, using the same techniques described previously. _____ feedings are not given through tubes inserted below the pylorus because such placement causes abdominal cramping and diarrhea. *(Bolus, Intermittent, Cyclic)*

2. _____ is a common disorder that develops when gastric contents flow upward into the esophagus. *(Esophageal diverticulum, Hiatal hernia, Gastroesophageal reflux disease)*

3. Administer _____ of water before and after medications and feedings and every 4 to 6 hours with continuous feedings to maintain tube patency. *(5 to 10 mL, 15 to 30 mL, 40 to 60 mL)*

4. The gastrointestinal tube used to relieve abdominal distention caused by problems after surgery, episodes of acute upper GI bleeding, or symptoms associated with intestinal obstruction, or for diagnostic purposes is _____ the one used for tube feeding. *(Smaller than, Larger than, The same size as)*

5. Signs and symptoms of _____ include foul breath, difficulty or pain when swallowing, belching, regurgitating, or coughing. Auscultation of the middle to upper chest may reveal gurgling sounds. *(Gastroesophageal reflux, Esophageal diverticula, Peptic ulcer disease)*

6. _____ occurs when the normal balance between factors that promote mucosal injury and factors that protect the mucosa is disrupted. The single greatest risk factor for the development of this disease is infection with the gram-negative bacterium *H. pylori*. *(Gastroesophageal reflux, Esophageal diverticula, Peptic ulcer disease)*

7. Clients with _____ are at greater risk for diabetes, heart disease, including hypertension, stroke, osteoarthritis, gallbladder disease, and some forms of cancer, including colorectal and kidney cancer. *(Esophageal cancer, Cancer of the stomach, Morbid obesity)*

Activity B *Mark each statement as either "T" (True) or "F" (False). Correct any false statements.*

1. **T F** Anorexia never requires medical intervention.

2. **T F** Weakness, weight loss, nutritional deficiency, dehydration, and electrolyte and acid-base imbalances may result from prolonged nausea and vomiting

3. **T F** In general, larger, more flexible tubes are used for feeding because they tend to be more easily tolerated by clients.

4. **T F** If a client's condition improves, a previously placed gastrostomy tube is removed and the opening requires surgical closure.

5. **T F** Tube feeding will always meet the fluid needs of the client.

6. **T F** A client with gastritis usually complains of epigastric fullness, pressure, pain, anorexia, nausea, and vomiting. When a bacterial or viral infection causes the gastritis, the client may experience vomiting, diarrhea, fever, and abdominal pain. Drugs, poisons, toxic substances, and corrosives can cause gastric bleeding.

7. **T F** Clients with peptic ulcer disease experience more discomfort when the stomach is empty than after eating food.

8. **T F** The nurse manages the care of clients having bariatric surgery as he or she would for clients having any other type of gastric surgery: however, clients have greater risk of complications related to their morbid obesity.

Activity C *Write the correct term for each description given below.*

1. A lack of appetite, which is a common symptom of many diseases. _____

2. A transabdominal opening into the stomach that provides long-term access for administering fluids and liquid nourishment. _____

3. The most common symptoms are epigastric pain or discomfort (dyspepsia), burning sensation in the esophagus (pyrosis), and regurgitation. _____

4. Never crush and administer this type of medication through any type of enteral feeding tube. _____

5. A protrusion of part of the stomach into the lower portion of the thorax. _____

6. Clients usually do not experience symptoms until the disease has progressed to interfere with swallowing and passage of food, leading to weight loss. _____

7. Most common among natives of Japan, as well as in African Americans and Latinos. _____

8. Defined as a body mass index (BMI) of 40 or higher or a body weight of more than 20% over ideal. _____

Activity D *Match the gastric tubes in Column A with their corresponding description in Column B:*

Column A

_____ 1. Nasogastric intubation

_____ 2. Orogastric intubation

_____ 3. Nasoenteric intubation

_____ 4. Gastrostomy

_____ 5. Jejunostomy

Column B

a. The tube passes through the nose, esophagus, and stomach to the small intestine.

b. The tube enters the stomach through a surgically created opening into the abdominal wall.

c. The tube enters the jejunum or small intestine through a surgically created opening into the abdominal wall.

d. The tube passes through the nose into the stomach via the esophagus.

e. The tube passes through the mouth into the stomach.

TABLE 45-1

Disorder	Non-medication Medical Management	Medications	Surgical Intervention
Gastroesophageal reflux disease (GERD)			
Esophageal diverticulum		N/A	
Hiatal hernia			
Chronic gastritis			N/A
Peptic ulcer disease (PUD)			
Cancer of the stomach			

Activity E *Identify the non-medication medical management, medications, and surgical interventions used to treat clients with the disorders of the upper gastrointestinal tract listed in Table 45-1.*

Activity F *Briefly answer the following questions.*

1. What types of issues can affect appetite?

_____

_____

_____

2. What serious signs and symptoms can occur as a result of nausea and vomiting?

_____

_____

_____

3. What is the focus of care for clients diagnosed with oral cancer?

_____

_____

_____

4. What equipment is kept at the client's bedside following oral surgery?

_____

_____

_____

5. Identify the functions of gastrointestinal intubation.

_____

_____

_____

6. Identify the causes of gastritis.

_____

_____

_____

7. What are the long-term goals of gastric bypass surgery?

_____

_____

_____

SECTION II: APPLYING YOUR KNOWLEDGE

Activity G *Give the rationale for the following questions:*

1. Why are older adults at increased risk for anorexia?

_____

_____

_____

2. Why would the use of a gastric sump tube be preferred to a non-vented tube?

_____

_____

_____

3. Why are intermittent, cyclic, or continuous feedings preferred to bolus feedings?

_____

_____

_____

4. Why is it essential to readminister the gastric contents after checking for residual?

_____

_____

_____

5. Why must the client be placed in semi-Fowler's position during and 30 to 60 minutes after an intermittent feeding, and at all times for a continuous feeding?

_____

_____

_____

6. Why is the client with peptic ulcer disease at high risk for developing pernicious anemia?

_____

_____

_____

Activity H *Answer the following questions related to caring for clients with disorders of the upper gastrointestinal tract.*

1. Identify the signs and symptoms of anorexia.

_____

_____

_____

2. How is nausea and vomiting medically managed?

_____

_____

_____

3. What are appropriate nursing assessments and goals when caring for a client with gastrointestinal intubation?

_____

_____

_____

4. How is a gastrostomy tube stabilized? What are the advantages and disadvantages of each method?

_____

_____

_____

5. Describe the post operative care following a gastrostomy.

_____

_____

6. What interventions will the nurse use to prevent infection when caring for a client with tube feeding?

_____

_____

_____

7. Describe the treatment options for esophageal cancer.

_____

_____

_____

8. What dietary guidelines will the nurse provide after roux-en-y gastric bypass surgery?

_____

_____

_____

Activity I *Think over the following questions. Discuss them with your instructor or peers.*

1. What high priority nursing diagnoses and interventions would you identify for clients diagnosed with anorexia?

_____

_____

2. What high priority nursing diagnoses and interventions would you identify for clients diagnosed with nausea and vomiting?

_____

_____

3. What high priority nursing diagnoses and interventions would you identify for a client following oral surgery?

_____

_____

4. What educational information about nutrition would you provide to a client diagnosed with esophageal cancer?

_____

_____

_____

SECTION III: GETTING READY FOR NCLEX

Activity J *Answer the following questions:*

1. The nurse assists the client experiencing nausea and vomiting to develop tolerance for fluids and foods. Which of the following nursing actions would help the client?

a. Advancing the diet slowly

b. Discouraging caffeinated or carbonated beverages

c. Recommending commercial over-the-counter beverages

d. Replacing dietary fat with medium-chain triglycerides (MCTs)

2. A nurse is preparing an intervention plan for a client who is receiving tube feedings after an oral surgery. Which of the following measures can prevent improper infusion and assist in preventing vomiting?

a. Consulting the physician and dietitian

b. Administering the feedings at room temperature

c. Changing the tube feeding container and tubing

d. Checking the tube placement and gastric residual prior to feedings

3. A client has diarrhea due to a high carbohydrate and electrolyte content of the fluid in the tube feeding. Which of the following nursing actions will be most appropriate?

a. Instructing the client to remain in a semi-Fowler's position

b. Consulting the physician about decreasing the infusion rate

c. Administering the tube feedings continuously

d. Maintaining the tube patency

4. The nurse needs to promote an easy passage of food to the stomach in an obese elderly client with hiatal hernia. Which of the following nursing actions in the care plan would help the client?

a. Encouraging frequent, small, well-balanced meals

b. Suggesting avoidance of foods that cause discomfort

c. Instructing to eat slowly and chew the food thoroughly

d. Instructing to avoid alcohol and tobacco products

5. A nurse is preparing an intervention plan for an older client who underwent an esophageal surgery. The client frequently reports problems of gastric distention. Which of the following aspects will be the most essential in his intervention plan?

a. Supporting the surgical incision for coughing and deep breathing

b. Avoiding oral nourishment until bowel sounds resume and are active

c. Turning him to perform deep breathing and coughing every two hours

d. Discouraging lying down immediately after eating

6. Which of the following measures will ensure tube patency and decrease the risk of bacterial infection as well as crusting or blockage of the tube?

a. Administering 10 to 40 ml of water before and after medications and feedings

b. Administering 15 to 30 ml of water before and after medications and feedings

c. Administering 30 to 40 ml of water before and after medications and feedings

d. Administering 5 to 10 ml of water before and after medications and feedings

7. The nurse needs to administer feedings to a client who has diarrhea due to gastroenteritis. Which of the following factors should the nurse consider?

a. Administer feedings at room temperature

b. Administer cold feedings

c. Administer bolus feedings

d. Administer intermittent feedings

8. The nurse is monitoring a client diagnosed with peptic ulcer disease. She is observing this nonsurgical client for any sign of medical complications. Which of the following assessment measures is the most useful?

   a. Assessing the client's bowel patterns and stool characteristics

   b. Evaluating the client's skin for signs of infections

   c. Evaluating the emotional status

   d. Assessing the vital signs and fluid status

9. After an esophageal surgery, a client exhibited the symptoms of dyspnea. What should a nurse do to minimize dyspnea?

   a. Ensure the intake of soft foods or high-calorie, high-protein semiliquid foods

   b. Advise avoidance of foods that contain significant air or gas

   c. Ensure frequent, small meals and discourage lying down immediately after eating

   d. Instruct to take liquid supplements between meals

10. Which of the following tubes is surgically inserted into the abdomen but goes to the small intestine?

    a. Orogastric tube

    b. Nasogastric tube

    c. Jejunostomy tube

    d. Gastrostomy tube

Caring for Clients with Disorders of the Lower Gastrointestinal Tract

Learning Objectives

1. List factors that contribute to constipation and diarrhea, and describe nursing management for clients with these problems.
2. Explain the symptoms of irritable bowel syndrome.
3. Contrast Crohn's disease and ulcerative colitis.
4. Describe the features of appendicitis and peritonitis.
5. Describe nursing management for a client with acute abdominal inflammatory disorders.
6. Describe the nurse's role as related to care measures for the client with intestinal obstruction.
7. Differentiate diverticulosis and diverticulitis.
8. Identify factors that contribute to the formation of an abdominal hernia.
9. Discuss nursing management for a client requiring surgical repair of a hernia.
10. Describe warning signs of colorectal cancer.
11. List common problems that accompany anorectal disorders.

SECTION I: ASSESSING YOUR UNDERSTANDING

Activity A *Fill in the blanks by choosing the correct word from the options given in parentheses.*

1. The _____ gastrointestinal tract includes the small and large intestines from the duodenum to anus. *(Upper, Lower, Terminal)*

2. _____ results from increased peristalsis, which moves fecal matter through the GI tract much more rapidly than normal. *(Constipation, Diarrhea, An impaction)*

3. Medical treatment for _____ includes applying anesthetic creams, ointments, or suppositories; taking sitz baths and analgesics; and preventing constipation. *(Anal fistula, Anorectal abscess, Anal fissure)*

4. _____ is a motility problem in which constipation and diarrhea are alternately present. *(Irritable bowel syndrome, Ulcerative colitis, Appendicitis)*

5. When _____ is present the abdomen feels rigid and boardlike as it distends with gas and intestinal contents and bowel sounds typically are absent. *(Ulcerative colitis, Appendicitis, Peritonitis)*

6. A _____ obstruction can occur when the intestine becomes adynamic from an absence of normal nerve stimulation to intestinal muscle fibers. *(Mechanical, Functional, Dysfunctional)*

7. _____ are sacs or pouches caused by herniation of the mucosa through a weakened portion of the muscular coat of the intestine or other structure. *(Fissures, Strictures, Diverticula)*

8. When a _____ is performed the protruding intestine is repositioned in the abdominal cavity and the defect in the abdominal wall is repaired. *(Herniorrhaphy, Hernioplasty, Herniation)*

9. Symptoms of a _____ lesion include dull abdominal pain and melena. *(Right-sided, Left-sided, Rectal)*

Activity B *Mark each statement as either "T" (True) or "F" (False). Correct any false statements.*

1. T F   Disorders of the lower GI tract usually affect movement of feces toward the anus, absorption of water and electrolytes, and elimination of dietary wastes.

2. T F   Irritable bowel syndrome causes inflammation of the bowel and changes in bowel tissue, and it increases the risk of colorectal cancer.

3. T F   Clients with an anorectal abscess experience pain that is aggravated by walking and sitting or other activities that increase intra-abdominal pressure such as coughing, sneezing, and straining to have a bowel movement.

4. T F   Treatment of peritonitis includes a nasogastric tube, IV fluids and electrolytes replacement, large doses of antibiotics, analgesics, and antiemetics. The perforation is surgically closed so that intestinal contents can no longer escape.

5. T F   Intestinal obstruction is more common in the large intestine.

6. T F   A volvulus is a telescoping of one part of the intestine into an adjacent part.

7. T F   Surgical intervention for an intestinal obstruction usually involves a section of the obstructed bowel being removed and then the proximal and distal sections are reconnected.

8. T F   Non-surgical treatment for a hernia includes wearing a truss, an apparatus that presses over the hernia and

prevents protrusion of the bowel. Alternately, some clients learn how to manually reduce the hernia themselves.

9. T F   Symptoms of a left-sided lesion include tenesmus, rectal pain, a feeling of incomplete evacuation after a bowel movement, alternating constipation and diarrhea, and bloody stools.

Activity C *Write the correct term for each description given below.*

1. This condition may result from insufficient dietary fiber and water, ignoring or resisting the urge to defecate, emotional stress, use of drugs that tend to slow intestinal motility, or inactivity. It may also stem from several disorders, either in the GI tract or systemically. _____

2. Refers to a cluster of symptoms that occur despite the absence of an identifiable disease process. Clients experience abdominal pain and cramping, bloating and flatus, as well as diarrhea and/or constipation, with or without the presence of mucus. _____

3. Antibiotics are prescribed to treat infection. A fistulotomy or fistulectomy are possible surgical options. _____

4. An obstruction that results from a narrowing of the bowel lumen with or without a space-occupying mass. _____

5. Medical management of this condition includes the client receiving nothing by mouth (NPO). IV fluids with electrolytes are administered to correct fluid and electrolyte imbalances, and antibiotics are ordered to treat infection. _____

6. Asymptomatic diverticula are called diverticulosis. When the diverticula become inflamed, this term is used. _____

7. Signs and symptoms include constipation alternating with diarrhea, flatulence, pain and tenderness in the LLQ, fever, and rectal bleeding. A palpable mass may be felt in the lower abdomen. _____

8. The protrusion of any organ from the cavity that normally confines it, the term most commonly is used to describe the protrusion of the intestine through a defect in the abdominal wall. _____

Activity D *Match the anorectal disorders in Column A with the corresponding descriptions listed in Column B.*

Column A

_____ **1.** Anal Fissure

_____ **2.** Anorectal Abscess

_____ **3.** Anal Fistula

_____ **4.** Hemorrhoids

_____ **5.** Pilonidal Sinus

Column B

a. An inflamed tunnel that develops when the healing of an anorectal abscess is inadequate in connecting the area of the original abscess with perianal skin; purulent material drains from the opening.

b. An infection in the hair follicles in the sacrococcygeal area above the anus.

c. A linear tear in the anal canal tissue.

d. An infection with a collection of pus in an area between the internal and external sphincters.

e. Dilated veins outside or inside the anal sphincter.

Activity E *Compare and contrast Crohn's Disease and Ulcerative Colitis based on the given criteria.*

Criteria	Crohn's Disease	Ulcerative Colitis
Description		
Predisposing and Contributing Factors		
Pathophysiology		
Complications		
Signs and Symptoms		
Non-gastrointestinal Signs and Symptoms		N/A
Medical Treatment		
Medication Therapy		
Surgical Treatment		

Activity F *Briefly answer the following questions:*

1. Describe a normal bowel pattern.

_____

_____

_____

2. What are the major problems associated with diarrhea?

_____

_____

_____

3. How is a pilonidal sinus surgically managed?

_____

_____

_____

4. Describe the signs and symptoms of internal and external hemorrhoids

_____

_____

_____

5. What is the pathophysiology of appendicitis?

_____

_____

_____

6. Identify common causes of peritonitis.

_____

_____

_____

7. What is the etiology of diverticula?

_____

_____

_____

8. How does a hernia develop?

_____

_____

_____

9. What are screening recommendations for colorectal cancer?

_____

_____

_____

SECTION II: APPLYING YOUR KNOWLEDGE

Activity G *Give rationale for each of the following questions:*

1. Why is constipation a common problem for older adults?

_____

_____

_____

2. Why would constipation be misinterpreted as diarrhea?

_____

_____

_____

3. Why would pain medication be withheld when a client is suspected to have appendicitis?

_____

_____

_____

4. Why does dehydration occur more slowly with a large bowel obstruction?

_____

_____

_____

5. Why is intestinal decompression initiated with an intestinal obstruction?

_____

_____

_____

6. Why is it crucial to monitor urine output when caring for a client with an intestinal obstruction?

_____

_____

_____

7. Why would a hernioplasty be performed in addition to a herniorrhaphy?

_____

_____

_____

8. Why is a strangulated hernia an emergency?

_____

_____

_____

Activity H *Answer the following questions related to caring for clients with disorders of the lower gastrointestinal tract.*

1. What educational information will the nurse provide related to the medical management of constipation?

_____

_____

_____

2. What situations indicate that medical intervention is required for the treatment of diarrhea? What treatments are indicated in these situations?

_____

_____

_____

3. What are the assessment findings with acute appendicitis?

_____

_____

_____

4. Describe the pathophysiology of peritonitis.

_____

_____

_____

5. What signs and symptoms associated with an intestinal obstruction?

_____

_____

_____

6. Describe the pathophysiology of diverticulitis.

_____

_____

_____

7. How are diverticulosis and diverticulitis medically and surgically managed?

_____

_____

_____

8. Identify the difference between a reducible, irreducible and strangulated hernia.

_____

_____

_____

Activity I *Think over the following questions. Discuss them with your instructor or peers.*

1. What high priority nursing diagnoses and interventions would you identify for the client with altered bowel elimination?

_____

_____

_____

2. Irritable bowel disease results in periods of flare ups and remissions. How would you assist the client in coping?

_____

_____

_____

3. Acute abdominal inflammatory disorders can be life threatening. What actions would you take to ensure early identification of the signs and symptoms associated with appendicitis and peritonitis?

_____

_____

_____

4. Describe the nursing management of an intestinal tube.

_____

_____

_____

SECTION III: GETTING READY FOR NCLEX

Activity J *Answer the following NCLEX style questions.*

1. The nurse should encourage a client with constipation to slowly increase the intake of dietary fiber up to _____ g/day.

2. Which of the following symptoms indicate that diarrhea is severe?
   a. Bowel sounds are hyperactive.
   b. Blood and mucus are passed with the stool.
   c. The client experiences tenesmus.
   d. The client has a fever.

3. When monitoring the food intake of a client with Crohn's disease, the nurse observes that the client does not eat most of the food served. The nurse learns that the client finds the food unappetizing. Which of the following steps should the nurse take to address this issue?
   a. Explain to the client the benefits of eating the prescribed food.
   b. Request the dietitian to suggest more acceptable food.
   c. Provide the client total parenteral nutrition and lipid infusions.
   d. Provide the client elemental diet formula and 5-ASA medications.

4. A client with ulcerative colitis, who experiences severe diarrhea, is prescribed a cleansing enema to relieve the symptoms. Which of the following interventions should the nurse consider at this stage?

a. Question the physician about the use of the cleansing enema.

b. Educate the client about the procedure of cleansing enema.

c. Position the client comfortably to receive the cleansing enema.

d. Instruct the client to visit the toilet before receiving the enema.

5. A client is assessed for surgery for herniation. Why is it important that the nurse ask if the client smokes?

a. Smoking increases the risk for development of malnutrition and diabetes.

b. Smoking interferes with lymphatic and venous blood flow.

c. The required medications are contraindicated in the presence of nicotine.

d. Sneezing and coughing due to smoking may increase intra-abdominal pressure.

6. Which of the following instructions should the nurse provide to a client who is asymptomatic of colonic cancer, but whose stool test results are positive for blood?

a. Add fiber to the diet

b. Undergo a colonoscopy

c. Use warm soaks

d. Use a stool softener

7. A nurse enters the room of a client with cramping, bloating and flatus, as well as diarrhea and/or constipation, with or without the presence of mucus. What condition do the client's symptoms represent?

a. Peritonitis

b. Irritable bowel syndrome

c. Ulcerative colitis

d. Appendicitis

8. A 55-year-old female client comes to the clinic for a physical examination. Which of the following screening tests would the nurse recommend the client have beginning at the age of 50 and every 10 years after?

a. Colonoscopy

b. Ultrasound of the kidney

c. Mammogram

d. Pap smear

9. A client is admitted to the hospital for a hemorrhoidectomy. Postoperatively, which of the following would a client's nurse be most concerned about?

a. Pain at the incision site.

b. White blood count of 6.5.

c. Client's refusal of a stool softener.

d. Excessive bloody drainage on the external gauze dressing.

10. Which of the following teaching strategies would the nurse plan for a client with an anal fissure?

a. Teach the client strategies to relieve diarrhea.

b. Instruct the client to not eat any fiber.

c. Teach the client how to insert a suppository.

d. Teach the client how to apply ice.

CHAPTER 47

Caring for Clients with Disorders of the Liver, Gallbladder, and Pancreas

Learning Objectives

1. Explain possible causes of jaundice.
2. List common findings manifested by clients with cirrhosis.
3. Discuss common complications of cirrhosis.
4. Identify the modes of transmission of viral hepatitis.
5. Discuss nursing management for clients with a medically or surgically treated liver disorder.
6. Identify factors that contribute to, signs and symptoms of, and medical treatments for cholecystitis.
7. Name techniques for gallbladder removal.
8. Summarize the nursing management of clients undergoing medical or surgical treatment of a gallbladder disorder.
9. Describe the treatment and nursing management of pancreatitis.
10. Describe the treatment of pancreatic carcinoma.
11. Explain the nursing management of clients undergoing pancreatic surgery.

SECTION I: ASSESSING YOUR UNDERSTANDING

Activity A *Fill in the blanks by choosing the correct word from the options given in parentheses.*

1. _____ accompanies many diseases that directly or indirectly affect the liver and is probably the most common sign of a liver disorder. *(Jaundice, Pallor, Cyanosis)*

2. Serum bilirubin levels increase when the liver cannot excrete bilirubin normally or there is excessive destruction of _____ *(RBCs, WBCs, Platelets)*

3. _____ may be performed to remove ascitic fluid. *(A balloon tamponade, Sclerotherapy, An abdominal paracentesis)*

4. Disorders of the _____ can affect both exocrine and endocrine functions. *(Liver, Gallbladder, Pancreas)*

5. Pancreatitis results in the accumulations of the enzymes _____ and _____. As the enzymes accumulate in the gland, they begin to digest the pancreatic tissue itself. *(Bilirubin and Bile salts, Amylase and Lipase, Albumin and Ammonia)*

6. _____ is usually the cause of chronic pancreatitis. *(Trauma, Infection, Alcohol)*

Activity B *Mark each statement as either "T" (True) or "F" (False). Correct any false statements.*

1. T F Poor function of the liver, gallbladder, and pancreas impairs the digestive process and the client's overall nutritional status.

2. T F Kupffer cells perform most of the liver's metabolic functions.

3. T F Treatment for ascites may include maintenance diuretic therapy and a sodium-restricted diet. The potassium-sparing diuretic furosemide (Lasix) may be

chosen because it specifically antagonizes the hormone aldosterone.

4. T F Hepatitis A is transmitted through the blood or sexual contact.

5. T F The most common liver malignancy is a primary malignancy which occurs in people with previous hepatitis B or D virus infections or cirrhosis.

6. T F Most pancreatic cancers are discovered late in the disease and invariably have a lethal prognosis.

Activity C *Write the correct term for each description given below.*

1. The hepatic duct joins with the cystic duct from the gallbladder to form this duct, which empties into the small intestine. _____

2. If a tumor is confined to a single lobe of the liver, this procedure may be attempted to remove primary malignant or benign tumors. _____

3. Occur more frequently in women than in men, particularly women who are middle-aged or have a history of multiple pregnancies, diabetes, and obesity or frequent weight changes. _____

4. Develops when there is reflux of bile and duodenal contents into the pancreatic duct, which activates the exocrine enzymes that the pancreas produces. _____

5. The most common complaint of clients is severe mid- to upper-abdominal pain, radiating to both sides and straight to the back. Nausea, vomiting, and flatulence usually are present. The client may describe the stools as being frothy and foul-smelling, a sign of steatorrhea. The symptoms worsen after the client eats fatty foods or drinks alcohol and are relieved when the client sits up and leans forward or curls into a fetal position. _____

6. A surgical procedure that involves removing the head of the pancreas, resecting the duodenum and stomach, and redirecting the flow of secretions from the stomach, gallbladder, and pancreas into the jejunum. _____

Activity D *Match the phases of hepatitis in Column A with their corresponding signs and symptoms in Column B.*

Column A

_____ 1. Incubation phase

_____ 2. Preicteric or prodromal phase

_____ 3. Icteric phase

_____ 4. Posticteric phase

Column B

a. Jaundice, pruritus, clay-colored or light stools, dark urine, fatigue, anorexia, and RUQ discomfort; symptoms of the preicteric phase may continue.

b. The virus replicates within the liver; the client is asymptomatic. Late in this phase the virus can be found in blood, bile, and stools (for hepatitis A). At this point, the client is considered infectious.

c. Liver enlargement, malaise, and fatigue; other symptoms subside; liver function tests begin to return to normal.

d. Nausea; vomiting; anorexia; fever; malaise; arthralgia; headache; right upper quadrant (RUQ) discomfort; enlargement of the spleen, liver, and lymph nodes; weight loss; rash; and urticaria.

Activity E *Table 47-1 lists the complications associated with cirrhosis. Provide the description for each and their related treatments.*

TABLE 47-1		
Complication	**Description**	**Treatments**
Portal hypertension		
Esophageal varices		
Ascites		
Hepatic encephalopathy		

Activity F *Briefly answer the following questions.*

1. What are the causes of hemolytic jaundice, hepatocellular jaundice, and obstructive jaundice?

_____

_____

_____

2. What are the causes of Laënnec's cirrhosis, postnecrotic cirrhosis, and cardiac cirrhosis?

_____

_____

_____

3. Acute hemorrhage from esophageal varices is life-threatening. Describe the care for an acute hemorrhage.

_____

_____

_____

4. How does ascites develop?

_____

_____

_____

5. Describe the treatment for hepatitis.

_____

_____

_____

6. Differentiate between the following terms: cholelithiasis, choledocholithiasis, and cholecystitis.

_____

_____

_____

7. Describe the signs and symptoms of cholecystitis.

_____

_____

_____

SECTION II: APPLYING YOUR KNOWLEDGE

Activity G *Give rationale for the following questions.*

1. Why do older adults need to be carefully screened for alcohol use?

_____

_____

_____

2. Why can disorders of the liver lead to coagulopathies?

_____

_____

_____

3. Why are metastatic liver tumors usually considered inoperable?

_____

_____

_____

4. Why does the client with pancreatitis usually receive nothing by mouth, and a nasogastric tube connected to suction?

_____

_____

_____

5. Why would a client with pancreatitis become hypotensive?

_____

_____

_____

6. Why is it important for the client with pancreatitis to remain on bed rest and receive adequate pain relief?

_____

_____

_____

Activity H *Answer the following questions related to caring for clients with disorders of the liver, gallbladder, and pancreas.*

1. How does jaundice develop?

   _____

   _____

   _____

2. Describe the pathophysiology of cirrhosis.

   _____

   _____

   _____

3. What are the signs and symptoms of cirrhosis?

   _____

   _____

   _____

4. Describe the medical and surgical management of cholecystitis.

   _____

   _____

   _____

5. Describe the medical management of pancreatitis.

   _____

   _____

   _____

Activity I *Think over the following questions. Discuss them with your instructor or peers.*

1. What high-priority nursing diagnoses and interventions would you identify for a client with hepatitis?

   _____

   _____

   _____

2. How would you provide support to a client diagnosed with pancreatic cancer?

   _____

   _____

   _____

3. How would you prepare a client who will be having a same-day surgery laparoscopic cholecystectomy?

   _____

   _____

   _____

4. A client taking multiple medications associated with liver disease does not understand their significance to the disorder. What educational information would you provide?

   _____

   _____

   _____

SECTION III: GETTING READY FOR NCLEX

Activity J *Answer the following NCLEX style questions.*

1. In a client who has undergone cholecystectomy, if more than _____ mL of bile drains within 24 hours, the nurse notifies the physician.

2. When assessing clients for chronic hepatitis, in which group of clients will the nurse observe the pain to be mild or absent?

   a. Women nearing menopause

   b. Children

   c. Young adults

   d. Older adults

3. Which of the following should a nurse instruct a client with symptomatic gallstones to avoid?

   a. Coffee and products containing caffeine

   b. Fruits and fruit juices

   c. Milk and milk products

   d. Potassium-rich foods

4. A client with pancreatitis experiences a seizure due to alcohol withdrawal. Which of the following interventions should a nurse consider to minimize the risk for injury in such a client?

   a. Initiate precautions by restraining the client

   b. Observe the client throughout the seizure

   c. Administer oxygen throughout the seizure

   d. Administer an analgesic during the seizure

5. When assessing a client for acute pancreatitis, which of the following symptoms will the nurse observe?

   a. Increased thirst and urination

   b. Hypertension and nausea

   c. Rapid breathing and pulse rate

   d. Frothy, foul-smelling stools

6. Which of the following dietary interventions should a nurse consider after the removal of the nasogastric tube in a client who has undergone surgery for a liver disorder?

   a. Provide small sips of clear liquids

   b. Provide small sips of fruit juice or soup

   c. Provide small meal of soft foods

   d. Provide meal of protein-rich foods

7. A nurse identifies that the skin of an elderly client with liver cancer is yellow. Which of the following is the cause of jaundice?

   a. Abnormally high concentration of bilirubin in the blood.

   b. Abnormally low concentration of bilirubin in the blood.

   c. Excessive production of RBCs.

   d. Excessive production of platelets.

8. A client who is experiencing alcohol withdrawal is diagnosed with cirrhosis of the liver. Which of the following physiological changes occurs in cirrhosis of the liver?

   a. The ability to metabolize hormones.

   b. Absorption of fat-soluble vitamins.

   c. Impaired ability to detoxify chemicals.

   d. Malabsorption of water-soluble vitamins.

9. A nurse is giving discharge instructions to a client with pancreatitis. Which of the following instructions is correct?

   a. Eat two meals a day.

   b. If alcohol abuse is known, limit alcohol to one drink per day.

   c. Follow written instructions for a high-carbohydrate, high-fat diet.

   d. Follow the written instructions for bland, low-fat calorie controlled diet.

10. A nurse is giving a presentation to a group of colleagues about the prevention of hepatitis transmission. Which of the following recommendations would the nurse suggest a healthcare worker use when working in the hospital?

   a. Perform handwashing even after removing gloves

   b. Wear a gown only if body fluids may be splashed

   c. Receive hepatitis A vaccine regardless of risk

   d. Perform CPR without a pocket mask

CHAPTER 48

Caring for Clients with Ostomies

Learning Objectives

1. Differentiate between ileostomy and colostomy.
2. Discuss preoperative nursing care of a client undergoing ostomy surgery.
3. List complications associated with ostomy surgery.
4. Discuss postoperative nursing management of a client with an ileostomy.
5. Describe the components used to apply and collect stool from an intestinal ostomy.
6. Cite reasons for changing an ostomy appliance.
7. Summarize how to change an ostomy appliance.
8. Explain how stool is released from a continent ileostomy.
9. Describe the two-part procedure needed to create an ileoanal reservoir.
10. Discuss various types of colostomies.
11. Explain ways in which clients with descending or sigmoid colostomies may regulate bowel elimination.

SECTION I: ASSESSING YOUR UNDERSTANDING

Activity A *Fill in the blanks by choosing the correct word from the options given in parentheses.*

1. An _____ refers to an opening between an internal body structure and the skin. *(Ostomy, Ileostomy, Colostomy)*

2. Irrigation for a single-barrel colostomy begins on the _____ postoperative day. *(1st or 2nd, 4th or 5th, 7th or 8th)*

3. In the usual surgical procedure for a conventional _____ the entire colon and rectum are removed. *(Ileostomy Single-barrel colostomy, Double-barrel colostomy)*

4. Clients with _____ always wear an appliance, which requires frequent emptying. *(A continent ileostomy, An ileoanal reservoir, An ileostomy)*

5. Following an ileostomy the rectal pack is removed after _____ *(1 to 2, 5 to 7 days, 10 to 14 days)*

6. After ileostomy surgery, the client is shown how to prepare the drainage pouch for a secure fit around the stoma, leaving an extra _____ inch in the appliance opening which provides room for stoma clearance and potential swelling. *(1/8, 1/2, 1)*

Activity B *Mark each statement as either "T" (True) or "F" (False). Correct any false statements.*

1. T F An ileostomy is an opening from the colon.

2. T F To reduce the risk for bowel incontinence, the nurse instructs the client to perform perineal exercises four to six times a day to reestablish anal sphincter control and enlarge the ileoanal reservoir.

3. T F Regular irrigations may control a sigmoid colostomy, and sometimes a descending colostomy, thus eliminating the need for the client to constantly wear an appliance.

4. T F About 6 months following the placement of a continent ileostomy the client or caregiver is required to empty the reservoir six or eight times daily.

5. T F When preparing to drain a continent ileostomy the catheter should be warmed to body temperature and the tip lubricated.

6. T F Natural methods are the most predictable for regulating the bowel.

Activity C *Write the correct term for each description given below.*

1. An opening on the exterior abdominal surface. _____

2. The collection device worn over a stoma. _____

3. When this procedure is performed, the stoma continually releases stool and gas. _____

4. A certified nurse who assists with marking placement of the stoma and collaborates with the surgeon regarding placement and the client's educational needs. _____

5. How a type of colostomy is described. _____

6. This type of ileostomy involves a two-part procedure. _____

Activity D *Match the type of colostomy in Column A with the appearance of feces in Column B.*

Column A

_____ **1.** Conventional and continent ileostomy

_____ **2.** Ascending and transverse colostomy

_____ **3.** Descending colostomy

_____ **4.** Sigmoid colostomy

Column B

a. Semiliquid
b. Formed
c. Liquid
d. Soft

Activity E *Listed are the various ileostomy and colostomy procedures. Differentiate the procedures by identifying characteristics of each type.*

Procedure	Description
Ileostomy	
Continent Ileostomy (Kock Pouch)	
Ileoanal Reservoir (Ileoanal Anastomosis)	
Colostomy	
Single-Barrel Colostomy	
Double-Barrel Colostomy	
Loop Colostomy	

Activity F *Briefly answer the following questions.*

1. Describe an appliance worn by an ostomate.

2. What issues with sexuality and reproduction may result from a colectomy?

3. What are the possible postoperative complications associated with ileostomy surgery?

4. Following a double-barrel colostomy, what essential information is recorded by the physician?

5. What is the benefit of a loop colostomy?

6. What interventions can the nurse use to promote adequate learning of the required information for ostomy care?

_____

_____

_____

SECTION II: APPLYING YOUR KNOWLEDGE

Activity G *Give rationale for the following questions.*

1. Why is a disposable, or temporary, appliance preferred in the immediate postoperative phase?

_____

_____

_____

2. Why would karaya gum be preferred over an adhesive in the immediate postoperative period?

_____

_____

_____

3. Why should clients with an ileostomy avoid enteric-coated products and some modified-release drugs?

_____

_____

_____

4. Why would clients with an ileostomy need B_{12} injections or intranasal B_{12}?

_____

_____

_____

5. Why is a double-barrel colostomy usually performed?

_____

_____

_____

Activity H *Answer the following questions related to caring for clients with ostomies.*

1. Describe a typical reusable appliance.

_____

_____

_____

2. What is the preoperative care for ileostomy surgery?

_____

_____

_____

3. What is the postoperative care for ileostomy surgery?

_____

_____

_____

4. Identify the steps for changing an appliance.

_____

_____

_____

5. Describe the irrigation process of a single-barrel colostomy.

_____

_____

_____

6. Describe the two stage procedure for an ileoanal reservoir.

_____

_____

_____

Activity I *Think over the following questions. Discuss them with your instructor or peers.*

1. When caring for an ostomy what interventions will you take to prevent bowel leaking from around the appliance?

_____

_____

_____

2. When caring for an ostomy what interventions will you take to promote skin integrity around the ostomy site?

_____

_____

_____

3. When caring for the client with an ostomy what interventions will you take to promote coping and a positive body image?

_____

_____

_____

SECTION III: GETTING READY FOR NCLEX

Activity J *Answer the following NCLEX style questions:*

1. Which of the following instructions should a nurse provide a client with an ileostomy when using the catheter?

  a. Avoid warming the catheter before inserting it into the ileal pouch.

  b. Report if there is resistance when the catheter reaches the nipple valve.

  c. Avoid coughing when the catheter is being inserted into the ileal pouch.

  d. Clean catheter with soapy water and store it in a plastic bag after use.

2. The nurse should urge a client with an ileoanal anastomosis to do perineal exercises four to six times a day for _____ repetitions.

3. Compounds containing aspirin are discontinued at least _____ week/s before ileostomy surgery.

4. The nurse has performed nasogastric decompression for a client who has undergone colostomy surgery. Which of the following related interventions should a nurse consider for this client?

  a. Inspect the swelling of joints.

  b. Inspect the bleeding wound.

  c. Monitor pulse pressure and rate.

  d. Measure the amount of fluids lost.

5. A client with an ileostomy wants to know why to avoid fibrous vegetables. What should be the nurse's response?

  a. They cause gas formation.

  b. They cause stomal obstruction.

  c. They are difficult to digest.

  d. They increase the risk of diarrhea.

6. Why should a nurse instruct a client with an ileostomy to avoid enteric-coated products?

  a. The coating prevents the absorption of the product.

  b. The coating adversely affects ileostomy.

  c. The coating affects the absorption of vitamins.

  d. The coating causes particularly strong odors.

7. Which of the following is an opening in the large bowel created by bringing a section of the large intestine out to the abdomen and fashioning a stoma?

  a. Continent ileostomy

  b. Colostomy

  c. Ileostomy

  d. Ileoanal reservoir

8. A client is visited by the dietician following a colostomy procedure. Which of the following is the primary nutrition concern for this type of client?

  a. Fiber.

  b. Small frequent meals.

  c. Chewing food thoroughly.

  d. Fluids and electrolytes.

9. A nurse is doing discharge teaching on a client with a colostomy. What would the nurse convey to the client regarding when is the best time to perform irrigation?

  a. After a meal.

  b. After a bowel movement.

  c. During a meal.

  d. Two hours before a meal.

10. The nurse is teaching a client about sexual modifications for clients with an ostomy. Which of the following strategies would the nurse suggest when anticipating sexual activity?

   a. Leave the stoma open to air and cover with a towel.

   b. Instruct the client to limit foods that activate the bowel.

   c. Bathe and apply a fresh pouch after having sex.

   d. Consult with members of a local ostomy group.

Introduction to the Endocrine System

Learning Objectives

1. Identify the chief function of the endocrine glands.
2. Describe the general function of hormones.
3. Explain the relationship between the hypothalamus and the pituitary gland.
4. Discuss the regulation of levels of hormones.
5. List endocrine glands and the hormones they secrete.
6. Name other organs that are not classified as endocrine glands but secrete hormones.
7. Outline information to include when taking the health history of a client with an endocrine disorder.
8. Describe physical assessment findings that suggest an endocrine disorder.
9. List examples of laboratory and diagnostic tests that identify endocrine disorders.
10. Discuss the nursing management of clients undergoing diagnostic tests to detect endocrine dysfunction.

SECTION I: ASSESSING YOUR UNDERSTANDING

Activity A *Fill in the blanks by choosing the correct word from the options given in parentheses.*

1. Hormones circulate in the blood until they reach _____ in target cells or other endocrine glands. *(Receptors, Exocrine glands, The nuclei)*

2. The _____ gland is attached to the thalamus in the brain. It secretes melatonin, which aids in regulating sleep cycles and mood. Melatonin is believed to play a role in hypothalamic–pituitary interaction. *(Thymus, Pineal, Thyroid)*

3. Insulin is a hormone released by _____. It lowers the level of blood glucose when it rises beyond normal limits. *(Alpha islet cells, Delta islet cells, Beta islet cells)*

Activity B *Mark each statement as either "T" (True) or "F" (False). Correct any false statements.*

1. T F   The pituitary gland is called the master gland because it regulates the function of other endocrine glands. The term is somewhat misleading, however, because the hypothalamus influences the pituitary gland.

2. T F   The thymus glands are four (some people have more than four) small, bean-shaped bodies, each surrounded by a capsule of connective tissue and embedded within the lateral lobes of the thyroid.

3. T F   Pancreatic polypeptide, a hormone secreted by delta islet cells, helps maintain a relatively constant level of blood sugar by inhibiting the release of insulin and glucagons.

4. T F   The ovaries produce the hormones estrogen and testosterone.

Activity C *Write the correct term for each description given below.*

1. Chemicals that accelerate or slow physiologic processes, secreted directly into the bloodstream by the endocrine glands. _____

2. The hormone-secreting cells of the pancreas which release insulin, glucagon, somatostatin, and pancreatic polypeptide. _____

3. A hormone released by alpha islet cells which raises blood sugar levels by stimulating glycogenolysis, the breakdown of glycogen into glucose, in the liver. _____

Activity D *Match the hypothalamic hormones given in Column A to their associated functions given in Column B.*

Column A

_____ 1. Thyrotropin-releasing hormone (TRH)

_____ 2. Corticotropin-releasing hormone (CRH)

_____ 3. Gonadotropin-releasing hormone (GnRH)

_____ 4. Growth hormone–releasing hormone (GHRH)

_____ 5. Somatostatin

_____ 6. Hypothalamic Dopamine

Column B

a. Triggers sexual development at the onset of puberty and continues to cause the anterior pituitary gland to secrete luteinizing hormone (LH) and follicle-stimulating hormone (FSH).

b. Inhibits the release of prolactin from the anterior pituitary gland.

c. Stimulates the release of thyroid-stimulating hormone (TSH) from the anterior pituitary gland.

d. Results in the release of somatotropin (growth hormone [GH]) from the anterior pituitary gland.

e. Causes the anterior pituitary gland to secrete adrenocorticotropic hormone (ACTH).

f. Inhibits GHRH and TSH and also blocks

the secretion of several gastrointestinal hormones, lowers the blood flow within the intestine, suppresses the release of insulin and glucagon from the pancreas, and suppresses the release of exocrine enzymes from the pancreas.

Activity E *Compare the following diagnostic tests used to evaluate endocrine function based on the given criteria.*

Diagnostic Test	Description/Purpose of Test
Hormone Levels	
Radiography, Computed Tomography, and Magnetic Resonance Imaging	
Radionuclide Studies	
Radioimmunoassay	
Nuclear Scan	

Activity F *Briefly answer the following questions.*

1. Describe the function of the hypothalamus.

_____

_____

_____

2. Describe a feedback loop.

_____

_____

_____

3. Identify fight-or-flight responses.

_____

_____

_____

SECTION II: APPLYING YOUR KNOWLEDGE

Activity G *Give rationale for the following questions.*

1. Why is a complete family history essential when obtaining a health history for a client related to endocrine disorders?

_____

_____

_____

2. Why is it essential to obtain a medication history for an older adult related to endocrine disorders?

_____

_____

_____

3. Why is the pancreas considered to be an exocrine and endocrine gland?

_____

_____

_____

4. Why does the nurse not palpate the thyroid repeatedly or forcefully?

_____

_____

_____

Activity H *Answer the following questions related to the endocrine system.*

1. Describe the thyroid gland and the hormones it secretes.

_____

_____

_____

2. Describe the adrenal glands and the hormones they secrete.

_____

_____

_____

3. Describe the organs that are not typically considered endocrine glands but secrete hormones, and the functions of the hormones these organs secrete.

_____

_____

_____

4. What assessment finding may the nurse identify when performing a physical examination on the client with an endocrine disorder?

_____

_____

_____

Activity I *Think over the following questions. Discuss them with your instructor or peers.*

1. How will you prepare clients for diagnostic testing related to the endocrine system?

_____

_____

_____

2. What information will you include in the health history for a client with an endocrine disorder?

_____

_____

_____

SECTION III: GETTING READY FOR NCLEX

Activity J *Answer the following questions.*

1. Which of the following can be performed to determine a client's general status and rule out disorders?
   a. A complete blood count
   b. A complete blood count and chemistry profile
   c. Chemistry profile
   d. Radiographs of the chest or abdomen

2. The nurse has to assess a client's mental and emotional status before he or she can begin therapy for treatment of an endocrine disorder. Which of the following can be tested to assess the client's mental and emotional status?

   a. Ability to respond to questions
   b. Motor function
   c. Sleep and awake cycles
   d. Facial expression

3. A nurse is obtaining the drug history of an older client before his diagnostic examination. Which of the following aspects is essential while obtaining the drug history?

   a. Consulting the physician
   b. Consulting a family member or the caregiver to confirm the client's diet history
   c. Consulting the institution's procedure manual
   d. Consulting a family member or the caregiver to confirm drugs the client is taking

4. A client, age 64, has complaints of frequent spells of fatigue and inability to sleep. She also reports hair loss and an allergy to seafood. Which of the following information is essential to consider before initiating a thyroid test for the client?

   a. Her age
   b. Complaints of fatigue and inability to sleep
   c. Allergy to seafood
   d. Hair loss

5. A nurse is collecting data about the diet history of a client who has low blood sugar. Which of the following would be an important consideration in the diet history?

   a. Consumption of health foods
   b. Consumption of sea salt and kelp
   c. Consumption of seafood
   d. Consumption of carbohydrates

6. Which one of the following is an appropriate nursing intervention for preparing a client for a CT scan?

   a. Consult the physician for the special preparation
   b. Provide general explanation to the client
   c. Inform client to temporarily eliminate salt from the diet
   d. Instruct the client to fast

7. What assessment findings, specific to the endocrine glands, should a nurse observe while inspecting the skin of a client during a physical examination?

   a. Skin breaks that heal quickly
   b. Excessive hair growth or loss
   c. Increased thickness
   d. Rashes with no underlying cause.

8. Which of the following hormones is released from the posterior pituitary gland?

   a. Antidiuretic hormone
   b. Thyroid-stimulating hormone
   c. Parathyroid hormone
   d. Prolactin

9. A nurse is teaching a client regarding a hormone that is released by beta islet cells in the pancreas. Which hormone is it?

   a. Progesterone
   b. Glucagon
   c. Insulin
   d. Parathormone

10. A nurse educator is giving a presentation on hypothalamic hormones. Which of the following hypothalamic hormones when stimulated is controlled by another hypothalamic hormone?

   a. Thyroid-stimulating hormone
   b. Corticotropin-releasing hormone
   c. Follicle-stimulating hormone
   d. Growth hormone–releasing hormone

CHAPTER 50

Caring for Clients with Disorders of the Endocrine System

Learning Objectives

1. Describe the physiologic effects of hyposecretion and hypersecretion of the pituitary, thyroid, parathyroid, and adrenal glands.
2. Describe the nursing management of clients with pituitary disorders.
3. Describe thyroid disorders and nursing management of clients with these disorders.
4. Compare the differences in physiologic effects, assessment findings, and management of disorders affecting the parathyroid glands.
5. Identify disorders of the adrenal glands and describe nursing management of clients with these disorders.
6. Identify symptoms of emergency conditions resulting from endocrine disorders.

SECTION I: ASSESSING YOUR UNDERSTANDING

Activity A *Fill in the blanks by choosing the correct word from the options given in parentheses.*

1. Growth hormone (GH) is overproduced when the pituitary gland is insensitive to feedback of _____ hormones. Overproduction may result from hypersecretion caused by hyperplasia. *(Stimulating, Sensitizing, Inhibiting)*

2. Tetany and severe hypoparathyroidism are treated immediately by the administration of IV _____ *(Calcium, Potassium, Phosphorus)*

3. Untreated hypothyroidism becomes a risk factor for _____ *(Diabetes, Coronary artery disease, Insomnia)*

4. _____ is an enlarged thyroid, usually with no symptoms of thyroid dysfunction. *(A nontoxic goiter, An endemic goiter, A nodular goiter)*

5. Clients with primary adrenal insufficiency require daily _____ replacement therapy for the rest of their lives. *(Growth hormone, Corticosteroid, Calcium)*

6. The cause of primary hyperaldosteronism may be a benign aldosterone-secreting adenoma of the _____. *(Adrenal glands, Thyroid gland, Parathyroid glands)*

7. Excessive secretion of _____ results in increased reabsorption of sodium and water and excretion of potassium by the kidneys. *(Mineralcorticoids, Aldosterone, Glucocorticoids)*

Activity B *Mark each statement as "T" (True) or "F" (False). Correct any false statements.*

1. **T F**   A disorder of any endocrine gland can profoundly affect the other endocrine glands, as well as many major body systems.

2. **T F**   If surgery or radiation therapy for treatment of acromegaly removes or destroys normal pituitary tissue, replacement therapy with thyroid hormone, corticosteroids, antidiuretic hormone (ADH), and sex hormones is necessary.

3. **T F**   Nephrogenic diabetes insipidus develops when there is insufficient ADH (also known as vasopressin) from the posterior pituitary gland.

4. **T F**   The most reliable thyroid function test to diagnose hyperthyroidism in an older adult is a serum T_3 level.

5. **T F**   Benign thyroid tumors are associated with voice changes, hoarseness, and difficulty swallowing.

6. **T F**   The only treatment for primary hyperparathyroidism is surgical removal of hypertrophied glandular tissue or of an individual tumor of one of the parathyroid glands.

7. **T F**   The adrenal medulla synthesizes and secretes the hormones known as corticosteroids. These include mineralocorticoids, glucocorticoids, and gonadocorticoids.

Activity C *Write the correct term for each description given below.*

1. The surgical treatment of choice for acromegaly (hyperpituitarism). _____

2. An enlarged thyroid gland. _____

3. Medications such as propylthiouracil (PTU, Propyl-Thyracil) and methimazole (Tapazole). _____

4. A surgery that involves partial removal of the thyroid gland. _____

5. A chronic form of thyroiditis believed to be an autoimmune disorder. _____

6. The main symptom of acute and sudden hypoparathyroidism. _____

7. Secondary adrenal insufficiency can result from discontinuation of this type of therapy. _____

8. Usually caused by a benign tumor. Hyperfunction causes the adrenal medulla to secrete the catecholamines epinephrine and norepinephrine excessively. _____

Activity D *Match these life-threatening endocrine conditions listed in column A with their signs and symptoms in column B.*

Column A

____ 1. Simmonds' disease (Panhypopituitarism)

____ 2. Thyrotoxic crisis (Thyroid storm)

____ 3. Myxedemic coma

____ 4. Acute adrenal crisis (Addisonian crisis)

Column B

a. Onset may be sudden or gradual. It may begin with anorexia, nausea, vomiting, diarrhea, abdominal pain, profound weakness, headache, intensification of hypotension, restlessness, or fever. The BP markedly decreases and shock develops. Without treatment the client's condition will deteriorate and death may occur from hypotension and vasomotor collapse.

b. The temperature may be as high as 106°F (41°C). The pulse rate is rapid, and cardiac dysrhythmias are common. The client may experience persistent vomiting, extreme restlessness with delirium, chest pain, and dyspnea.

c. The gonads and genitalia atrophy. Because of the impaired pituitary stimulus, the thyroid and adrenals fail to secrete adequate hormones. Signs and symptoms of hypothyroidism, hypoglycemia, and adrenal insufficiency are apparent. The client ages prematurely and becomes extremely cachectic.

d. A client with hypothyroidism experiencing infection, trauma, or excessive chills, or taking narcotics, sedatives, or tranquilizers, can lapse into this condition. Signs of this life-threatening event are hypothermia, hypotension, and hypoventilation.

Activity E *For the endocrine disorders listed in Table 50-1, identify the hormones involved and compare and contrast the signs and symptoms.*

Activity F *Briefly answer the following questions.*

1. Describe Simmonds' Disease (Panhypopituitarism).

_____

_____

_____

2. What are nursing priorities when caring for the client with acromegaly?

_____

_____

_____

3. Describe the nursing management of Simmonds' disease?

_____

_____

_____

TABLE 50-1		
Disorder	**Hormone Involvement**	**Signs and Symptoms**
Anterior Pituitary		
Gigantism		
Dwarfism		
Acromegaly (Hyperpituitarism)		
Posterior Pituitary		
Diabetes Insipidus (DI)		
Syndrome of Inappropriate Antidiuretic Hormone secretion (SIADH)		
Thyroid		
Hyperthyroidism		
Hypothyroidism		
Parathyroid		
Hyperparathyroidism		
Hyporparathyroidism		
Adrenal Cortex		
Adrenal Insufficiency		
Cushing's Syndrome		
Adrenal Medulla		
Pheochromocytoma		

4. Describe the function of antidiuretic hormone (ADH), also called vasopressin.

_____

_____

_____

5. Describe the medical management of syndrome of inappropriate antidiuretic hormone.

_____

_____

_____

6. Describe the signs and symptoms of a goiter.

_____

_____

_____

7. What conditions may cause acute adrenal crisis?

_____

_____

_____

8. What is the nursing management of pheochromocytoma?

_____

_____

_____

SECTION II: APPLYING YOUR KNOWLEDGE

Activity G *Give rationale for the following questions.*

1. Why are thyroid disorders difficult to diagnose?

_____

_____

_____

2. Why might hyperthyroidism be overlooked in an older adult?

_____

_____

_____

3. Why are antithyroid medications avoided during pregnancy?

_____

_____

_____

4. Why is a client receiving antithyroid medication instructed to report sore throat, fever, chills, headache, malaise, weakness, or unusual bleeding or bruising?

_____

_____

_____

5. Why is hypothyroidism difficult to identify in the older client?

_____

_____

_____

Activity H *Answer the following questions related to caring for clients with disorders of the endocrine system.*

1. How is the treatment for neurogenic diabetes insipidus different from nephrogenic diabetes insipidus?

_____

_____

_____

2. Describe the nursing management of the client with SIADH.

_____

_____

_____

3. What are potential complications of thyroid surgery?

_____

_____

_____

4. Describe the pathophysiology of thyroiditis.

_____

_____

_____

5. Describe the nursing management for a client with hyperparathyroidism.

_____

_____

_____

6. How is hypoparathyroidism medically managed?

_____

_____

_____

7. Describe the medical and surgical management of Cushing's syndrome/Cushingoid syndrome.

_____

_____

_____

8. What are the signs and symptoms of hyperaldosteronism?

_____

_____

_____

Activity I _Think over the following questions. Discuss them with your instructor or peers._

1. You are caring for a client diagnosed with SIADH. What signs and symptoms will you closely monitor?

_____

_____

_____

2. What high priority nursing diagnoses and interventions will you identify for the client with hypothyroidism?

_____

_____

_____

3. You are providing post operative care to a client who has undergone a total thyroidectomy. What high priority assessment and interventions will you identify?

_____

_____

_____

4. Your client is diagnosed with pheochromocytoma. What priority interventions will you implement to care for this client?

_____

_____

_____

5. Your client is diagnosed with Cushingoid syndrome secondary to corticosteroid therapy. The client is receiving corticosteroids to prevent organ transplant rejection and it will not be discontinued. What interventions will you implement to assist the client in dealing with the issues associated with Cushingoid syndrome?

_____

_____

_____

SECTION III: GETTING READY FOR NCLEX

Activity J _Answer the following questions:_

1. Which of the following post-operative nursing actions should the nurse perform when a client with acromegaly has nasal packing?

a. Detect the signs of increased intracranial pressure and meningitis.

b. Detect the presence of cerebrospinal fluid.

c. Detect the signs of hypoglycemia.

d. Detect the presence of striae.

2. Which of the following should the nurse advise a client with diabetes insipidus in order to reduce fluid loss?

a. Remain in air-conditioned areas during hot and humid weather.

b. Avoid any activity.

c. Emphasize compliance with drug therapy.

d. Avoid a high-protein diet.

3. Which of the following are the signs of fluid overload?

a. Weakness

b. Headache

c. Pulmonary congestion

d. Weight gain without edema

4. Which of the following is the most reliable thyroid function test to diagnose hyperthyroidism in an older adult?
   a. Serum T_4 level
   b. Glucose tolerance test
   c. Cosyntropin
   d. Iodine tolerance test

5. Which of the following is the most common adverse reaction during initial therapy with a thyroid replacement?
   a. Allergy
   b. Signs of hyperthyroidism
   c. Weight loss
   d. Bones become demineralized

6. Which of the following group of clients should be assessed for pheochromocytoma?
   a. Clients with hypertension that is difficult to control
   b. Clients with high blood glucose levels
   c. Clients who take more than two medicines to control their blood pressure
   d. Clients with either primary or secondary adrenal insufficiency

7. A client is admitted to the hospital with Addison's disease. When discharging the client, the nurse reviews discharge instructions on nutrition. Which of the following discharge instructions are important for the client with Addison's disease regarding nutrition?
   a. Eat a diet high in protein, low in refined carbohydrates
   b. Consume two meals per day
   c. Eat foods high in potassium
   d. Drink less than 1 L of fluid per day

8. A nurse is taking care of a client with a parathyroid disorder. Which of the following nutrients does a client with hypoparathyroidism need more of?
   a. Potassium
   b. Calcium
   c. Magnesium
   d. Sodium

9. The nurse is assessing a client who exhibits spontaneous spasm of the fingers or toes, mouth twitching or jaw tightening when he taps the cheek anteriorly to the earlobe. What sign does the nurse identify to document in the chart that is consistent with tetany?
   a. Lhermitte's sign
   b. Trousseau's sign
   c. Chvostek's sign
   d. Bulge sign

10. A nurse is teaching a client about signs and symptoms of thyrotoxic crisis. Which of the following signs and symptoms below are indicative of thyrotoxic crisis?
   a. Chest pain
   b. Bradycardia
   c. Altered level of consciousness
   d. Hypothermia

CHAPTER 51

Caring for Clients with Diabetes Mellitus

Learning Objectives

1. Define and distinguish the two types of diabetes mellitus.
2. Identify the three classic symptoms of diabetes mellitus.
3. Name three laboratory methods used to diagnose diabetes mellitus.
4. Describe the methods used to treat diabetes mellitus.
5. Discuss the nursing management of the client with diabetes mellitus.
6. Explain the source of ketones and cause of diabetic ketoacidosis.
7. List three main goals in the treatment of diabetic ketoacidosis.
8. Identify two physiologic signs of hyperosmolar hyperglycemic nonketotic syndrome.
9. Describe the treatment of hyperosmolar hyperglycemic nonketotic syndrome.
10. Explain the cause and treatment of hypoglycemia.
11. Differentiate between the symptoms of hypoglycemia and hyperglycemia.
12. Describe common chronic complications of diabetes mellitus.

SECTION I: ASSESSING YOUR UNDERSTANDING

Activity A *Fill in the blanks by choosing the correct word from the options given in parentheses.*

1. Although no age group is exempt from diabetes, the American Diabetes Association (2007) indicates that _____ of affected people acquire the disease as adults. *(70% to 80%, 75% to 80%, 90% to 95%)*

2. The onset for rapid-acting insulin is _____ minutes. *(1 to 2, 5 to 15, 20 to 30)*

3. All clients with _____ diabetes must rely on insulin therapy. *(Type 1, Type 2, Type 1 and Type 2)*

4. The buildup of subcutaneous fat at the site of repeated injections that eventually interferes with insulin absorption in the tissue is called _____ . *(Lipoatrophy, Lipohypertrophy, Liposuction)*

5. _____ and _____ are described as being "insulin releasers" because they stimulate the pancreas to secrete more insulin. *(Thiazolidinediones and biguanides, Alpha-glucosidase inhibitors and thiazolidinediones, Sulfonylureas and meglitinides)*

6. _____ refers to the progressive decrease in renal function that occurs with diabetes mellitus. *(Sensory neuropathy, Diabetic nephropathy, Motor neuropathy)*

Activity B *Mark each statement as True (T) or False (F). Correct any false statements.*

1. T F Diabetes mellitus is a metabolic disorder of the pancreas that affects carbohydrate, fat, and protein metabolism. This disease is reaching epidemic proportions in the United States.

2. T F   Type 2 diabetes is considered an autoimmune disorder.

3. T F   Glargine (Lantus) can be mixed with either rapid acting or short acting insulin in the same syringe.

4. T F   Regular insulin is the only type of insulin that may be administered by intravenous route.

5. T F   Biguanides and thiazolidinediones delay the digestion of carbohydrates.

Activity C *Write the correct term for each description given below.*

1. A syndrome that includes obesity, especially in the abdominal area; high blood pressure (BP); elevated triglyceride, low-density lipoprotein, and blood glucose levels; and a low high-density lipoprotein level. _____

2. An elevated blood glucose level. _____

3. This system buffers ketones. _____

4. The peak for Lantus insulin. _____

5. The breakdown of subcutaneous fat at the site of repeated injections. _____

6. Always a potential adverse reaction when administering medications for diabetes. _____

7. Clients may not experience any visual changes for some time. When symptoms do occur, clients report blurred vision, no vision in spotty areas, or seeing debris floating about the visual field. _____

Activity D *Match the diagnostic tests in Column A with their descriptions given in Column B.*

Column A

____ **1.** Glucometer testing

____ **2.** Glycosylated hemoglobin (hemoglobin A1c)

____ **3.** Urine screening

____ **4.** Oral glucose tolerance test

____ **5.** Postprandial glucose

____ **6.** Fasting blood glucose

Column B

a. Blood specimen is obtained after 8 hours of fasting. In the nondiabetic client the glucose level will be between 70 and 110 mg/dL.

b. Normally contains no detectable glucose or ketones; in diabetes, one or both may be present.

c. The results of this test reflect the amount of glucose that is stored in the hemoglobin molecule during its life span of 120 days. Normally, the level is less than 7%. According to the American Diabetes Association, 7% is the equivalent of an average blood glucose level of 150 mg/dL. Amounts of 8% or greater indicate that control of the client's blood glucose level has been inadequate during the previous 2 to 3 months.

d. Measures capillary blood glucose from blood sampled from a finger stick. Ideally, blood sugar should measure 90 to 130 mg/dL before meals and <180 mg/dL 1 to 2 hours after meals.

e. A diet high in carbohydrates is eaten for 3 days. Client then fasts for 8 hours. A baseline blood sample is drawn, and a urine specimen is collected. An oral glucose solution is given and time of ingestion recorded. Blood is drawn at 30 minutes and 1, 2, and 3 hours after the ingestion of glucose solution. Urine is collected simultaneously. In the nondiabetic client, the glucose returns to normal in

2 to 3 hours and urine is negative for glucose.

f. Blood sample is taken 2 hours after a high-carbohydrate meal. In the nondiabetic client, the glucose level will be between 70 and 110 mg/dL

Activity E *Compare and contrast the signs and symptoms and treatments for acute complications of diabetes.*

Acute complication	Signs and symptoms	Treatment
Diabetic ketoacidosis (DKA)		
Hyperosmolar hyperglycemic nonketotic syndrome (HHNKS)		
Hypoglycemia		

Activity F *Briefly answer the following questions.*

1. Incidence of diabetes is increased among which ethnic groups?

   _____

   _____

   _____

2. What is the criterion to identify people with pre-diabetes?

   _____

   _____

   _____

3. How can individuals with pre-diabetes avoid or delay the onset of type 2 diabetes?

   _____

   _____

   _____

4. Identify the three functions of insulin.

   _____

   _____

   _____

5. Name three methods used for diet control and weight management with the diabetic client.

   _____

   _____

   _____

6. Identify and describe the three important properties of insulin.

   _____

   _____

   _____

7. Describe the procedure for mixing two types of insulin in a syringe.

   _____

   _____

   _____

8. How does diabetic nephropathy result in swelling of the hands and feet?

   _____

   _____

   _____

SECTION II: APPLYING YOUR KNOWLEDGE

Activity G *Give rationale for the following questions.*

1. Why does exercise reduce blood sugar levels in type 2 diabetes?

   _____

   _____

2. Why is a client with type 1 diabetes more likely to develop ketoacidosis and a client with type 2 diabetes more likely to develop hyperosmolar hyperglycemic nonketotic syndrome?

   _____

   _____

   _____

3. Why do infection, failure to eat, vomiting, and stress increase the risk of ketosis?

_____

_____

_____

4. Why do clients with diabetes often develop skin, urinary tract, and vaginal infections?

_____

_____

_____

5. Why might human insulin be preferred to pork or beef insulin?

_____

_____

_____

6. Why are clients with type 2 diabetes not offered the option of a pancreas transplant?

_____

_____

_____

7. Why are steroids not used to prevent rejection of islet cell transplantation?

_____

_____

_____

Activity H *Answer the following questions related to caring for clients with diabetes mellitus.*

1. Differentiate between type I and type II diabetes.

_____

_____

_____

2. How does ketoacidosis result in type 1 diabetes?

_____

_____

_____

3. Describe the pathophysiology of type 2 diabetes.

_____

_____

_____

4. The three classic signs of diabetes are polyuria, polydipsia, and polyphagia. What causes these three signs to develop in the diabetic client?

_____

_____

_____

5. Differentiate between an insulin pen, jet injector, and insulin pump and describe how each distributes insulin.

_____

_____

_____

6. Compare and contrast motor, sensory, and autonomic neuropathy.

_____

_____

_____

7. In addition to neuropathy, nephropathy, and retinopathy, what other vascular changes occur with diabetes?

_____

_____

_____

Activity I *Think over the following questions. Discuss them with your instructor or peers.*

1. Your client is a brittle diabetic; what signs and symptoms would you expect to see if the client is experiencing a hypoglycemic reaction? What treatment would you provide?

_____

_____

_____

2. Your neighbor asks you to provide assistance to their spouse, who is diabetic. You take a glucometer reading and the results are 360 mg/dL. What symptoms would you expect this person to be exhibiting? What treatment would you provide? What signs and symptoms would indicate further medical intervention is required?

_____

_____

_____

3. What educational information would you provide about foot care to a diabetic client?

_____

_____

_____

4. A diabetic client describes visual changes they are experiencing. How would you advise them?

_____

_____

_____

5. A client asks you how they can reduce their risk of long-term complications associated with diabetes. What educational information would you provide?

_____

_____

_____

SECTION III: GETTING READY FOR NCLEX

Activity J *Answer the following questions.*

1. A client with type 1 diabetes mellitus is advised pancreas and islet cell transplantation. Which of the following is the goal of this transplantation?
   a. Cholesterol reduction
   b. Muscle tone improvement
   c. Blood circulation improvement
   d. Insulin independence

2. Which of the following actions should the nurse take into consideration when a client with diabetes mellitus is on the hospital unit?
   a. Insert an indwelling urinary catheter
   b. Stock quick-acting carbohydrates
   c. Arrange for an insulin pump
   d. Administer insulin through IV route

3. Which of the following nursing actions helps the nurse to detect evidence of albuminuria when caring for a client with diabetic neuropathy?
   a. Check the urine with a test strip a
   b. Monitor blood glucose and hemoglobin A1c results.
   c. Check the postprandial glucose test results a
   d. Check the fasting blood glucose test results.

4. Which of the following instructions related to nutrients should the nurse give elderly diabetic clients who are not treated with medication?
   a. Avoid saturated fat
   b. Maintain consistency in carbohydrate intake
   c. Avoid sugar
   d. Avoid overeating

5. Which of the following are effects of using oral antidiabetic drugs in conjunction with insulin therapy in some clients with insulin-dependent diabetes?
   a. Increased response to leptin
   b. Reduced insulin requirement
   c. Fewer allergic reactions
   d. Consistency in blood glucose level

6. The client with diabetes is advised to maintain hygiene and take precautions against infections. Which of the statements are true about infections in diabetes?
   a. The elevated blood glucose reduces bacterial growth.
   b. Infection in a diabetic client cannot be treated.
   c. Infection increases the demand for insulin.
   d. The high glucose in the blood protects the client from infection.

7. A nurse is taking care of a client with diabetes who is experiencing diabetic ketoacidosis (DKA). The nurse knows that DKA is a type of what acid-base imbalance?

   a. Metabolic acidosis

   b. Respiratory acidosis

   c. Metabolic alkalosis

   d. Respiratory alkalosis

8. A nurse is taking care of a client with hyperosmolar hyperglycemic nonketotic syndrome. Which of the following is a priority area for the nurse in evaluating a client with hyperosmolar hyperglycemic nonketotic syndrome?

   a. Skin color

   b. Hydration status

   c. Temperature

   d. Response to diet

9. A nurse finds that before lunch a diabetic client is having signs of hypoglycemia. The accucheck is 54. How many grams of carbohydrates should the nurse give immediately to the client?

   a. 20 grams

   b. 15 grams

   c. 10 grams

   d. 5 grams

10. A nurse draws up 10 units of regular acting insulin to give to a client who has been diabetic for 10 years. What does the nurse do prior to giving the insulin to the client to prevent a medication error?

    a. Check the client's last glucose level drawn and inform the physician of the result.

    b. Inform the diabetic educator that the client needs education.

    c. Assume the client knows what the insulin is for and why it is to be given.

    d. Have another nurse check the amount and type of insulin drawn up against the order.

Introduction to the Reproductive System

1. Name the major external structures of the female reproductive system.
2. Name and give the functions of four internal female reproductive structures.
3. Discuss the process of ovulation.
4. Explain the physiologic changes that lead to menstruation.
5. List at least five types of reproductive data that are obtained when taking a female's health history.
6. Discuss the purpose for the cytologic test known as a Papanicolaou test.
7. Review the instructions the nurse provides for a client who is scheduling a gynecologic examination and Papanicolaou test.
8. Name diagnostic tests used for diagnosing disorders of the female reproductive system.
9. Describe the anatomy and physiology of the breast.
10. Explain the differences between a clinical breast examination and breast self-examination.
11. Discuss the advantages of a mammographic examination.
12. Name three techniques for performing a breast biopsy.
13. Identify the major external structures of the male reproductive system.
14. Name and give the functions of the chief internal male reproductive structures.
15. List three accessory structures of the male reproductive system.
16. Explain the terms: erection, emission, and ejaculation.
17. List at least five types of reproductive data that are obtained when taking a male's health history.
18. Name techniques for physically assessing male reproductive structures.
19. List methods that are used to diagnose prostate cancer.
20. Name two tests for determining infertility problems in males.

SECTION I: ASSESSING YOUR UNDERSTANDING

Activity A *Fill in the blanks by choosing the correct word from the options given in parentheses.*

1. _____ causes the mature follicle to rupture, thereby releasing an ovum from the ovary. *(Luteinizing hormone, Follicle-stimulating hormone, Growth hormone)*

2. _____ is a test that is used mainly to detect early cancer of the cervix and secondarily to determine estrogen activity as it relates to menopause or endocrine abnormalities. *(Endometrial smear, Papanicolaou test, Culdoscopy)*

3. _____ is performed when results from a Pap test are positive or questionable. *(Cervical biopsy, Endometrial smear, Culdoscopy)*

4. _____ refers to the manual palpation of the breast performed by a physician, nurse, or physician's assistant that is performed during a client's gynecologic examination, before a mammogram, or during an annual physical examination. *(Mammography, Breast self-examination, Clinical breast examination)*

5. The _____ lie within the scrotum and are responsible for spermatogenesis, or sperm production, and secretion of testosterone. *(Ductus deferens, Epididymis, Testes)*

6. The _____ loops through the inguinal canal and into the pelvic cavity before it descends to the prostate gland. The wall of the ductus deferens contains smooth muscle that moves sperm along the ductal pathway. *(Spermatic cord, Testes, Epididymis)*

Activity B *Mark each statement as either "T" (True) or "F" (False). Correct any false statements.*

1. T F Diagnosing cancer of the endometrium is accomplished by dilatation of the cervix and curettage of the endometrium.

2. T F Culdoscopy is an examination of the interior of the abdomen using a special endoscope called a laparoscope, which is inserted through a small incision located one-half inch below the umbilicus. A culdoscopy is used to detect an ectopic pregnancy, to perform a tubal ligation, to obtain ovarian tissue for biopsy, and to detect pelvic abnormalities.

3. T F An abdominal ultrasonography aids in visualizing soft tissue by recording the reflection of sound waves. An abdominal ultrasound detects pelvic abnormalities such as tumors and the size and location of fetal and placental tissue.

4. T F The ductus deferens collects the spermatocytes from the seminiferous tubules.

5. T F Erection refers to a state in which the penis becomes elongated and rigid, facilitating its insertion into the female vagina. Erection takes place as a result of parasympathetic nerve activity.

6. T F The movement of sperm mixed with fluid from the seminal vesicles and prostate gland into the urethra is called ejaculation, a process mediated via the sympathetic nervous system.

Activity C *Write the correct term for the descriptions given below.*

1. When the reproductive system becomes active and functional. _____

2. The anterior pituitary hormone known as follicle-stimulating hormone (FSH) initiates this monthly. _____

3. Begins about 2 weeks after ovulation; usually lasts 4 to 5 days, with a normal loss of 30 to 60 mL of blood. _____

4. Age of the first menstruation. _____

5. A procedure used to visualize the cervix and vagina. A speculum is inserted into the vagina, and the surface areas are examined with a light and magnifying lens. _____

6. The testes are subdivided into lobules containing coiled _____. Within the tubules, spermatocytes (immature spermatozoa) form.

Activity D *Match the examination procedures and diagnostic tests performed to evaluate the male genitourinary tract, given in Column A, with their descriptions given in Column B.*

Column A

___ 1. Transrectal Ultrasonography (TRUS)

___ 2. Cystoscopy

___ 3. Needle Biopsy of Prostatic Tissue

___ 4. Testicular Biopsy

___ 5. Digital Rectal Examination (DRE)

___ 6. Fertility studies

___ 7. Transillumination

___ 8. Prostate-Specific Antigen (PSA)

___ 9. Cultures

Column B

a. Obtained to diagnose a definitive cancer of the prostate when other assessment findings like digital rectal examination and prostate-specific antigen (PSA) appear suspiciously abnormal. The biopsy is obtained via the perineal or rectal approach.

b. Evaluates spermatozoa production for diagnosing infertility problems or testicular malignancy.

c. A test in which a lubricated probe is inserted into the rectum to obtain a view of the prostate gland from various angles. The test is indicated in cases in which the prostate gland is enlarged or the blood level of prostate-specific antigen is elevated.

d. An illuminated optical instrument is inserted into the urinary meatus to inspect the bladder, prostate, and urethra. This aids in evaluating the degree of encroachment by the prostate on the urethra.

e. Performed to assess the prostate for size as well as evidence of tumor. Yearly examinations are recommended for men older than 40 to 50 years of age.

f. A blood test that detects prostate cancer.

g. Obtained from urethral secretions, skin lesions, or urine. Prostatic fluid can be expressed during a DRE and also sent.

h. Includes a semen analysis to determine sperm count, sperm motility, and abnormal sperm. Other laboratory tests may include measuring the level of plasma LH, which is necessary for the release of testosterone from the testes.

i. Shining a light through the scrotum provides clues about the density of scrotal tissue.

Activity E *Provide the description and purpose of the following diagnostic tests used to evaluate the female breasts.*

Diagnostic Test	Description	Purpose
Mammography		
Ultrasonography		
Breast Biopsy		
Incisional Biopsy *(description only)*		
Excisional Biopsy *(description only)*		
Aspirational Biopsy *(description only)*		

Activity F *Briefly answer the following questions.*

1. Provide a description for each of the major female external structures; mons pubis, vaginal orifice, Bartholin glands, labia majora, labia minora, clitoris, fourchette, and hymen.

_____

_____

_____

2. Describe the procedure for a gynecological examination.

_____

_____

_____

3. What instructions will the nurse provide to a client scheduling a Papanicolaou test?

_____

_____

_____

4. What is a hysterosalpingogram? What is it used for?

_____

_____

_____

5. What are the recommendations for breast examinations by the American Cancer Society (ACS)?

_____

_____

_____

6. How does the scrotum maintain the temperature of the testes at 3 degrees cooler than body temperature?

_____

_____

_____

SECTION II: APPLYING YOUR KNOWLEDGE

Activity G _Provide rationale for the following questions._

1. Why is routine douching of the vagina discouraged?

_____

_____

_____

2. Why does the endometrium become thick and vascular during ovulation?

_____

_____

_____

3. Why is it important that each gynecologic specimen sent to the laboratory be marked with the date of the beginning of the client's last menstrual period (LMP)?

_____

_____

_____

4. Why are breast self-examinations (BSE) encouraged even though they play a small role in the detection of breast cancer?

_____

_____

_____

5. Why may the older male experience difficulty with urination?

_____

_____

_____

Activity H _Answer the following questions related to the reproductive system._

1. Identify the internal female structures and describe their function.

_____

_____

_____

2. Describe the process of fertilization and implantation.

_____

_____

_____

3. What are the recommendations by the American Cancer Society for the Papanicolaou test? What are additional recommendations for testing?

_____

_____

_____

4. Provide a description and identify the major function of the female breasts.

_____

_____

_____

5. Describe the external structures of the male reproductive system.

_____

_____

_____

6. Describe the accessory structures of the male reproductive system.

_____

_____

_____

Activity I *Think over the following questions. Discuss them with your instructor or peers.*

1. A married couple is trying to conceive and asks your advice about how to increase their chances of conception. Based on your knowledge of the female and male reproductive systems, how would you advise them?

_____

_____

_____

2. A male client is being seen by the physician about erectile dysfunction. What information is significant for you to obtain about the client's history and reproductive health?

_____

_____

_____

3. A female client is being seen by the physician about irregular menstruation. What essential information will you obtain about the client's history and reproductive health?

_____

_____

_____

SECTION III: GETTING READY FOR NCLEX

Activity J *Answer the following questions.*

1. Why is rupturing of the hymen not considered a confirmation of loss of virginity?
   a. Because the hymen is not affected by any sexual activity
   b. Because the hymen can be perforated during physical activity, insertion of a tampon, or pelvic examination.
   c. Because the hymen is ruptured the first time a person urinates.
   d. Because the hymen is very delicate and may be ruptured even when running or doing strenuous exercises.

2. Which of the following assessments does a nurse obtain to ensure a thorough baseline history of a client?
   a. Age of menarche, the first menstruation
   b. Accident history
   c. Mother's past menstruation patterns
   d. Frequency of sexual activities

3. Which of the following reasons should a nurse provide a client when asked about the purpose of a Papanicolaou test?
   a. It is used to detect early breast cancer.
   b. It is used to detect early cancer of the cervix.
   c. It is used to detect the fertility status of the woman.
   d. It is used to detect early stages of an STD.

4. A client who is scheduled for an endometrial biopsy expresses concerns about the procedure as she is apprehensive of "being operated" on. How can the nurse relieve her anxiety?
   a. The nurse should inform her that this test will not require her to be under anesthetic influence for a long period.
   b. The nurse should inform her that this test will be performed under general anesthesia and she will be pain free.
   c. The nurse should inform her that this test will be performed under the care of expert physicians and nurses.
   d. The nurse should inform her that this procedure may be performed without anesthesia in the physician's office.

5. The nurse monitors a client who has gone through an endoscopic examination. Following a culdoscopy, what does a nurse need to observe for in this client?
   a. The nurse observes the client for any discomfort in the shoulders.
   b. The nurse observes the client for the signs of internal bleeding and the symptoms of shock.
   c. The nurse observes the client for changes in skin color and for any rise in body temperature.
   d. The nurse observes the quantity and frequency of urinary output.

6. What is the function of the prolactin hormone?

   a. Prolactin promotes the production of milk from elements in the blood.

   b. Prolactin stimulates the development of alveoli.

   c. Prolactin stimulates increased production of tubules and ducts.

   d. Prolactin promotes the growth and development of the breasts' fatty tissue.

7. During a physical examination of the male reproductive system, how does the nurse assist the examiner to gather clues about the density of scrotal tissue?

   a. Through a digital rectal examination

   b. By externally inspecting the size of the scrotum

   c. Through transillumination

   d. Through a scrotal radiography

8. When men age, what is the effect of prostate gland enlargement?

   a. It compromises the ability to fertilize ova

   b. It compromises erectile function

   c. It compromises urination

   d. It compromises sperm production

9. A male nurse is teaching a client about the scrotum and the ability of sperm to be effective in fertility. The nurse teaches the client that the sperm is contained in the testes and that its temperature is regulated by which of the following?

   a. Penis and surrounding structures

   b. Bladder tone

   c. Structure of the scrotum

   d. Smooth and skeletal muscles in the scrotum

10. A nurse identifies a client with an abnormal lab test that screens for prostate cancer. What is the test that the client will receive to screen for prostate cancer?

    a. PAS

    b. APS

    c. PSA

    d. PCA

CHAPTER 53

Caring for Clients with Disorders of the Female Reproductive System

Learning Objectives

1. Describe at least four conditions that deviate from normal menstrual patterns.
2. Describe the purpose of and how to keep a menstrual diary.
3. Give two examples of disorders characterized by amenorrhea and oligomenorrhea.
4. Discuss therapeutic techniques and nursing management for menstrual disorders.
5. List several physiologic consequences of menopause.
6. Give reasons for and against hormone replacement therapy.
7. Name four infectious and inflammatory conditions common in women and one cause for each.
8. Describe the signs and symptoms that differentiate three types of vaginal infections.
9. Discuss methods that may help prevent vaginal infections or their recurrence.
10. Describe the technique for inserting vaginal medications.
11. Name at least four aspects of nursing care for clients with pelvic inflammatory disease.
12. Give at least two suggestions that can help women avoid toxic shock syndrome.
13. List four structural abnormalities of the female reproductive system and their effects on fertility or sexuality.
14. Discuss methods the nurse can use to help a client select an appropriate treatment for endometriosis.
15. List three problems experienced by women who develop vaginal fistulas, and related nursing management.
16. Give examples of appropriate information when teaching a client to use a pessary.
17. Explain the term *carcinoma in situ* and how it applies to the prognosis of women with gynecologic malignancies.
18. Identify the most common reproductive cancers and methods for early diagnosis.
19. Discuss nursing diagnoses and potential complications among clients who undergo a hysterectomy and nursing interventions important to include in their care.
20. Give two reasons that explain the high lethality associated with ovarian cancer.
21. Name three possible causes of vaginal cancer.
22. Discuss the nursing management of and appropriate discharge instructions for a client who has a radical vulvectomy for vulvar cancer.

SECTION I: ASSESSING YOUR UNDERSTANDING

Activity A *Fill in the blanks by choosing the correct word from the options given in parentheses.*

1. Treatment of _____ includes IV fluids to support circulation while combating the infection with IV antibiotic therapy. Potent

adrenergic drugs are given to counteract peripheral vasodilation and maintain renal perfusion. Oxygen is given to promote aerobic metabolism at the cellular level. *(Vaginitis, Pelvic inflammatory disease, Toxic shock syndrome)*

2. _____ is a condition in which tissue with a cellular structure and function resembling that of the endometrium is found outside the uterus. *(Endometriosis, Vaginal fistula, Pelvic organ prolapse)*

3. A _____ is an unnatural opening between two structures. *(Prolapse, Fistula, Abscess)*

4. A _____ is a firm, doughnut-shaped or ring device which may be inserted in the upper vagina to reposition and give support to the uterus when surgery cannot be done or the client declines surgery. *(Kegel, Pessary, Colporrhaphy)*

5. A _____ (also called myoma) is a benign uterine growth principally consisting of smooth muscle and fibrous connective tissue. Myomas, which are the most common tumor in the female pelvis, often are referred to as fibroid tumors. *(Leiomyoma, Endometriosis, Vaginal Fistula)*

6. A localized malignancy is referred to as _____. *(Premalignant, Non-malignant, Carcinoma in situ)*

7. Cancer of the _____ is relatively rare. It usually occurs in women older than 60 years of age, but cases among younger women have arisen recently. This type of cancer is highly curable when diagnosed in an early stage. *(Ovaries, Cervix, Vulva)*

Activity B *Mark each statement as either "T" (True) or "F" (False). Correct any false statements.*

1. T F   Douches and local or systemic antibiotics are the treatment of choice for acute cervicitis. Chronic cervicitis is treated with electrocautery.

2. T F   If surgical repair of a vaginal fistula is possible, it is performed after inflammation and edema have disappeared. Until then, symptomatic treatment to reduce the risk for infection and manage skin excoriation is provided.

3. T F   Clients with rectocele may experience stress incontinence—a little urine seeps every time the woman coughs, sneezes, laughs, bears down, or strains. Cystitis results from the stagnation of urine in the bladder.

4. T F   An enterocele is the downward displacement of the cervix anywhere from low in the vagina to outside the vagina.

5. T F   Symptoms of a uterovaginal prolapse include backache, pelvic pain, fatigue, and a feeling that "something is dropping out," especially when lifting a heavy object, coughing, or standing for prolonged periods.

6. T F   An ovarian cyst is a membranous sac filled with fluid, cells, or both. Ovarian cysts, which are benign, are filled with fluid. Benign ovarian tumors are noncancerous growths of solid tissue.

7. T F   Only a small percentage of clients with malignant tumors of the ovary survive 5 or more years despite intensive treatment.

Activity C *Write the correct term for each description given below.*

1. This hormone deficiency causes thinning of the vaginal walls, breast and uterine atrophy, and loss of bone density. The risks of heart disease and stroke increase with reduction in this hormone. _____

2. Hospitalization with complete bed rest often is necessary. Parenteral or oral antibiotics are administered as soon as culture and sensitivity tests are obtained. Intravenous (IV) fluids are ordered if the client is dehydrated, and antipyretics are used if the temperature is elevated. A ruptured pelvic abscess requires emergency surgery. _____

3. Severe dysmenorrhea and copious menstrual bleeding are typical symptoms. The client may experience dyspareunia and pain on defecation. Rupture of a chocolate cyst results in severe abdominal pain that can mimic other abdominal pathologies such as appendicitis or bowel obstruction. _____

TABLE 53-1

Disorder	Description	Signs and Symptoms	Treatment
Premenstrual syndrome (PMS), in the extreme called premenstrual dysphoric disorder (PMDD)			
Dysmenorrhea			
Amenorrhea			N/A
Oligomenorrhea			
Premature ovarian failure (POF)			N/A
Polycystic ovarian syndrome			
Menorrhagia			
Metrorrhagia			

4. They result in the continuous drainage of urine or feces from the vagina. The vaginal wall and the external genitalia become excoriated and often infected. The client may not void through the urethra because urine does not accumulate in the bladder. _____

5. These exercises are also known as pelvic floor strengthening exercises. They are recommended when there is stress incontinence.

_____

6. When symptoms exist, menorrhagia is most common. There can be a feeling of pressure in the pelvic region, dysmenorrhea, anemia (from loss of blood), and malaise.

_____

7. The incidence of this type of cancer is higher among women infected with HPV, a sexually transmitted microorganism, and among those who use a pessary but neglect to remove and clean it. _____

Activity D *Compare the infectious and inflammatory disorders given below in terms of their pathophysiology and signs and symptoms.*

Disorder	Pathophysiology	Signs and Symptoms
Vaginitis		
Cervicitis		
Pelvic inflammatory disease (PID)		
Toxic shock syndrome (TSS)		

Activity E *Compare the disorders listed in Table 53-1 in terms of their description, signs and symptoms, and treatment.*

Activity F *Briefly answer the following questions.*

1. What is a menstrual diary? What is it used for?

_____

_____

_____

2. What is the nurse's role when caring for the client with a menstrual disorder?

_____

_____

_____

3. Describe the treatment for infectious vaginitis.

_____

_____

_____

4. Describe the types of uterine displacements. What are the typical causes?

_____

_____

_____

5. What are the signs and symptoms of cervical and endometrial cancer?

_____

_____

_____

6. What is an important role of the nurse in the prevention and early diagnosis of cervical and endometrial cancer?

_____

_____

_____

7. Describe the medical and surgical management of an ovarian cyst.

_____

_____

_____

SECTION II: APPLYING YOUR KNOWLEDGE

Activity G *Give rationale for the following questions.*

1. If hormone replacement therapy (HRT) is indicated for the treatment of menopause, why it is prescribed in the lowest appropriate dose for a relatively short time?

_____

_____

_____

2. Why are low dose androgens given to women who are menopausal?

_____

_____

_____

3. Why are women taking HRT instructed to contact the physician if tenderness, pain, swelling, or redness occurs in the legs?

_____

_____

_____

4. Why are older women predisposed for development of vaginitis?

_____

_____

_____

5. Historically, why has ovarian cancer been so lethal?

_____

_____

_____

6. Why are client with HPV and herpes simplex virus type 2 at lifelong risk for genital cancer?

_____

_____

_____

Activity H *Answer the following questions related to caring for the client with disorders of the female reproductive system.*

1. Describe the process of menopause.

_____

_____

_____

2. Describe the pathophysiology of endometriosis.

_____

_____

_____

3. What are the treatment options for endometriosis?

_____

_____

_____

4. Describe the pathophysiology of pelvic organ prolapse.

_____

_____

_____

5. What are the instructions for use of a pessary?

    _____

    _____

    _____

6. What are the risk factors associated with cervical and endometrial cancer?

    _____

    _____

    _____

7. What preventative measures are recommended for women at high risk for ovarian cancer?

    _____

    _____

    _____

Activity I *Think over the following questions. Discuss them with your instructor or peers.*

1. A client asks you how to prevent vaginal infections. What educational information will you provide?

    _____

    _____

    _____

2. What high priority nursing diagnoses and interventions will you identify for the client undergoing a hysterectomy?

    _____

    _____

    _____

3. What educational information will you provide to the client undergoing a hysterectomy?

    _____

    _____

    _____

4. What nutritional information will you provide to the client with premenstrual syndrome?

    _____

    _____

    _____

SECTION III: GETTING READY FOR NCLEX

Activity J *Answer the following questions.*

1. Vaginal candidacies are suspected in a young woman who complains of severe vaginal itching. Which of the following nursing actions should be performed first when assisting in the collection of a vaginal smear for microscopic examination?

    a. Inspect the external genitalia

    b. Don gloves

    c. Wash hands

    d. Label the specimen

2. Women infected with human papilloma virus (HPV) are at risk for which of the following?

    a. Uterine fibroids

    b. Cervical cancer

    c. Ovarian cysts

    d. Hemorrhagic

3. A client has been advised to use a pessary to provide support to the uterus. The nurse educates the client about pessary management and the precautions related to its use. In which of the following situations should the client report to the physician?

    a. Regarding a Pap test of the client

    b. Regarding the maintenance of a pessary

    c. When a white or yellow discharge from the vagina develops

    d. Regarding a culture and sensitivity test of vagina

4. A client has been diagnosed with thrombophlebitis. The nurse needs to closely monitor the client for detecting, managing, and minimizing the risk for thrombophlebitis development. Which of the following nursing actions will help a nurse minimize the occurrence of thrombophlebitis in the client?

    a. Give warm sitz baths after sutures have been removed

    b. Apply an air or egg crate mattress to the bed

    c. Administer prescribed analgesics liberally

    d. Assess for and report calf pain or calf tenderness

5. Which of the following are the advantages of a vaginal hysterectomy over an abdominal hysterectomy?

   a. Fewer complications

   b. Increased recovery time

   c. Radical hysterectomy can even be done laparoscopically

   d. No pain

6. Chronic cervicitis is treated with _____.

7. A client diagnosed with a vaginal fistula is at risk for low self-esteem. Which of the following would be an appropriate recommendation for the client?

   a. Wear disposable, absorbent incontinence briefs

   b. Avoid the use of commercial deodorizers at home

   c. Abstain from sexual intercourse

   d. Avoid frequent douches

8. PID is an infection of the pelvic organs, excepting the uterus. The nurse's role in caring for a client hospitalized with PID includes which of the following?

   a. The nurse inquires if the client has douched within the last 48 hours

   b. The nurse advises a douche every hour prior to being examined

   c. The nurse avoids administering analgesics

   d. The nurse avoids washing the perineal area

9. Why should a nurse educate women to have regular gynecologic examinations and Pap tests?

   a. It helps decide the mode of surgical treatment.

   b. It is the best cure for most infections.

   c. It increases the potential for an early diagnosis.

   d. It is an inexpensive test.

10. A client is asking the nurse questions about the diagnosis of endometriosis. The nurse teaches the client that endometrial tissue is found outside the uterus and that the major symptom that a client experiences is which of the following?

   a. Pain

   b. Infection

   c. Minimal bleeding

   d. Cramping

CHAPTER 54

Caring for Clients with Breast Disorders

Learning Objectives

1. List four signs and symptoms that are common in breast disorders.
2. Name two infectious and inflammatory breast disorders and explain how they are acquired.
3. Discuss health teaching that may help prevent or eliminate infectious and inflammatory breast disorders.
4. Compare and contrast two benign breast disorders.
5. Name groups at high risk for developing breast cancer.
6. List common signs and symptoms of breast cancer.
7. Describe four methods for treating cancer, including six surgical techniques used to remove a malignant breast tumor.
8. Give two criteria that are used when selecting a mastectomy procedure.
9. Name a serious complication of breast cancer treatment.
10. Discuss the nursing management of clients who undergo surgical treatment for breast cancer.
11. List four sites to which breast cancer commonly metastasizes.
12. Describe three elective cosmetic breast procedures for clients with a mastectomy.
13. Describe three cosmetic breast procedures that women with nondiseased breasts may elect.

SECTION I: ASSESSING YOUR UNDERSTANDING

Activity A *Fill in the blanks by choosing the correct word from the options given in parentheses.*

1. The breasts' primary function is the production of milk, a process referred to as _____ *(Gestation, Lactation, Ovulation)*

2. Signs and symptoms of _____ include fever and malaise, breast tenderness, pain, and redness. The breast later becomes swollen, firm, and hard. A crack in the nipple or areola develops, and the axillary lymph nodes enlarge. *(Mastitis, Breast abscess, Fibroadenoma)*

3. _____ is a benign breast condition that affects women primarily between the ages of 30 and 50 years. *(Mastitis, Fibroadenoma, Fibrocystic breast disease)*

4. One in _____ women develops breast cancer. *(Five, Eight, Ten)*

5. Side effects of _____ include nausea, vomiting, changes in taste, alopecia (hair loss), mucositis, dermatitis, fatigue, weight gain, and bone marrow suppression. *(Radiation, Chemotherapy, Radial breast mastectomy)*

6. _____ are most commonly involved in metastasis. Skeletal and pulmonary systems may also be involved (in that order). In addition, metastases may be found in the brain and liver. (*Lymph nodes, Cardiac tissue, Skin tissue*)

Activity B *Mark each statement as either "T" (True) or "F" (False). Correct any false statements.*

1. T F   A breast abscess is a localized collection of pus in breast tissue.

2. T F   There is a correlation between fibrocystic breast disease and breast cancer.

3. T F   A fibroadenoma, a benign tumor, is a single nodule that grows slowly in non-pregnant women until it reaches a fixed, stable size. It usually does not enlarge and regress with each menstrual cycle, like those in fibrocystic breast disease, and is not considered precancerous.

4. T F   Mammography detects breast lesions earlier than they can be palpated.

5. T F   Radiation therapy is never given after a modified radical mastectomy.

6. T F   Side effects of radiation therapy include bone marrow depression, granulocytopenia, anemia, nausea and vomiting, hypotension, dermatitis, malaise, diarrhea, and stomatitis.

Activity C *Write the correct term for each description given below.*

1. It is most common in women who are breast-feeding. Although inflammation can occur at any time, it is most common during the 2nd or 3rd week postpartum. _____

2. Most frequently occurs as a complication of postpartum mastitis. Purulent exudate accumulates in a confined, local area of breast tissue. The client is usually started on intravenous (IV) antibiotic therapy and may require incision, drainage, and packing. _____

3. This condition may produce no symptoms. However, many women report having tender or painful breasts and feeling one or more often multiple lumps within breast tissue. The symptoms are most noticeable just before menstruation and usually abate during menstruation. _____

4. A solid, benign breast mass composed of connective and glandular tissue. This type of breast lesion usually occurs in women during late adolescence and early adulthood, but occasionally it is found in older women. _____

5. Soft-tissue swelling from accumulated lymphatic fluid that occurs in some women after they have undergone breast cancer surgery. The condition, a consequence of removing or irradiating the axillary lymph nodes, is evidenced by temporary or permanent enlargement of the arm and hand on the side of the amputated breast. _____

6. The migration of cancer cells from one part of the body to another. Malignant cells are spread by direct extension, through the lymphatic system, bloodstream, and cerebrospinal fluid. _____

Activity D *Match the surgical procedures for breast cancer given in Column A with their descriptions in Column B.*

Column A

____ **1.** Lumpectomy

____ **2.** Partial or segmental mastectomy

____ **3.** Simple or total mastectomy

____ **4.** Subcutaneous mastectomy

____ **5.** Modified radical mastectomy

____ **6.** Radical mastectomy

Column B

a. The breast, the axillary lymph nodes, and pectoralis major and minor muscles are removed. In some instances, sternal lymph nodes are also removed.

b. The tumor and some breast tissue and some lymph nodes are removed.

c. The breast, some lymph nodes, the lining over the chest muscle, and the pectoralis minor muscle are removed.

d. All breast tissue is removed, but the skin and nipple are left intact.

e. Only the tumor is removed; some axillary lymph nodes may be excised at the same time for microscopic examination.

f. All breast tissue is removed. No lymph node dissection is performed.

Activity E *Compare and contrast the following cosmetic breast procedures.*

Cosmetic Breast Procedure	Description
Breast Reconstruction	
Artificial Implants	
Autogenous Tissue	
Reduction Mammoplasty	
Opposite Breast Reduction	
Mastopexy (Breast lift)	
Breast Augmentation	

Activity F *Briefly answer the following questions.*

1. Describe the pathophysiology of mastitis.

2. What is the cause of fibrocystic disease?

3. How does breast cancer spread to distant areas?

4. What are the signs and symptoms of breast cancer?

5. What is the treatment for breast cancer?

6. What options are available for women at increased risk of developing breast cancer?

SECTION II: APPLYING YOUR KNOWLEDGE

Activity G *Give rationale for the following questions.*

1. Why are clients diagnosed with a breast abscess placed in contact isolation precautions?

2. Why are the arms and shoulders of the client with a breast abscess supported on pillows?

3. Why might older women mistake changes in their breasts associated with aging for signs of breast cancer?

4. Why can lymphedema be a serious complication following breast cancer surgery?

5. Why are antiemetics and anxiolytic medications administered before chemotherapy?

6. Why would taking nonsteroidal anti-inflammatory drugs (NSAIDs) be beneficial to the client at risk for the development of breast cancer?

_____

_____

_____

Activity H *Answer the following questions related to caring for clients with breast disorders.*

1. What educational information will the nurse provide to the client with mastitis?

_____

_____

_____

2. What educational information will the nurse provide to the client with fibrocystic breast disease?

_____

_____

_____

3. What are the risk factors associated with breast cancer?

_____

_____

_____

4. What instructions will the nurse provide to the client with fibroadenoma?

_____

_____

5. What information must the nurse commonly address with clients following breast cancer surgery?

_____

_____

_____

6. Identify the action/purpose of each of the following medications used in the treatment of breast cancer:
   Antiestrogen drug; Aromatase inhibitors (AIs); Antiprogestin drug; Androgen therapy; Single or combined antineoplastic agents.

_____

_____

_____

Activity I *Think over the following questions. Discuss them with your instructor or peers.*

1. You are providing post operative instruction to a client following breast cancer surgery. What information will you provide about post operative arm exercises?

_____

_____

_____

2. What high priority nursing diagnoses and intervention will you identify for the client with infectious and inflammatory breast disorders?

_____

_____

_____

3. What educational information will you provide to the client following breast cancer surgery?

_____

_____

_____

4. What high priority nursing diagnoses and interventions will you identify for the client following breast cancer surgery?

_____

_____

_____

SECTION III: GETTING READY FOR NCLEX

Activity J *Answer the following questions.*

1. Which of the following adverse reactions may occur when a client is taking danzol (Danocrine) for fibrocystic breast disease?

   a. Nausea

   b. Confusion

   c. Amenorrhea

   d. Hypotension

2. Which of the following findings would confirm that a female client has mastitis? Choose all that apply.

   a. A crack in the nipple or the areola

   b. Multiple lumps within the breast tissue

   c. Flat and soft breasts

   d. Breast tenderness, without any sensation or pain

3. Which of the following is a reason for providing early discharge instructions and making arrangements for home care for clients undergoing mastectomy?

   a. The adverse effects of mastectomy are immediate.

   b. The wound of the surgery is highly contagious and the client should exercise isolation precautions immediately after the procedure.

   c. Most clients are not hospitalized long after a mastectomy.

   d. The suicidal tendencies in women undergoing a mastectomy are high.

4. Which of the following suggestions should a nurse give breast-feeding mothers to prevent or eliminate mastitis and breast abscess?

   a. Offer the opposite breast at each feeding to their infants.

   b. Minimize frequent nursing of the infants.

   c. Avoid breast-feeding.

   d. Avoid bathing or showering regularly.

5. Which of the following nursing interventions would a nurse perform to avoid maceration from irritating drainage or wound compresses in a client with a breast abscess?

   a. Apply zinc oxide to the surrounding skin.

   b. Use a binder to hold the dressing in place.

   c. Support the arm and the shoulder with pillows.

   d. Instruct the client not to shave the axillary hair on the side with the abscess.

6. Which of the following is the primary sign of breast cancer?

   a. A bloody discharge from the nipple

   b. A dimpling of the skin over the lesion

   c. A retraction of the nipple

   d. A painless mass in the breast

7. When a nurse is educating a group of women about the risks of breast cancer, she includes which of the following common risk factor?

   a. Older than 30 years of age

   b. Family history of breast cancer

   c. African-American heritage

   d. Early menopause

8. Which diagnostic study is recommended for high risk clients in addition to mammography?

   a. Breast biopsy

   b. MRI

   c. Ultrasound

   d. CT scan

9. A client is undergoing sentinel lymph node mapping. A nurse explains that this new technique reduces the likelihood of which complication?

   a. Wound dehiscence

   b. Lymphedema

   c. Excessive scarring

   d. Cellulitis

10. A nurse is working with a client who has undergone chemotherapy for breast cancer. The client is experiencing body image disturbances. Which of the following symptoms would contribute to this psychosocial issue?

   a. Fatigue

   b. Vomiting

   c. Alopecia

   d. Nausea

CHAPTER 55

Caring for Clients with Disorders of the Male Reproductive System

Learning Objectives

1. Give four examples of structural disorders that affect the male reproductive system.
2. Explain the technique and purpose for performing testicular self-examination.
3. List three infectious or inflammatory conditions and how they are acquired.
4. Discuss two erectile disorders and explain their effects on fertility and sexuality.
5. Identify two methods for treating erectile dysfunction.
6. Describe nursing care for a client being treated for erectile dysfunction.
7. Explain how prostatic hyperplasia compromises urinary elimination, and the symptoms it produces.
8. Discuss the nursing management of a client undergoing a prostatectomy.
9. Compare and contrast three male reproductive cancers in terms of age of onset, incidence, and treatment outcomes.
10. List home care instructions after a vasectomy.

SECTION I: ASSESSING YOUR UNDERSTANDING

Activity A *Fill in the blanks by choosing the correct word from the options given in parentheses.*

1. _____ refers to an inability to retract the foreskin (prepuce). The condition is often caused by congenitally small foreskin; however, chronic inflammation at the glans penis and prepuce secondary to poor hygiene or infection also are etiologic factors. *(Phimosis, Paraphimosis, Torsion)*

2. Medical treatment for _____ consists of bed rest, scrotal elevation, analgesics, anti-inflammatory agents, and comfort measures such as local cold applications. Antibiotic therapy is initiated to eliminate the infectious agent. *(Phimosis and paraphimosis, Epididymis and orchitis, Hydrocele and Spermatocele)*

3. _____ is a condition in which the penis becomes engorged and remains persistently erect without any sexual stimulation. *(Phimosis, Paraphimosis, Priapism)*

4. When the number of nonmalignant cells in the prostate gland increases it is called _____ *(A spermatocele, Benign prostatic hyperplasia, A hydrocele)*

5. Because residual urine is a good culture medium for bacteria, symptoms of _____ (inflammation of the bladder) may develop with benign prostatic hyperplasia. *(Cystitis, Epididymis, Orchitis)*

6. _____ cancer is second to skin cancer in frequency among American men. It ranks second as the cause of deaths from cancer. About 1 American male in 6 will be diagnosed with this type of cancer, and 1 in 35 will die of the disease. *(Prostatic, Testicular, Penile)*

7. A _____ is a surgical attempt to reverse an elective sterilization by restoring patency and continuity to the vas deferens. It may take from 3 to 6 months after reversal procedures before sperm counts and motility are normal. Lack of success usually is the result of either scar formation or sperm leakage from the surgical connection. *(Vasectomy, Transurethral needle ablation, Vasovasostomy)*

Activity B *Mark each statement as either "T" (True) or "F" (False). Correct any false statements.*

1. T F Torsion is a condition in which one or both testes fail to descend into the scrotum.

2. T F Circumcision is recommended for phimosis and paraphimosis to relieve these conditions permanently; if surgery is not indicated, the client is instructed to wash under the foreskin daily and seek care if he cannot retract the tissue.

3. T F Hydrocele, spermatocele, and varicocele all present as a swelling of the scrotum but in each case, the conditions are somewhat different.

4. T F When using ice for treatment of scrotal swelling the nurse places the ice bag on top of the scrotum directly against the skin.

5. T F Common causes of erectile dysfunction (ED) include neurologic disorder such as spinal cord injury, perineal trauma, testosterone insufficiency, side effects of drug therapy, atherosclerosis, hypertension, and complications of diabetes mellitus. ED also may be related to anxiety or depression.

6. T F With priapism, if the erection lasts longer than 6 hours, the tissue may be sufficiently damaged to result in impotence.

Activity C *Write the correct term for each description given below.*

1. Clients report a sudden, sharp testicular pain, with visible local swelling. The pain may be so severe that nausea, vomiting, chills, and fever occur. The condition may follow severe exercise, but it also may occur during sleep or after a simple maneuver such as crossing the legs. _____

2. A strangulation of the glans penis from an inability to replace the retracted foreskin. If the condition continues, severe edema and urinary retention may occur. _____

3. The underlying etiology of this disorder usually is a vascular problem, a medical condition that causes blood to thicken, or a side effect of medications, including those prescribed to treat impotence. _____

4. The client notices that it takes more effort to void. Eventually, the urinary stream narrows and has decreased force. The bladder empties incompletely. As residual urine accumulates, the client has the urge to void more often and nocturia occurs. _____

5. In the early stage of benign prostatic hyperplasia the progression of prostatic enlargement is monitored with this periodic examination. _____

6. This minor surgical procedure involves the ligation of the vas deferens and results in permanent sterilization by interrupting the pathway that transports sperm.

_____

Activity D *Match the options for treating erectile dysfunction in Column A with their descriptions in Column B.*

Column A	Column B
____ 1. Sildenafil (Viagra) phosphodiesterase inhibitors	a. An injection site is selected on either of the lateral sides of the penis. The prescribed medication is injected into erectile tissue at a 90-degree angle.
____ 2. Apomorphine (Uprima) a dopamine agonist	

_____ **3.** Papaverine
(Pavatine)
with phentola-
mine (Regitine)
or alprostadil
(Caverject).

_____ **4.** A vacuum
device

_____ **5.** Surgically
implanted
penile prosthesis

b. One type contains a
saline reservoir that is
pumped to fill the
implant when sexual
activity is desired, and
the other type
maintains the penis in
a semierect state at
all times.

c. Administered as a
nasal spray and acts
within 15 to 25
minutes of administra-
tion. This medication
is safer for men with
coronary artery
disease.

d. Facilitates penile
erection by producing
smooth muscle
relaxation in the cor-
pora cavernosa, facili-
tating an inflow of
blood. These
drugs are taken 1/2
hour to 1 hour
before sexual
activity. They
have no erectile
effect without
sexual
stimulation.

e. The device is used
to engorge the penis
with blood.
A constricting
attachment
prohibits the
outflow of
blood to sustain
the erection.

Activity E _Compare and contrast prostatic, testicular, and penile cancer based on the criteria
listed in Table 55-1._

Activity F _Briefly answer the following
questions:_

1. Describe the treatment for cryptorchidism.

_____

_____

_____

2. What are the recommendations for testicular
self-examination?

_____

_____

_____

3. How does the nurse instruct the client with
prostatitis?

_____

_____

_____

4. What are the signs and symptoms of epididymis and orchitis?

_____

_____

_____

5. What conditions must be met for erectile dysfunction to be considered pathologic?

_____

_____

_____

6. How are physical origins of erectile dysfunction differentiated from psychological origins?

_____

_____

_____

TABLE 55-1

Type of Cancer	Pathophysiology and Etiology	Signs and Symptoms	Treatment
Cancer of the prostate			
Cancer of the testes			
Cancer of the penis			

7. Describe the action of the following medications used to treat benign prostatic hyperplasia: alpha-adrenergic blockers, androgen hormone inhibitors, and saw palmetto.

_____

_____

_____

SECTION II: APPLYING YOUR KNOWLEDGE

Activity G *Give the rationale for the following questions.*

1. Why is cryptorchidism treated when the child is between 1 to 2 years of age?

_____

_____

_____

2. Why does the American Cancer Society not currently recommend regular testicular examinations, except in the case of those with specific testicular risk factors?

_____

_____

_____

3. Why is surgery immediately performed when torsion is present?

_____

_____

_____

4. Why does a varicocele usually require surgery whereas a hydrocele and spermatocele usually do not?

_____

_____

_____

5. Why is it important to differentiate epididymitis from testicular torsion?

_____

_____

_____

6. Why does the nurse need to obtain a thorough medication record when evaluating a client with erectile dysfunction (ED)?

_____

_____

_____

7. Why is a client sterile after a transurethral resection of the prostate (TURP)?

_____

_____

_____

Activity H *Answer the following questions related to caring for clients with disorders of the male reproductive system.*

1. Describe the pathophysiology, signs and symptoms, and treatment for prostatitis.

_____

_____

_____

2. Describe the etiology of epididymis and orchitis.

_____

_____

_____

3. What processes are necessary for an erection?

_____

_____

_____

4. What are possible complications that can occur following a penile implant?

_____

_____

_____

5. Describe the options for treating priapism.

_____

_____

_____

6. Identify the purpose and types of surgeries used to treat benign prostatic hyperplasia.

_____

_____

_____

7. Describe the use of PSA screening in prostatic cancer.

_____

_____

_____

Activity I *Think over the following questions. Discuss them with your instructor or peers.*

1. What home care instructions will you provide to the client following a vasectomy?

_____

_____

_____

2. What high priority nursing diagnoses and interventions will you identify for a client following a transurethral resection of the prostate (TURP)?

_____

_____

_____

3. A client asks you what the signs and symptoms are for testicular cancer. What would you tell him?

_____

_____

_____

4. A client asks how to perform a testicular self-examination. How would you instruct him?

_____

_____

_____

5. What high priority nursing diagnoses and intervention would you identify for the client following a radical prostatectomy with a bilateral orchiectomy?

_____

_____

_____

SECTION III: GETTING READY FOR NCLEX

Activity J *Answer the following questions:*

1. A client with phimosis is not a candidate for surgery. Which of the following suggestions should a nurse give the client?
    a. Apply a skin cream and try retracting the tissue.
    b. Wash under the foreskin daily and seek care if he cannot retract the tissue.
    c. Apply warm soaks to the foreskin.
    d. Take sitz baths regularly until the tissue retracts.

2. Which of the following would a nurse suggest for a client with an inflammation of the prostate gland?
    a. Treat the client and also his sexual partners.
    b. Avoid standing for long periods and foods that cause diarrhea.
    c. No masturbation or sexual intercourse until treated.
    d. Avoid foods that may cause acidity.

3. Which of the following nursing interventions are required for a client undergoing antibiotic treatment for epididymitis and orchitis?
    a. Use an alcohol rub to keep the scrotum dry.
    b. Apply a skin cream.
    c. Elevate the scrotum to relieve the pain.
    d. Limit alcohol intake to 2 drinks per week.

4. Which of the following nursing interventions are advised for clients with prostate cancer to avoid an infection related to the home-care of a Foley catheter?
    a. Boil the leg bag regularly in a solution of hot water and vinegar for 15 minutes during the cleaning.
    b. Disinfect several inches of the catheter with alcohol or any other antiseptic agent before the insertion.
    c. Clean the leg bag by using soap and water and then rinse it with a 1:7 solution of vinegar and water.
    d. Open the connections between the leg bag and the catheter only once in 15 days to reduce the risks of microbial entry.

5. Which of the following suggestions should a nurse give a client with a prostate cancer to deal with his impotency?

    a. Abstain from any sexual activity.

    b. Demonstrate sexual feelings in ways other than intercourse.

    c. Practice sexual intercourse at least two to three times daily until successful.

    d. Perform pelvic floor retraining exercises.

6. Which of the following factors increase the risk of prostate cancer?

    a. A low-fat diet

    b. Alcohol and caffeine consumption

    c. Living an inactive lifestyle

    d. Smoking habits

7. A nurse is called to the playground near her house in relation to an adolescent who experienced intense pain in his testicle after riding his bike. The nurse suspects which of the following problems has occurred?

    a. Torsion of the spermatic cord

    b. Cryptorchidism

    c. Phimosis

    d. Spermatocele

8. A male client is having trouble with erections and comes to the clinic to be seen by the doctor. The doctor diagnoses the client with erectile dysfunction. The nurse provides education regarding the disorder and teaches the client that erectile dysfunction can be caused by which of the following?

    a. Obsessive compulsive disorder

    b. Complications of STIs

    c. Side effects of drug therapy

    d. Spinal stenosis

9. A client is learning how to maintain optimum bladder function. Which of the following strategies identifies the method of pressing on the bladder while seated on the toilet?

    a. Valsalva maneuver

    b. Kegel maneuver

    c. Pelvic floor maneuver

    d. Credé's maneuver

10. A nurse teaches a male client how to perform a testicular self exam in an effort to identify lumps that may be present in the testes. What does the nurse teach the client regarding normal testes size?

    a. Both testes should be the same size

    b. One testis is usually larger than the other

    c. One testis usually has a lump; the other does not

    d. Both testes usually have lumps

CHAPTER 56

Caring for Clients with Sexually Transmitted Infections

1. Name five common sexually transmitted infections (STIs) and identify those that are curable.
2. List five STIs that by law must be reported.
3. Give two reasons why statistics on reportable STIs are not totally accurate.
4. Discuss several factors contributing to the transmission of STIs.
5. Give two reasons why women acquire STIs more often than men.
6. Name the most common and fastest-spreading STI.
7. Explain two ways STIs are spread.
8. Discuss methods that are helpful in preventing STIs.
9. Discuss information that is important to teach clients about using condoms.
10. Name the type of the infectious microorganism that causes each of the common STIs.
11. Identify complications that are commonly associated with each of the most common STIs.

SECTION I: ASSESSING YOUR UNDERSTANDING

Activity A *Fill in the blanks by choosing the correct word from the options given in parentheses.*

1. Untreated _____ can cause sterility in infected women; infected pregnant women can transmit the microorganism to their infants during birth. *(Chlamydia, Herpes infection, Genital warts)*

2. The incidence of _____ in the United States has been increasing for the past 6 years, especially among homosexual men, women, newborns of infected mothers, and African Americans. *(Chlamydia, Gonorrhea, Syphilis)*

3. One in five people older than 12 years of age is infected with the virus that causes _____; at the current rate of infection, approximately 40% to 50% of Americans may be infected by the year 2025. *(Genital herpes, Chancroid, Genital warts)*

4. One fourth of the people in the United States carry the virus for _____ and are infectious but do not manifest symptoms. *(Genital herpes, Gonorrhea, Genital warts)*

5. _____ causes approximately 10% of cases of heart disease in clients older than 50 years of age. *(Syphilis, Chlamydia, Gonorrhea)*

Activity B *Mark each statement as either "T" (True) or "F" (False). Correct any false statements.*

1. T F Some STIs such as acquired immunodeficiency syndrome, hepatitis, and skin infestations with lice and mites are spread by sexual transmission as well as additional routes.

2. T F Reporting of new STI cases is the responsibility of the client or their partner.

3. T F Chlamydia, gonorrhea, and syphilis are STIs not reportable by law.

4. T F Herpes recurs because after the initial infection, the virus remains dormant in the ganglia of the nerves that supply the area. When the virus is active, shedding viral particles are infectious.

5. T F HPV infection is associated with uterine cervical abnormalities, which may lead to cervical and other pelvic reproductive types of cancer. However, the strains of HPV that cause genital warts are different than those that cause cervical cancer.

Activity C *Write the correct term for each description given below.*

1. The study of the occurrence, distribution, and causes of human diseases. _____

2. The most common and fastest-spreading bacterial STI in the United States. The number of new cases totals 2.8 million per year.

_____

3. Tissue irritation, which may be permanent despite successful eradication of the bacteria, puts those with this type of infection at greater risk for acquiring other STIs, such as AIDS. _____

4. The second most frequently reported communicable disease in the United States. Its highest incidence occurs in the 15- to 24-year-old age group. _____

5. A highly contagious STI that is controllable but not curable. Presently, at least 50 million people in the United States are affected.

_____

6. Anyone can become infected, but people with AIDS as well as others with an immunodeficiency are particularly susceptible._____

Activity D *Match the STIs in Column A with their usual treatments in Column B.*

Column A

____ **1.** Chlamydia

____ **2.** Gonorrhea

____ **3.** Syphilis

____ **4.** Herpes infection

____ **5.** Genital warts

Column B

a. A single dose of parenterally administered penicillin G (Pfizerpen, Wycillin) is used to treat primary and secondary symptoms. Those with tertiary symptoms may require 3 doses of penicillin at one-week intervals to prevent complications.

b. If treatment is necessary, either type responds to the antiviral drugs acyclovir (Zovirax), valacyclovir (Valtrex), and famciclovir (Famvir)

c. Antimicrobial drugs, such as a single oral dose of azithromycin (Zithromax) or a 7-day regimen of doxycycline (Vibramycin), erythromycin (E-Mycin), ofloxacin (Floxin), or levofloxacin (Levaquin) are used for treatment.

d. A single intramuscular dose of a broad-spectrum cephalosporin such as ceftriaxone (Rocephin) or oral dosing with cefixime (Suprax). Coinfection with chlamydia is common; therefore, the client is also given appropriate treatment for this infection simultaneously.

e. The physician may prescribe podofilox (Condylox) solution or gel, or imiquimod (Aldara) cream for self-application. Physician-administered treatment involves surgical excision with scalpel or scissors, laser therapy, electrocautery (heat), cryotherapy (freezing) with liquid nitrogen, local applications of chemicals, or parenteral administration of natural or recombinant interferon.

Activity E *Identify the causative organisms, modes of transmission and signs and symptoms for the following STIs.*

	Causative Organism and Mode of Transmission	Signs and Symptoms
Chlamydia		
Gonorrhea		
Syphilis		
Herpes Infection		
Genital Warts		
Granuloma inguinale		
Chancroid		
Lymphogranuloma venereum		

Activity F *Briefly answer the following questions.*

1. Identify the pathogens that cause STIs.

2. Identify the possible reasons for the disproportionate reporting of higher incidences of STIs among racial and ethnic minorities.

3. When testing for gonorrhea in women, why is the speculum moistened with water instead of lubricant?

4. Besides AIDS, what are the five most common STIs?

5. Out of the five most common STIs, which ones are curable?

SECTION II: APPLYING YOUR KNOWLEDGE

Activity G *Give the rationale for the following questions.*

1. Why is the term "sexually transmitted infections" increasingly used rather than "sexually transmitted diseases"?

2. Why is it difficult to determine the exact incidence of STI infection?

3. Why do STIs occur more often in women?

4. Why might an older adult be at risk for acquiring or not receiving treatment for an STI?

5. Why does the Centers for Disease Control (CDC) recommend annual screening for chlamydia in all sexually active women younger than 26 years of age and in women with new or multiple sexual partners?

6. Why is it a common practice to test clients for chlamydia and gonorrhea as well as syphilis?

_____

_____

_____

Activity H *Answer the following questions related to caring for clients with sexually transmitted infections.*

1. Identify the factors that contribute to the high incidence of STIs.

_____

_____

_____

2. What complications may occur as a result of untreated gonorrhea?

_____

_____

_____

3. What questions will the nurse ask when obtaining a sexual history?

_____

_____

_____

4. How will the nurse instruct the client to reduce the risk of STIs?

_____

_____

_____

5. How does the nurse instruct the client with HSV-2 infections?

_____

_____

_____

6. How does the nurse instruct the client with HPV?

_____

_____

_____

Activity I *Think over the following questions. Discuss them with your instructors or peers.*

1. A client requests information about the proper use of condoms. How will you instruct them?

_____

_____

_____

2. What high priority nursing diagnoses and interventions will you identify for the client diagnosed with an STI?

_____

_____

_____

3. What information will you provide to the client diagnosed with an STI?

_____

_____

_____

SECTION III: GETTING READY FOR NCLEX

Activity J *Answer the following questions:*

1. Which of the following reasons would make a client who was treated successfully for a chlamydia infection at a greater risk for acquiring AIDS?
   a. The tissue irritation may be permanent, despite successful eradication of the bacteria.
   b. The immune system is already compromised.
   c. The bacterium *Chlamydia trachomatis* causes AIDS.
   d. The bacterium *Chlamydia trachomatis* continues to live inside the cells it has infected.

2. A male client, living in an underdeveloped country, is diagnosed with chlamydia, acquired through an ophthalmic infection by autoinoculation. Which of the following are the symptoms experienced by the client?

   a. Testicular pain

   b. Anal infection

   c. Granulation of the cornea and blindness

   d. Sore throat with an infected pharynx

3. Which of the following STIs are curable?

   a. Chlamydia and gonorrhea

   b. Gonorrhea and herpes

   c. Herpes and venereal warts

   d. AIDS and syphilis

4. A client with the herpes simplex virus type 2 (HSV-2) undergoes a viral shedding. Which of the following statements is true when caring for a client with HSV-2?

   a. An outbreak of the HSV-2 infection is often self-limiting and hence a treatment may be unnecessary.

   b. Antiviral IV drugs are recommended to prevent viral shedding.

   c. Topical applications of the antiviral drugs are recommended for clinical benefits.

   d. Use of alcohol, peroxide, witch hazel, and warm air from a hair dryer are recommended to keep the lesions dry.

5. Which of the following instructions would a nurse give a client undergoing treatment for an HSV-2 infection?

   a. Have an annual Papanicolaou smear to detect cervical cancer.

   b. Have an annual mammogram to detect breast cancer.

   c. Increase the frequency of breast self-examination for early detection of any breast disorders.

   d. Undergo an HIV detection test every six months.

6. A nurse in a clinic is giving a talk to colleagues on sexually transmitted infections. She is trying to find statistics on certain STIs but is unable to locate accurate numbers on some of them. What is the rationale for not being able to find statistics on STIs such as genital herpes, hepatitis B, and venereal warts?

   a. Clients don't seek treatment because of embarrassment.

   b. Healthcare providers and laboratories are not required by law to report.

   c. Healthcare providers are afraid to report these statistics.

   d. Reporting is up to the client, not the provider.

7. Which of the following sexually transmitted infections is caused by *Treponema pallidum*?

   a. Herpes

   b. Venereal warts

   c. Gonorrhea

   d. Syphilis

8. A nurse is teaching a client in the doctor's office about genital warts. Which of the following is the best discharge instruction to give to a client with genital warts?

   a. Advise all sexual contacts to be examined and treated.

   b. It is acceptable to have intimate contact when a wart is present.

   c. Use a condom only when the lesion is present; otherwise no condom necessary.

   d. Suggest application of an antibiotic cream to sexual partner after intimate contact.

9. Of the following antibiotics, which one is used to treat chlamydia?

   a. Acyclovir

   b. Ciprofloxacin

   c. Tetracycline

   d. Ceftriaxone

10. A nurse goes to a high school to teach students about reducing the risk of sexually transmitted infections. Which of the following is the best answer for providing information on the prevention of STIs?

    a. Have monogamous sex with an infected partner.

    b. Abstain from sexual activities.

    c. Wash any areas where there has been indirect contact with semen or vaginal mucus.

    d. Avoid protected sex until you and sexual partners have completed treatment.

CHAPTER 57

Introduction to the Urinary System

Learning Objectives

1. Name the parts of the urinary system.
2. Define the primary functions of the kidneys and other structures in the urinary system.
3. List tests performed for the diagnosis of urologic and renal system diseases.
4. Identify laboratory tests performed to diagnose urologic and renal system diseases.
5. Discuss nursing management for a client undergoing diagnostic evaluation of the urinary tract.

SECTION I: ASSESSING YOUR UNDERSTANDING

Activity A *Fill in the blanks by choosing the correct word from the options given in parentheses.*

1. The two _____ are paired, bean-shaped organs located in the upper abdomen on either side of the vertebral column. The blood supply to each consists of a renal artery and renal vein. The renal artery arises from the aorta and the renal vein empties into the vena cava. *(Kidneys, Ureters, Bladders)*

2. The _____ contains calyces (pyramids), cone-shaped structures that open to the renal pelvis, a large funnel-like structure in the center of the kidney. The renal pelvis then empties into the ureter, which carries urine to the bladder for storage. *(Medulla, Bladder, Pelvic floor muscles)*

3. _____ is a radiologic study used to evaluate the structure and function of the kidneys, ureters, and bladder. It locates the site of any urinary tract obstructions and is helpful in the investigation of the causes of flank pain, hematuria, or renal colic. It is based on the ability of the kidneys to excrete a radiopaque dye in the urine. *(A biopsy, An intravenous pyelogram, A cystogram)*

4. Severe pain in the back, shoulder, or abdomen following a biopsy can indicate _____ *(Infection, Bleeding, Distention)*

5. A _____ is performed to evaluate bladder and sphincter function. This noninvasive procedure measures the time and rate of voiding, the volume of urine voided, and the pattern of urination. Results are compared with normal flow rates and urinary patterns. Results vary by age and sex. *(Uroflowmetry, Postvoid residual, Cystometrogram)*

6. _____ evaluates the bladder tone and capacity. *(Uroflowmetry, Cystometrogram, Urinalysis)*

Activity B *Mark each statement as either "T" (True) or "F" (False). Correct any false statements.*

1. T F The kidneys receive 50% of the total cardiac output.

2. T F In general, adult bladders hold 100 to 200 mL of urine.

3. T F The urethra is a hollow tube that begins at the kidney neck and ends at the external meatus.

4. T F A cystogram evaluates abnormalities in bladder structure and filling through the instillation of contrast dye and radiography.

5. T F Urinary tract infection is a contraindication to a cystogram or voiding cystourethrogram.

Activity C *Write the correct term for each description given below.*

1. Form a sling that supports the bladder and urethra, rectum, and some reproductive organs. _____

2. May result secondary to an overdistended bladder or other problems, and may cause infections. _____

3. Clients receive this type of medication following a cystoscopy. _____

4. Taken to diagnose cancer, assess prostatic enlargement, diagnose and monitor progression of renal disease, and assess and evaluate treatment of renal transplant rejection.

_____

5. A diagnostic test similar to a cystogram except the client is instructed to void (the urine contains the radiopaque dye), and a rapid series of x-rays are taken. _____

6. Measures the amount of urine left in the bladder after voiding; provides information about bladder function. _____

Activity D *Match the diagnostic tests related to renal disorders listed in Column A with their descriptions in Column B.*

Column A

_____ **1.** Radiography

_____ **2.** Ultrasonography

_____ **3.** Computed Tomography Scan and Magnetic Resonance Imaging

_____ **4.** Angiography

_____ **5.** Cystoscopy

Column B

a. Uses include identification of renal cysts or obstruction sites, assistance in needle placement for renal biopsy or nephrostomy tube placement, and drainage of a renal abscess.

b. Used to identify the cause of painless hematuria, urinary incontinence, or urinary retention. It is useful in the evaluation of structural and functional changes of the bladder.

c. Provides details of the arterial supply to the kidneys, specifically the location and number of renal arteries (multiple vessels to the kidney are not unusual) and the patency of each renal artery.

d. May be obtained to diagnose renal pathology, determine kidney size, and evaluate tissue densities with or without contrast material.

e. Performed to show the size and position of the kidneys, ureters, and bony pelvis as well as any radiopaque urinary calculi (stones), abnormal gas patterns (indicative of renal mass), and anatomic defects of the bony spinal column (indicative of neuropathic bladder dysfunction).

Activity E *Compare the following laboratory tests, their purpose, and how to perform the test.*

Test	Purpose	How to Perform Test
Urinalysis		
Urine Culture and Sensitivity		
24-Hour Urine Collection		
Urine Specific Gravity		
Urine Osmolality		
Urine Protein Test		
Creatinine Clearance Test		
Blood Urea Nitrogen (BUN)		

Activity F *Briefly answer the following questions.*

1. Describe the nephrons of the kidneys.

2. What usually prevents the backflow of urine?

3. What causes the urge to urinate?

4. What can occur if the bladder muscles are impaired?

5. During a physical examination, how does the nurse assess for kidney pain?

6. If the client is being discharged the day after a biopsy what instruction will the nurse provide?

SECTION II: APPLYING YOUR KNOWLEDGE

Activity G *Give rationale for the following questions.*

1. Why are periodic, small amounts of protein in the urine not considered a problem?

2. Why would glucose be excreted in the urine?

3. Why would older adults be at risk for drug toxicity?

4. Why would older adults be at risk for dehydration?

5. Why might the physician inject a minute amount of contrast and wait 5 to 10 minutes before proceeding?

6. Why is an intravenous pyelogram scheduled prior to a barium test or gallbladder series using contrast material?

Activity H *Answer the following questions related to the urinary system.*

1. Describe the structures and function of the urinary system.

2. Explain the process of urine formation.

3. How is an intravenous pyelogram performed?

_____

_____

_____

4. What post procedure care will the nurse provide following an intravenous pyelogram?

_____

_____

_____

Activity I *Think over the following questions. Discuss them with your instructor or peers.*

1. Your client is scheduled for an intravenous pyelogram. What instructions would you provide?

_____

_____

_____

2. What high-priority nursing diagnoses and intervention would you identify for the client being evaluated for renal dysfunction?

_____

_____

_____

3. You need to obtain a clean-catch midstream urine specimen. How would you instruct the client?

_____

_____

_____

SECTION III: GETTING READY FOR NCLEX

Activity J *Answer the following questions.*

1. The nurse should physically examine a client who experiences difficulty in voiding. Which of the following methods should the nurse use to assess the kidneys for tenderness or pain?

  a. By auscultating the abdomen for bruits.

  b. By lightly striking the fist at the costovertebral angle.

  c. By palpating the suprapubic area.

  d. By percussing the area over the bladder.

2. A female client, age 52 and of Spanish descent, is suspected to have a renal disorder. She has been asked to undergo a diagnostic test. However, she is nervous and worried before the test. Which of the following patient teaching techniques may be used by the nurse to help the client overcome her anxiety?

  a. Use simple language with client or significant others.

  b. Administer sedative medications as ordered.

  c. Explain in detail all the technicalities about the test.

  d. Tell her about the risk factors of the test.

3. After an angiography procedure, a pressure dressing to the femoral area of the client has been applied. As part of the post-procedure care, why should the nurse assess the client's pressure dressing frequently?

  a. To note frank bleeding.

  b. To note hematoma formation.

  c. To check for signs of arterial occlusion.

  d. To assess peripheral pulses.

4. A client who underwent a biopsy is due to be discharged from the hospital. The nurse instructs him to complete the prophylactic antibiotic therapy and to notify the physician about any signs or symptoms of systemic infections. Which of the following instructions should the nurse offer the client to prevent bleeding, which may result after a biopsy?

  a. Increase fluid intake.

  b. Refrain from taking nephrotoxic drugs.

  c. Take sedative medications.

  d. Maintain limited physical activity.

5. A client who undergoes a retrograde pyelogram is transferred to post procedure care. At this stage, the nurse should monitor for signs of pyelonephritis in the client. Which of the following measures should the nurse take when she observes signs of pyelonephritis?

  a. Report them to the physician.

  b. Advise the client to take bed rest.

  c. Observe further for signs of bleeding.

  d. Monitor pressure dressing to note any frank bleeding.

6. Before cystoscopy, the nurse checks for signs of fever and chills in the client because they may indicate:

   a. Bleeding

   b. A urinary infection

   c. A systemic infection

   d. A urinary tract disorder

7. Which of the following should the nurse closely monitor in older clients with renal dysfunction?

   a. Decreased urine output

   b. Urine discoloration

   c. Signs of ketonuria

   d. Signs of nephrotoxicity

8. A female client comes in to deposit a 24-hour urine specimen. However, the client says she may have lost some urine in the process because she was very sleepy when she was trying to void in the morning. Which of the following appropriate actions should the nurse take in such a case?

   a. Accept the sample and send it to laboratory for testing.

   b. Discard the test and ask the client to rec-ollect urine afresh.

   c. Send it to the laboratory but also inform the lab technician of the lapse.

   d. Refrigerate the sample for 24 hours and then send it to the laboratory for the test.

9. The nurse should monitor for signs of arterial occlusion in a client after an angiography. Which of the following should help the nurse observe for signs of arterial occlusion in the client?

   a. Palpate the pulses in the legs and feet of the client every hour.

   b. Monitor and document the intake and output.

   c. Assess the pressure dressing.

   d. Obtain a 24-hour urine specimen.

10. The kidneys receive _____ % of cardiac output?

Caring for Clients with Disorders of the Kidneys and Ureters

Learning Objectives

1. Differentiate pyelonephritis and glomerulonephritis.
2. Name problems the nurse manages when caring for clients with glomerulonephritis.
3. Explain the pathophysiology and associated renal complications of polycystic disease.
4. Give examples of conditions that predispose to renal calculi.
5. Identify methods for eliminating small renal calculi and larger stones.
6. Discuss the nursing management of a client with a nephrostomy tube.
7. Describe conditions that cause a ureteral stricture.
8. Explain the classic triad of symptoms associated with renal cancer.
9. Discuss problems the nurse manages when caring for a client with a nephrectomy.
10. Differentiate acute and chronic renal failure.
11. Explain pathophysiologic problems associated with chronic renal failure.
12. Describe sources of organs for kidney transplantation.
13. Identify nursing methods for managing pruritus.
14. Explain the purposes and methods of dialysis.
15. Discuss nursing assessments performed when caring for clients undergoing dialysis.

SECTION I: ASSESSING YOUR UNDERSTANDING

Activity A *Fill in the blanks by choosing the correct word from the options given in parentheses.*

1. Laboratory findings for _____ include urine findings of proteinuria, sediment, casts, and red and white blood cells. The urinary creatinine clearance is reduced. Serum electrolyte changes indicate nephron dysfunction. *(Pyelonephritis, Acute glomerulonephritis, Chronic glomerulonephritis)*

2. _____ is performed by inserting a fine wire into the ureter by means of a cystoscope. A laser beam passes through it and repeated bursts of the laser reduce the stone to a fine powder, which is then passed in the urine. *(Laser lithotripsy, Extracorporeal shock wave lithotripsy, Ureteral stent placement)*

3. _____ disorders usually are obstructive problems in structures below the kidney(s) that have damaging repercussions for the nephrons above. *(Prerenal, Intrarenal, Postrenal)*

4. During the _____ phase of acute renal failure, symptoms of fluid volume excess develops, which leads to edema,

hypertension, and cardiopulmonary complications. *(Initiation, Oliguric, Diuretic)*

5. Chronic renal failure is associated more often with _____ conditions or is a complication of systemic diseases such as diabetes mellitus and disseminated lupus erythematosus. *(Prerenal, Intrarenal, Postrenal)*

6. In _____, the kidneys are so extensively damaged that they do not adequately remove protein by-products and electrolytes from the blood and do not maintain acid–base balance. *(Acute renal failure, Pyelonephritis, Chronic renal failure)*

7. _____ is a neurologic condition believed to be caused by cerebral edema. The shift in cerebral fluid volume occurs when the concentrations of solutes in the blood are lowered rapidly during dialysis. Decreasing solute concentration lowers the plasma osmolality. Water then floods the brain tissue. *(Disequilibrium syndrome, Uremic frost, Azotemia)*

Activity B *Mark each statement as either "T" (True) or "F" (False). Correct any false statements.*

1. T F Give drugs excreted by the kidney with caution to those with renal disease. If the drug is deemed necessary, it may be given in lower than normal doses.

2. T F No specific treatment exists for acute glomerulonephritis. Treatment is guided by the symptoms and the underlying abnormality.

3. T F The severity of the pain caused by renal calculi is usually equally proportional to the size of the stone.

4. T F Intrarenal disorders are non-neurologic conditions that disrupt renal blood flow to the nephrons, affecting their filtering ability. This is the most common type of acute renal failure (ARF).

5. T F The initiation phase of acute renal failure is associated with the excretion of less-than-adequate urinary volumes.

6. T F The recovery phase of acute renal failure lasts 10 to14 days and always results in complete recovery of the renal system.

7. T F The dialyzer is the solution used during dialysis that has a composition similar to normal human plasma.

8. T F Peritoneal dialysis uses the peritoneum, the semipermeable membrane lining the abdomen, to filter fluid, wastes, and chemicals. The dialysate is similar in composition to normal plasma but made hypertonic by dextrose.

Activity C *Write the correct term for each description given below.*

1. The chief abnormality of pyelonephritis. _____

2. Laboratory findings include proteinuria (primarily as albumin in the urine) and an elevated anti-streptolysin O titer from the recent streptococcal infection. There is decreased hemoglobin, slightly elevated BUN and serum creatinine levels, and an elevated erythrocyte sedimentation rate. _____

3. An accumulation of nitrogen waste products in the blood; evidenced by elevated BUN, serum creatinine, and uric acid levels. _____

4. Distention of the renal pelvis which may result from complete obstruction caused by renal calculi. _____

5. Refers to the death of cells in the collecting tubules of the nephrons where reabsorption of water, electrolytes, and excretion of protein wastes and excess metabolic substances occurs. _____

6. In end-stage renal disease the skin becomes the excretory organ for the substances the kidney usually clears from the body and a precipitate may form on the skin. _____

7. A procedure for cleaning and filtering the blood. It substitutes for kidney function when the kidneys cannot remove the nitrogenous waste products and maintain adequate fluid, electrolyte, and acid–base balances. _____

8. This syndrome is characterized by headache, disorientation, restlessness, blurred vision, confusion, and seizures. The symptoms are self-limiting and disappear within several hours after dialysis as fluid and solute concentrations equalize. The syndrome can be prevented by slowing the dialysis process to allow time for gradual equilibration of water. _____

Activity D *Match the congenital and obstructive disorders in Column A with the descriptions in Column B.*

Column A

_____ **1.** Adult polycystic disease

_____ **2.** Urolithiasis

_____ **3.** Ureteral stricture

_____ **4.** Kidney tumor

Column B

a. Calculi traumatize the walls of the urinary tract and irritate the cellular lining, causing pain as violent contractions of the ureter develop to pass the stone along. If a stone totally or partially obstructs the passage of urine beyond its location, pressure increases in the area above the stone. The pressure contributes to pain, and urinary stasis promotes secondary infection.

b. The incidence is higher in older adults, which suggests chronic exposure to a carcinogen whose metabolites involve renal excretion. It is possible that the cause is initiated through exposure to an environmental toxin or volatile solvent.

c. The incidence is higher among those with chronic ureteral stone formation. Recurrent inflammation and infection cause scar tissue to accumulate in the ureter. This condition may also result from congenital anomalies or conditions that mechanically compress the ureter, such as pregnancy or tumors in the abdomen or upper urinary tract.

d. This is inherited as an autosomal dominant disorder. The disorder is characterized by the formation of multiple bilateral kidney cysts, which interfere with kidney function and eventually lead to renal failure. The fluid-filled cysts cause great enlargement of the kidneys, from their normal size of a fist to that of a football. As the cysts enlarge, they compress the renal blood vessels and cause chronic hypertension. Bleeding into cysts causes flank pain.

Activity E *Compare the infectious and inflammatory diseases of the kidney based on the following criteria.*

Disease	Pathophysiology	Signs and Symptoms
Pyelonephritis		
Acute Glomerulonephritis		
Chronic Glomerulonephritis		

Activity F *Briefly answer the following questions.*

1. What is extracorporeal shock wave lithotripsy?

_____

_____

_____

2. What are the signs and symptoms of renal cancer?

_____

_____

_____

3. Identify the four phases of acute renal failure.

_____

_____

_____

4. Describe the diuretic phase of acute renal failure.

_____

_____

_____

5. What signs and symptoms occur with chronic renal failure?

_____

_____

_____

6. Describe the process of hemodialysis.

_____

_____

_____

7. How does the nurse assess a vascular access devise?

_____

_____

_____

8. Compare the advantages and disadvantages of an arteriovenous fistula and an arteriovenous graft.

_____

_____

_____

SECTION II: APPLYING YOUR KNOWLEDGE

Activity G *Give rationale for the following questions.*

1. Why does the nurse encourage an oral intake of 3000mL – 4000mL of fluid for the client with pyelonephritis?

_____

_____

_____

2. Why is it important that the client with glomerulonephritis receive adequate carbohydrates in their diet?

_____

_____

_____

3. Why is a low RBC volume detected through complete blood counts with chronic glomerulonephritis?

_____

_____

_____

4. Why can neurological symptoms occur during the oliguric phase of acute renal failure?

_____

_____

_____

5. Why would a chest radiography and echocardiography be pertinent with a diagnosis of chronic glomerulonephritis?

_____

_____

_____

6. Why does urine have a very low specific gravity with acute renal failure?

_____

_____

_____

7. Why are blood samples taken before and after dialysis?

_____

_____

_____

Activity H *Answer the following questions related to caring for the client with disorders of the kidneys and ureters.*

1. Describe the pathophysiology of pyelonephritis.

_____

_____

_____

2. What are the medical management goals of chronic glomerulonephritis?

_____

_____

_____

3. What surgical treatment options are available for the treatment of calculi that are large or complicated by obstruction, ongoing UTI, kidney damage, or constant bleeding?

_____

_____

_____

4. Describe the treatment options for renal cancer.

_____

_____

_____

5. Describe the electrolyte and blood component changes that occur with chronic renal failure.

_____

_____

_____

6. How are acute and chronic renal failure medically and surgically managed?

_____

_____

_____

7. What are the options for vascular access with hemodialysis?

_____

_____

_____

8. Describe the process of peritoneal dialysis.

_____

_____

_____

Activity I *Think over the following questions. Discuss them with your instructor or peers.*

1. What high priority nursing diagnoses and interventions would you identify for a client with chronic glomerulonephritis?

_____

_____

_____

2. What educational information related to diet would you provide to the client with renal calculi?

_____

_____

_____

3. What high priority nursing diagnoses and interventions would you identify for a client with renal cancer?

_____

_____

_____

4. Your client is informed they will need dialysis and asks you to explain the difference between hemodialysis and peritoneal dialysis and the process for each. What educational information will you provide?

_____

_____

_____

SECTION III: GETTING READY FOR NCLEX

Activity J *Choose the best answer for each of the following questions:*

1. Why must a nurse measure the intake and output, and recommend a daily fluid intake of approximately 3000 to 4000 mL for a client with pyelonephritis?

   a. To determine the client's response to the therapy

   b. To flush out the infectious microorganisms from the urinary tract

   c. To determine the location of discomfort

   d. To detect any evidence of changes

2. Mrs. Rutte is being treated for acute pyelo-nephritis and will undergo laboratory tests. These tests are expected to help determine the client's BUN, creatinine, and serum electrolyte levels. Why should the nurse evaluate these test results?

   a. To determine the severity of the disorder

   b. To determine the location of discomfort

   c. To identify signs of fluid retention

   d. To determine the client's response to therapy

3. The nurse has been asked to prepare an intervention plan for a client, age 70, admitted for treatment of renal calculi. He complains of frequent pain due to increased pressure in the renal pelvis, and is frightened of the excruciating pain. Which of the following measures can the nurse include in the client's nursing care plan?

   a. Administer prescribed nephrotoxic drugs.

   b. Observe aseptic principles when changing dressings.

   c. Advise against protein restriction.

   d. Encourage ambulation and liberal fluid intake.

4. A female client, age 66, is admitted following a nephrolithotomy. One of her laboratory tests reveals a urinary tract infection. Which would be the best nursing action in her case?

   a. Administer IV fluids and blood transfusions.

   b. Administer narcotic analgesics as prescribed.

   c. Encourage fluid intake of 3000 mL/day.

   d. Suggest taking herbs or spices to increase food palatability.

5. A client has undergone a nephrectomy and is placed under observation after a urethral catheter insertion. As part of the nursing care plan, the nurse records the color of drainage from each tube and catheter. Which of the following is the reason for this?

   a. To restore and maintain intravascular volume.

   b. To provide a means for further comparison and evaluation.

   c. To avoid interference with wound drainage.

   d. To prevent pain related to obstruction.

6. A client is undergoing peritoneal dialysis. Which of the following is a major complication of the procedure that the nurse should monitor for?

   a. Internal hemorrhage

   b. Ecchymosis

   c. Hydronephrosis

   d. Peritonitis

7. While planning for proportionate distribution of restricted fluid volumes, what is the reason for a nurse to ensure that the client is actively involved during the development of the plan?

   a. Promotes the client's compliance with therapy

   b. Minimizes the chances of adverse effects

   c. Promotes a strict food and fluids intake habit

   d. Raises the self-esteem of the client

8. Mr. Scott has been diagnosed with renal failure and is admitted for dialysis. Which of the following is the nurse's responsibility as the client undergoes dialysis?

   a. Keeping dialysis supplies in a clean area

   b. Inspecting the catheter insertion site for signs of infection

   c. Weighing the client before and after the procedure

   d. Washing hands before and after handling the catheter

9. A client is admitted for postoperative assessment and recovery after surgery for a kidney tumor. The nurse needs to assess for signs of urinary tract infection. Which of the following measures can be used to help detect urinary tract infection?

   a. Encourage the client to breathe deeply and cough every 2 hours.

   b. Monitor temperature every 4 hours.

   c. Splint the incision when repositioning the client.

   d. Irrigate tubes as ordered.

10. A nurse is taking care of a client with acute renal failure. The client is in what stage when reduced blood flow to the nephrons to the point of acute tubular necrosis is noted?

   a. Recovery phase

   b. Initiation phase

   c. Oliguric phase

   d. Diuretic phase

CHAPTER 200

Caring for Clients with Disorders of the Bladder and Urethra

Learning Objectives

1. Explain urinary retention and appropriate nursing management.
2. Discuss urinary incontinence and appropriate nursing management.
3. Describe the pathophysiologic changes seen in cystitis, interstitial cystitis, and urethritis.
4. Explain the symptoms associated with bladder stones.
5. Discuss the cause and treatment of urethral strictures.
6. Identify the most common early symptom of a malignant tumor of the bladder, and outline treatment and nursing care.
7. Describe various types of urinary diversion procedures.
8. Identify components of a teaching plan for a client having a urinary diversion procedure.

SECTION I: ASSESSING YOUR UNDERSTANDING

Activity A *Fill in the blanks by choosing the correct word from the options given in parentheses.*

1. _____ urinary retention requires immediate catheterization. *(Acute, Chronic, Delayed)*

2. Usually, clients with bladder stones are told to increase their _____ intake significantly, consume a moderate protein intake, and limit sodium. *(Calcium, Fluid, Carbohydrate)*

3. Urethral strictures are treated by _____ *(Urethroplasty, Litholapaxy, Dilatation)*

4. Small, superficial tumors may be removed by resection or _____ with a transurethral resectoscope. *(Fulguration, Dilatation, Litholapaxy)*

5. _____ exercises increase muscle tone to assist bladder emptying and bladder training. *(Kegel, Credé, Valsalva)*

Activity B *Mark each statement as either "True" (T) or "False" (F). Correct any false statements.*

1. T F Urinary incontinence is the inability to urinate or effectively empty the bladder.

2. T F It is essential that the nurse explain the importance of taking the full course of antibiotic therapy to clients diagnosed with cystitis and urethritis.

3. T F Large bladder stones develop in clients who are immobile and in those with chronic urinary retention and urinary stasis.

4. **T F** A diet that is adequate in calcium and low in oxalate is followed in the case of uric acid stones.

5. **T F** When a client is diagnosed with urinary stones, the nurse filters the urine for stones by straining all urine through gauze or wire mesh. If solid material is found, it is sent in a labeled container to the laboratory for analysis.

6. **T F** Up to 85% of men experience erectile dysfunction after urinary diversion. Women may have painful intercourse and lack lubrication.

Activity C *Write the correct term for each description given below.*

1. This procedure uses a stone-crushing instrument and is suitable for small and soft stones. It is performed under general anesthesia. _____

2. Only clients who have type II absorptive hypercalciuria, approximately half of all clients with hypercalciuria, need to limit intake of this substance. _____

3. Often the first sign of bladder cancer, and the reason clients seek medical attention. _____

4. The bladder and lower third of both ureters are removed. _____

5. A method of bladder training that combines scheduled voiding with prompting and praising. _____

Activity D *Match the terms related to voiding dysfunction in Column A to their descriptions in Column B.*

Column A

____ 1. Neurogenic bladder

____ 2. Residual urine

____ 3. Urinary retention

____ 4. Urinary incontinence

____ 5. Cystostomy

Column B

a. Urine retained in the bladder after the client voids.

b. Acute symptoms are the sudden inability to void, distended bladder, and severe lower abdominal pain and discomfort. A chronic condition may not produce symptoms because the bladder has stretched

over time and accommodates large volumes without producing discomfort.

c. A bladder that does not receive adequate nerve stimulation.

d. A catheter inserted through the abdominal wall directly into the bladder.

e. May result from either bladder or urethral dysfunction (or both). The bladder can contract without warning, fail to accommodate adequate volumes of urine, or fail to empty completely and become overstretched, or the urethral sphincters may fail to hold urine in the bladder.

Activity E *Compare the following infectious and inflammatory disorders of the bladder and urethra based on the following criteria.*

Disorder	Pathophysiology	Signs and Symptoms
Cystitis		
Interstitial cystitis (IC)		
Urethritis		

Activity F *Briefly answer the following questions.*

1. Describe how the following medications can improve bladder retention, emptying, and control: anticholinergic drugs, tricyclic antidepressant medications, pseudoephedrine, and estrogen.

_____

_____

_____

2. What problems may interfere with the success of a bladder training program? What interventions would the nurse implement?

_____

_____

_____

3. What are the effects when incontinence can not be avoided? What interventions would the nurse implement?

_____

_____

_____

4. What is involved in the nursing management of interstitial cystitis (IC)?

_____

_____

_____

5. Describe the nursing management implemented to prevent urethritis for the client with an indwelling urinary catheter.

_____

_____

_____

6. Describe the etiology of a urethral stricture.

_____

_____

_____

SECTION II: APPLYING YOUR KNOWLEDGE

Activity G _Provide rationale for the following questions._

1. Why is permanent catheterization avoided?

_____

_____

_____

2. Why is it necessary to clamp the tubing if a large volume of urine is returned during catheterization?

_____

_____

_____

3. Why is it important to carefully assess the older client and the conditions that may contribute to incidents of incontinence?

_____

_____

_____

4. Why may cranberry juice or vitamin C be recommended for a client diagnosed with cystitis?

_____

_____

_____

5. Why would a client with bladder cancer exhibit symptoms of anemia?

_____

_____

_____

Activity H _Answer the following questions that relate to caring for clients with disorders of the bladder and urethra._

1. What options may be used to treat urinary retention?

_____

_____

_____

2. A client with chronic urinary retention will be managed using intermittent catheterization. Describe the procedure that will be used.

_____

_____

_____

3. How is bladder training accomplished for a client with an indwelling catheter?

_____

_____

_____

4. What complications can result from a urethral stricture?

_____

_____

_____

5. Describe the medical treatment options for bladder cancer.

_____

_____

_____

6. Describe the two types of urinary diversions.

_____

_____

_____

Activity I _Think over the following questions. Discuss them with your instructor or peers._

1. Your client has functional incontinence. What high priority nursing diagnoses and interventions would you identify?

_____

_____

_____

2. How would you instruct the client to use Credé or Valsalva voiding?

_____

_____

_____

3. Which clients would you identify as being at risk for urinary incontinence?

_____

_____

_____

4. What high priority diagnoses and interventions would you identify for the client with an infection of the bladder or urethra?

_____

_____

_____

5. What educational information would you provide to the client caring for a stoma and urinary ostomy?

_____

_____

_____

SECTION III: GETTING READY FOR NCLEX

Activity J _Choose the best answer for the following questions._

1. Which of the following is a critical task of a nurse during the ureterosigmoidostomy procedure for treating a malignant tumor?

   a. Inspecting for bleeding or cyanosis

   b. Assessing the client's allergy to iodine

   c. Inspecting for symptoms of peritonitis

   d. Checking for signs of electrolyte losses

2. A nurse needs to assess a client who is undergoing urinary diversion. Which of the following assessments is essential for the client?

   a. The client's knowledge about effects of the surgery on his sexual function

   b. The client's medical history of allergy to iodine or seafood

   c. The client's knowledge about the effects of the surgery on his nervous control

   d. The client's occupational and environmental health hazards

3. A male client recently undergoes a surgical procedure for malignant tumor. As a result of the surgery, his urine is diverted to a stomal pouch. What should the nurse suggest so that he remains odor free?

   a. Eating spicy foods

   b. Eating eggs, asparagus, or cheese

   c. Drinking cranberry juice

   d. Drinking tea, coffee, and colas

4. While managing a client after a medical or surgical procedure for bladder stones, when should the nurse notify the physician?

   a. When the temperature rises above 101° F

   b. When the temperature rises above 98°F

   c. When the temperature rises above 100°F

   d. When the temperature rises above 99°F

5. A client who underwent litholapaxy surgery for removing bladder stones wants to know how long the urethral catheter needs to stay in place. Which of the following is the correct response?

   a. The catheter should remain in place for 7 days.

   b. The catheter should remain in place for 1 to 2 days.

   c. The catheter should remain in place for 2 to 3 days.

   d. The catheter should remain in place for 3 to 4 days.

6. Which of the following is the most important factor in the nursing management of clients who undergo treatment for malignant tumor following the urinary diversion procedure?

   a. Placement of IV and central venous pressure lines

   b. Administering cleansing enemas

   c. Observing for leakage of urine or stool from the anastomosis

   d. Assessing the client's ability to manage self-catheterization

7. The nurse is instructed to perform preoperative preparation for the management of a client with malignant tumors. Which of the following is the most important factor of the nursing management plan?

   a. Insertion of an ostomy pouch

   b. Maintaining the integrity of the urinary diversion procedure

   c. Assessing for symptoms of peritonitis

   d. Insertion of a nasogastric tube

8. A female client experiences trauma to her urinary tract during an accident. Which of the following factors should the nurse consider while assessing the client?

   a. Assessment of sexual habits

   b. Assessment and recognition of abnormal findings

   c. Assessment of allergies to sea food

   d. Assessment of insurance coverage

9. A client complains of urinary discomfort and a burning sensation while urinating. A urethral smear shows evidence of urethritis, and the client is prescribed antibiotics and instructed to drink 2L-3L of water daily. For which of the following reasons is the client advised to drink the specified amount of water?

   a. It will help him overcome urinary incontinence.

   b. It will promote renal blood flow and flush bacteria from the urinary tract.

   c. It will help him eliminate urinary odors.

   d. It will provide relief from pain and discomfort as a result of urinary tract infection.

10. A nurse in a physician's office is explaining the procedures that a physician can perform to assist with urinary control. The client has questions about the procedure that involves the placement of small amounts of collagen in urethral walls to aid the closing pressure. What is this procedure called?

    a. Bladder augmentation

    b. Retropubic suspension

    c. Implantation of an artificial sphincter

    d. Periurethral bulking

CHAPTER 60

Introduction to the Musculoskeletal System

Learning Objectives

1. Describe major structures and functions of the musculoskeletal system.
2. Discuss elements of the nursing assessment of the musculoskeletal system.
3. Identify common diagnostic and laboratory tests used in the evaluation of musculoskeletal disorders.
4. Discuss the nursing management of clients undergoing tests for musculoskeletal disorders.

SECTION I: ASSESSING YOUR UNDERSTANDING

Activity A *Fill in the blanks by choosing the correct word from the options given in parentheses.*

1. The human body has _____ bones. *(206, 260, 620)*

2. _____ build bones; these cells secrete bone matrix (mostly collagen), in which inorganic minerals, such as calcium salts, are deposited. *(Osteocytes, Osteoblasts, Osteoclasts)*

3. A layer of tissue called _____ covers the bones (but not the joints). *(Epiphyses, Periosteum, Diaphyses)*

4. A _____ is the junction between two or more bones. *(Joint, Ligament, Tendon)*

5. _____ are cordlike structures that attach muscles to the periosteum of the bone. *(Joints, Bursae, Tendons)*

6. _____ are small sacs filled with synovial fluid. They reduce friction between areas, such as tendon and bone and tendon and ligament. *(Cartilage, Bursae, Muscles)*

Activity B *Mark each statement as either "T" (True) or "F" (False). Correct any false statements.*

1. T F The musculoskeletal system consists of bones, muscles, joints, tendons, ligaments, cartilage, and bursae.

2. T F Cancellous bony tissue covers bones and is found chiefly in the long shafts, or diaphyses, of bones in the arms and legs.

3. T F The process of ossification and calcification transforms the blast cells into mature bone cells, called osteocytes, which are involved in maintaining bone tissue.

4. T F Yellow bone marrow, found primarily in the sternum, ileum, vertebrae, and ribs, manufactures blood cells and hemoglobin.

5. T F Ligaments consisting of fibrous tissue connect two adjacent, freely movable bones. They help protect the joints by stabilizing their surfaces and keeping them in proper alignment. In some instances, ligaments completely enclose a joint.

6. T F Smooth muscles are found mainly in the walls of certain organs or cavities of the body, such as the stomach, intestine, blood vessels, and ureters. Cardiac muscle is found only in the heart.

7. T F Lordosis is an exaggerated convex curvature of the thoracic spine (humpback).

Activity C *Write the correct term for each description given below.*

1. Bone cells involved in the destruction, resorption, and remodeling of bone.

   _____

2. These types of muscles are voluntary muscles; impulses that travel from efferent nerves of the brain and spinal cord control their function. They promote movement of the bones of the skeleton. _____

3. The space between is the joint cavity, which is enclosed by a fibrous capsule lined with synovial membrane. This membrane produces fluid, which acts as a lubricant.

   _____

4. A firm, dense type of connective tissue that consists of cells embedded in a substance called the matrix. The matrix is firm and compact, thus enabling it to withstand pressure and torsion. The primary functions are to reduce friction between articular surfaces, absorb shocks, and reduce stress on joint surfaces. _____

5. Lateral curvature of the spine.

   _____

6. Intake recommendations of this nutrient are set at 1000 mg/day for adults younger than 50 years of age and 1200 mg/day for those over age 50. _____

Activity D *Match the blood test findings listed in Column A with the conditions they may indicate in Column B.*

Column A

____ 1. Elevated alkaline phosphatase level and increased serum phosphorus level

Column B

a. May indicate Paget's disease and metastatic cancer.

b. May indicate osteomalacia, osteoporosis, and bone tumors.

____ 2. Elevated acid phosphatase level

____ 3. Decreased serum calcium level

____ 4. Elevated serum uric acid level

____ 5. Elevated antinuclear antibody level

c. May indicate bone tumors and healing fractures.

d. May indicate lupus erythematosus.

e. May indicate gout.

Activity E *Compare the diagnostic tests of the musculoskeletal system based on the following criteria.*

Test	Purpose	How Test is Performed
Imaging Procedures		
Arthrogram		
Arthroscopy		
Arthrocentesis		
Synovial Fluid Analysis		
Bone Densitometry		
Bone Scan		
Electromyography		
Biopsy		

Activity F *Briefly answer the following questions.*

1. Describe the functions of the musculoskeletal system.

   _____

   _____

   _____

2. Describe the types of involuntary muscles.

   _____

   _____

   _____

3. Which results of a 24-hour urine test would be significant to the musculoskeletal system?

   _____

   _____

   _____

4. How are the activities of smooth and cardiac muscles controlled?

_____

_____

_____

5. What is the purpose of hyaline cartilage that covers diarthrodial joints?

_____

_____

_____

6. Identify non-dairy sources of calcium.

_____

_____

_____

7. How are vitamin K, magnesium, and potassium related to bone health?

_____

_____

_____

SECTION II: APPLYING YOUR KNOWLEDGE

Activity G *Provide rationale for the following questions.*

1. Why do older adults lose as much as 1 to 2 cm of height every two decades?

_____

_____

_____

2. Why are older adults at higher risk for skeletal fractures?

_____

_____

_____

3. Why do older adults experience a greater amount of bone mass loss?

_____

_____

_____

4. Why should the nurse consult with the physician before applying a cold pack to a recent injury?

_____

_____

_____

5. Why is a swollen body part elevated above heart level?

_____

_____

_____

6. Why is vitamin D intake necessary for bone health?

_____

_____

_____

Activity H *Answer the following questions related to the musculoskeletal system.*

1. Identify the classification of bones and provide examples of each.

_____

_____

_____

2. Describe bone composition and the process of bone remodeling.

_____

_____

_____

3. Describe how skeletal muscles contract and relax.

_____

_____

_____

4. Describe the tendon attachments to a bone.

_____

_____

_____

5. What information is included in a general assessment of the musculoskeletal system?

_____

_____

_____

6. What information does the nurse gather if the client has experienced a traumatic injury to the musculoskeletal system?

_____

_____

_____

Activity I *Think over the following questions. Discuss them with your instructor or peers.*

1. A client over age 50 asks you how they can maintain their bone health and prevent loss of bone mass. What educational information would you provide?

_____

_____

_____

2. A client is brought in to the emergency department with a traumatic injury to the right ankle; there is no obvious deformity. What assessments and interventions would be appropriate for this client? What diagnostic tests would you anticipate?

_____

_____

_____

3. Your client is scheduled for an arthroscopy. What pre and post procedure care would you provide?

_____

_____

_____

SECTION III: GETTING READY FOR NCLEX

Activity J *Answer the following questions.*

1. An older female client experiences a musculoskeletal injury to her hip. Which of the following methods would help a nurse identify any swelling in the client?
   a. Asking questions of the client to assess the severity of pain
   b. Palpating the muscles and joints
   c. Asking the client to move the injured area as much as possible
   d. Observing the client for any involuntary movements

2. When instructed, the nurse collects ___-hour urine samples for analysis to determine levels of uric acid and calcium excretion.

3. Which of the following methods would best help the nurse determine the degree of a traumatic musculoskeletal injury?
   a. Palpating the injured area to assess the extent of pain experienced by the client
   b. Applying force to the client's extremity and asking the client to push back as much as possible
   c. Encouraging the client to move the injured area as much as possible
   d. Comparing structures and assessment findings on one side of the body with those on the opposite side

4. A client undergoes arthrography for an examination of the knee. What information should the nurse provide to the client?
   a. Expect crackling or clicking noises in the joint for up to 2 days.
   b. Expect fever, nausea, and vomiting for up to 2 days.
   c. Avoid dairy products for up to 2 days.
   d. Avoid potassium-rich foods for up to 2 days.

5. The nurse needs to detect the presence of ischemia in a client with tissue injury. Which of the following signs and symptoms may indicate the presence of ischemia?
   a. Signs of fatigue
   b. Signs of respiratory depression
   c. Absence of a peripheral pulse
   d. Heavy swelling in the injured area

6. Which of the following measures should be taken by the nurse to help relieve edema in a client with tissue injury?

   a. Massaging the swollen body part

   b. Taking a prescribed analgesic

   c. Applying a cold pack to the swollen body part

   d. Keeping the swollen body part above the level of the heart

7. Which of the following practices would delay the decline in muscle strength and bone mass in older adults?

   a. Maintaining an active lifestyle

   b. Maintaining a low-activity lifestyle

   c. Maintaining an adequate calcium intake after the age of 35

   d. Reducing the calcium intake after the age of 60

8. An elderly client has undergone electromyography tests to evaluate muscle weakness and deterioration. The client complains of slight pain after the tests. Which of the following nursing interventions would help relieve the client's discomfort?

   a. Administering topical analgesics to the area where the needle electrodes were inserted

   b. Massaging the area where the needle electrodes were inserted

   c. Applying a cold pack to the area where the needle electrodes were inserted

   d. Applying warm compresses to the area where the needle electrodes were inserted

9. A client recovering from a fractured knee wants to know if there are any non-dairy sources of calcium that are absorbed well by the body. Which one of the following food items should the nurse suggest to enable the client to meet his daily calcium intake requirement?

   a. Green leafy vegetables

   b. Canned salmon with bones

   c. Broccoli

   d. Calcium-fortified orange juice

10. A nurse is assessing a client on the musculoskeletal floor and identifies symptoms of weak pulses, dusky color in the ankles, and 3+ local edema. Which of the following does the nurse suspect to be an issue with this client?

    a. Problems with circulation

    b. Problems with sensation

    c. Problems with mobility

    d. Problems with pain

Caring for Clients Requiring Orthopedic Treatment

Learning Objectives

1. Differentiate types of casts.
2. Discuss the nursing management for a client with a cast.
3. State the reasons for using splints or braces.
4. Identify the principles for maintaining traction and describe nursing care for the client in traction.
5. Differentiate between closed reduction and open reduction and between internal fixation and external fixation.
6. Describe nursing care for the client with a fracture reduction.
7. Identify the reasons for performing orthopedic surgery.
8. Discuss the nursing management for a client undergoing orthopedic surgery.
9. Describe the positioning precautions after a conventional total hip replacement.
10. Explain the nursing needs of the client undergoing total knee replacement.
11. Discuss amputation, including reasons it may be performed and appropriate nursing management of the client.

SECTION I: ASSESSING YOUR UNDERSTANDING

Activity A *Fill in the blanks by choosing the correct word from the options given in parentheses.*

1. _____ provides support, controls movement, and prevents additional injury. (*A reduction, A brace, Traction*)

2. In a _____ reduction, the bone is restored to its normal position by external manipulation. (*Closed, Open, Internal*)

3. In _____ fixation, the surgeon inserts metal pins into the bone or bones from outside the skin surface and then attaches a compression device to the pins. (*Internal, Closed, External*)

4. _____, death of bone tissue, occurs when there is diminished or absent blood supply. (*Subluxation, Avascular necrosis, Hemorrhage*)

5. Following an amputation, pain may result from a stump _____, which is formed when the cut ends of nerves become entangled in the healing scar. (*Hematoma, Neuroma, Causalgia*)

6. A _____ amputation is planned when a client has severe infection and gangrene. The guillotine method is first used, and then a few days later, after the infection is treated and the client is stable, a more definitive, closed amputation is done. (*Open, Closed, Staged*)

Activity B *Mark each statement as either "T" (True) or "F" (False). Correct any false statements.*

1. T F A cylinder cast encircles the trunk from about the nipple line to the iliac crests.

2. T F Reducing a fracture involves restoring proper alignment to the injured bone.

3. T F For traction to achieve its purpose, it requires counter traction, a force opposite to the mechanical pull. Counter traction usually is supplied by the client's own weight.

4. T F Skeletal traction is achieved by applying devices to the skin that indirectly affect the muscles or bones.

5. T F Clients with knee replacements have the amount of flexion and the frequency of use increased daily while hospitalized. The goal is for the client to have the ability to bend the knee 90° by discharge. The amount of flexion for clients with hip replacements should never exceed 30° in a CPM machine.

6. T F Unless an amputation is an emergency, the client is treated for any disorder that may influence healing such as uncontrolled diabetes mellitus, dehydration, infection, electrolyte imbalances, poor nutrition, or chronic respiratory disorders.

7. T F Phantom pain is a feeling that the amputated portion of the limb still remains.

Activity C *Write the correct term for each description given below.*

1. This type of cast surrounds one or both legs and the trunk. It may be strengthened by a bar that spans a casted area between the legs. _____

2. This is used to relieve muscle spasm, align bones, and maintain immobilization. The two most common types are skin and skeletal. _____

3. When this type of reduction is performed (in the operating room) the bone is surgically exposed and realigned. _____

4. Dislocation of the artificial joint. _____

5. A _____ machine promotes healing and flexibility in the knee and hip joint and increases circulation to the operative area.

6. In a _____ amputation (flap amputation), skin flaps cover the severed bone end.

Activity D *Match the methods to treat the fractures given in Column A with their correct descriptions in Column B.*

Column A

_____ **1.** Short leg cast

_____ **2.** Short arm cast

_____ **3.** Body cast

_____ **4.** Long arm cast

_____ **5.** Hip spica cast

_____ **6.** Long leg cast

_____ **7.** Shoulder spica cast

_____ **8.** Walking cast

Column B

a. Extends from below the elbow to the palmar crease and is secured around the base of the thumb. If the thumb is also casted, it is referred to as a thumb spica or gauntlet cast.

b. Extends from the upper level of the axillary fold to the proximal palmar crease. The elbow is usually immobilized at a right angle.

c. Extends from below the knee to the base of the toes. The foot is flexed at a right angle in a neutral position.

d. Extends from the junction of the upper and middle third of the thigh to the base of the toes. The knee may be slightly flexed.

e. A short or long leg cast reinforced for strength.

f. Encircles the trunk.

g. A body cast that encloses the trunk and the shoulder and elbow.

h. Encloses the trunk and a lower extremity. A double hip spica cast includes both legs.

Activity E *Identify the risk factors and interventions for the potential complications following joint replacement surgery.*

Complication	Risk Factors	Interventions
Dislocation of Prosthesis		
Infection		
Neurovascular Compromise		
Deep Vein Thrombosis		

Activity F *Briefly answer the following questions.*

1. Describe the purpose of a cast window.

_____

_____

_____

2. What is the purpose of a bivalve cast?

_____

_____

_____

3. Describe skin care once a cast is removed and limb care following cast removal from an extremity.

_____

_____

_____

4. What conditions must be met for the use of a splint?

_____

_____

_____

5. Describe the proper application of a splint.

_____

_____

_____

6. Describe reasons for orthopedic surgery.

_____

_____

_____

7. What interventions are used preoperatively to prevent excessive bleeding?

_____

_____

_____

8. What factors help the surgical team decide at which level to amputate the arm or leg?

_____

_____

_____

SECTION II: APPLYING YOUR KNOWLEDGE

Activity G *Give rationale for the following questions.*

1. Why is a cast applied from the joint above the break to the one below it? Why is the joint slightly flexed?

_____

_____

_____

2. Why do some fractures not require a cast?

_____

_____

_____

3. Why are the palms of healthcare personnel used when repositioning a wet cast?

_____

_____

_____

4. Why is Buck's extension or another form of skin traction applied if surgery can not be performed right away?

_____

_____

_____

5. Why are porous-coated cementless joint components used with an artificial joint (prosthesis)?

_____

_____

_____

Activity H *Answer the following questions related to caring for clients requiring orthopedic treatment.*

1. Describe the advantages and disadvantages of a plaster and fiberglass cast.

_____

_____

_____

2. When is an open reduction required? When is internal fixation used?

_____

_____

_____

3. What are general nursing measures following a reduction?

_____

_____

_____

4. Explain the precautions following a total hip replacement to prevent subluxation.

_____

_____

_____

5. What are the discharge planning needs for the client following a joint replacement?

_____

_____

_____

6. What conditions may necessitate an amputation?

_____

_____

_____

7. What factors influence an amputee's rehabilitation?

_____

_____

_____

Activity I *Think over the following questions. Discuss them with your instructor or peers.*

1. How will you manage care for the client in traction?

_____

_____

2. What high priority nursing diagnoses and interventions will you identify for the client following a total knee replacement?

_____

_____

_____

3. What steps will you take to provide pin care?

_____

_____

_____

4. What priority nursing diagnoses and interventions would you identify for the client following a traumatic amputation?

_____

_____

_____

SECTION III: GETTING READY FOR NCLEX

Activity J *Answer the following questions.*

1. A cylinder cast needs to be applied to a client with a fracture. What is the role of the nurse during the procedure?

   a. Gently massage the arm or the leg.

   b. Hold the arm or the leg in place.

   c. Provide intense heat or a cast dryer to speed the evaporation.

   d. Compress the cast on a hard surface for better support.

2. Which of the following factors should the nurse emphasize while teaching a client with a cast on the lower extremities?

   a. The importance of following a regular diet.

   b. The use of prescribed analgesics to manage the pain.

   c. Instructions about ambulating with the crutches.

   d. The importance of regular exercise.

3. A client with a skeletal traction reports a throbbing pain. Which of the following actions should the nurse take to relieve the pain?

   a. Administer antibiotics

   b. Elevate the extremity

   c. Petal cast edges with waterproof tape

   d. Massage the area of pain

4. It is important for the nurse to maintain proper pin care for which of the following methods of treating a fracture?

   a. Closed reduction

   b. Open reduction

   c. External fixation

   d. Internal fixation

5. A client who has a musculoskeletal problem is being discharged after a few days of hospital care. Why should the nurse consider factors related to the home environment while determining a plan for the continued rehabilitation of the client?

   a. To include additional care for clients who lack the basic amenities at home.

   b. To determine the client's access to the nearest drugstore.

   c. To modify the client's living arrangements or other accommodation changes.

   d. To determine if the client would continue with the self-care.

6. Fill in the blank: Clients with calcium-related disorders should take other drugs _____hours after calcium carbonate.

7. Which of the following may reduce the risk of excessive bleeding in a client who is scheduled to undergo an orthopedic surgery?

   a. Withholding aspirin before the surgery.

   b. Withholding antacids before the surgery.

   c. Encouraging the intake of red meat before the surgery.

   d. Avoiding excess fluid intake before the surgery.

8. A client who underwent an amputation a week ago still feels an itching sensation or a dull pain in the missing limb. Which of the following nursing actions would help the client in getting relief?

   a. Seek an additional prescription for an analgesic from the physician.

   b. Advice the client to meet a psychiatrist.

   c. Discuss with the physician the possibility of a surgical removal of the nerve endings at the end of the stump.

   d. Discuss the phenomenon of phantom pain with the client.

9. A nurse is assisting a client who is scheduled for surgery for a leg amputation. What are the pre-surgery nursing management strategies utilized to assist the client?

   a. Evaluate pain level and discomfort

   b. Evaluating the client's mental acceptance

   c. Evaluate bleeding and hemorrhage

   d. Evaluate client for risk of infection

10. A nurse evaluates a client for postoperative complications following joint replacement surgery. Upon discharge, the nurse teaches the client that the risk of infection is present for how long after surgery?

    a. Two weeks

    b. One month

    c. Three months

    d. Six months

Caring for Clients with Traumatic Musculoskeletal Injuries

Learning Objectives

1. Differentiate strains, contusions, and sprains.
2. Define joint dislocations.
3. Discuss the nursing management of various types of sports or work related injuries.
4. Identify the stages of bone healing after a fracture.
5. Describe the signs and symptoms of a fracture.
6. Explain the nursing management for clients with various types of fractures.
7. Discuss methods used to prevent complications associated with fractures.
8. Discuss potential complications associated with a fractured hip.

SECTION I: ASSESSING YOUR UNDERSTANDING

Activity A *Fill in the blanks by choosing the correct word from the options given in parentheses.*

1. A _____ is confined to the soft tissues and does not affect the musculoskeletal structure. Many small blood vessels rupture, causing ecchymosis or a hematoma. *(Strain, Contusion, Sprain)*

2. A test that elicits tingling, numbness, and pain, known as _____, may be used to diagnose carpal tunnel syndrome. *(Tinel's sign, Phalen's sign, Turner's sign)*

3. A _____ injury occurs with twisting of the knee or repeated squatting. *(Tendon, Ligament, Meniscal)*

4. Rupture of the _____ occurs secondary to trauma. As the client engages in an activity, the calf muscle contracts suddenly while the foot is grounded firmly in place. There is often a loud pop, and the client experiences severe pain and inability to plantar flex the affected foot. *(Rotator cuff, Achilles tendon, Collateral knee ligaments)*

5. Usually a hip fracture affects the _____ end of the femur. This type of fracture commonly results from a fall and occurs more frequently in older adults with osteoporosis. *(Proximal, Medial, Distal)*

Activity B *Mark each statement as either "T" (True) or "F" (False). Correct any false statements.*

1. T F Areas most subject to sprains are the wrist, elbow, knee, and ankle. Sprains result from sudden, unusual movement or stretching about a joint, common with falls or other accidental injuries.

2. T F The pain from tendonitis tends to be more prominent at night and early in the morning.

3. T F The lateral or medial collateral knee ligaments provide stability to forward and backward movements.

4. T F Treatment of ligament and meniscal injuries depends upon the extent of the injury. Initial treatment involves immobilizing the joint and limiting weight bearing.

5. T F About 1 year of healing must pass before bone regains its former structural strength, becomes well consolidated and remodeled (re-formed), and possesses fat and marrow cells.

Activity C *Write the correct term for each description given below.*

1. Results from excessive stress, overuse, or over-stretching. Small blood vessels in the muscle rupture, and the muscle fibers sustain tiny tears. The client experiences inflammation, local tenderness, and muscle spasms._____

2. A sprain of the cervical spine. _____

3. The client flexes the wrist for 30 seconds to determine if pain or numbness occurs, a positive sign for carpal tunnel syndrome. _____

4. Made up of a complexity of muscles and tendons that connect the proximal humerus, clavicle, and scapula, which in turn connect with the sternum (clavicle) and ribs (scapula). _____

5. For torn menisci, the surgeon removes the damaged cartilage. _____

6. A break in the continuity of a bone. _____

Activity D *Match the terms in Column A with their correct descriptions in Column B.*

Column A

____ **1.** Dislocation

____ **2.** Subluxation

____ **3.** Compartment syndrome

____ **4.** Palsy

____ **5.** Volkmann's contracture

Column B

a. A partial dislocation.

b. Decreased sensation and movement.

c. A clawlike deformity of the hand resulting from obstructed arterial blood flow to the forearm and hand.

d. When the articular surfaces of a joint are no longer in contact.

e. A condition in which a structure such as a tendon or nerve is constricted in a confined space.

Activity E *Describe these common complications of fractures and appropriate interventions based on the following criteria.*

Complication	Description	Intervention
Shock		
Fat embolism		
Pulmonary embolism		
Compartment syndrome		
Delayed bone healing		
Infection		
Avascular necrosis		

Activity F *Briefly answer the following questions.*

1. Describe the pathophysiology of a sprain and avulsion fracture.

_____

_____

_____

2. Describe the nursing care for a dislocation.

_____

_____

_____

3. Provide the names and locations of the common types of tendonitis that commonly occur as a result of repeated sports and/or work activities.

_____

_____

_____

4. How do injuries to the ligaments of the knee occur? What are the signs and symptoms?

_____

_____

_____

5. How do rotator cuff injuries often occur? What are the signs and symptoms of a rotator cuff injury?

_____

_____

_____

SECTION II: APPLYING WHAT YOU KNOW

Activity G *Give the rationale for the following questions.*

1. Why is a dislocation immobilized following a manipulation?

2. Why are older adults more prone to skeletal fractures?

3. Why do multiple injuries often accompany fractures of the femur?

4. Why are fractures of the femur initially treated with some form of traction?

5. Why are hip fractures a serious problem for older adults?

Activity H *Answer the following questions related to caring for clients with traumatic musculoskeletal injuries.*

1. Describe the medical management of a sprain.

2. Describe the signs and symptoms of a dislocation.

3. Describe the medical and surgical management of tendonitis.

4. What are the signs and symptoms of a fracture?

5. What is the nursing care for a client with a fracture?

6. Describe the assessments findings with a femur fracture.

7. What is the nursing management for a client with a femur fracture?

Activity I *Think over the following questions. Discuss them with your instructor or peers.*

1. You are working at a community health fair. What information would you provide to clients for prevention of sports or work related injuries?

2. Your client returns from surgery for treatment of a hip fracture. What high priority nursing diagnoses and interventions would you identify?

_____

_____

_____

3. You witness an individual take a fall; they complain of pain in their ankle. How would you assist the individual until additional assistance arrives?

_____

_____

_____

4. Your client is postoperative following musculoskeletal surgery. The client does not want to participate in any activities that involve movement. What educational information would you provide?

_____

_____

_____

SECTION III: GETTING READY FOR NCLEX

Activity J *Answer the following questions.*

1. A female client informs the nurse that she overstretched her arm muscles when lifting a heavy suitcase, and now experiences inflammation, some tenderness, and muscle spasms. Which of the following problems is she most likely to have?

   a. Strain

   b. Contusion

   c. Sprain

   d. Avulsion fracture

2. Which of the following measures should the nurse strongly recommend to a client recovering from a ruptured Achilles tendon to help regain mobility, strength, and the full range of motion?

   a. Regular use of NSAIDs

   b. Vigorous exercise

   c. Physical therapy

   d. Non-medical interventions, such as yoga

3. A graphic designer, who spends hours working on the computer, complains of a slight pain in her right hand. The client describes the pain to be more prominent at night and early in the morning. The condition is not yet serious. Which of the following measures should the nurse suggest to the designer to help alleviate the pain?

   a. Flexing the affected wrist

   b. Shaking the affected hand

   c. Using surgical intervention

   d. Applying physical therapy

4. Which of the following symptoms should the nurse specifically monitor while assessing a client with a femoral neck fracture?

   a. Severe pain at the site of the fracture

   b. Bleeding from joint capsules

   c. Muscle spasms

   d. Crepitus at the site of the fracture

5. Fill in the blank: In a client who has undergone an orthopedic surgery, it is necessary for the nurse to auscultate the lung sounds every ___ hours.

6. The nurse positions a client who is being treated for a fracture. Why should care be taken to position the client's joints in an anatomic alignment?

   a. To prevent deep vein thrombosis

   b. To facilitate the lung expansion and prevent the pooling of secretions

   c. To prevent the escalation of the pain and swelling

   d. To prevent damage to the peripheral nerves and the blood vessels

7. Which of the following symptoms should the nurse closely monitor for in a client with a compartment syndrome in the upper arm?

   a. Epicondylitis

   b. Carpal tunnel syndrome

   c. Volkmann's contracture

   d. Ganglion cyst

8. A client is monitored for complications after having surgery to repair a fracture. Which of the following symptoms would indicate an arterial obstruction in the affected area?
   a. Rapid capillary refill
   b. Warm skin
   c. Cool skin
   d. Numbness

9. A client who is treated for a meniscal injury to the knee is advised prolonged immobility. To help prevent skin breakdown and infections, the nurse should instruct the client to increase the intake of which of the following?
   a. Protein
   b. Fiber
   c. Calcium
   d. Liquid

10. A physician is discussing the care of the client with a certain type of fracture with the nurse. Which type of fracture is defined as a fracture in which damage also involves the skin or mucous membranes?
    a. Pathologic
    b. Compression
    c. Depressed
    d. Compound

63

Caring for Clients with Orthopedic and Connective Tissue Disorders

1. Explain the difference between rheumatoid arthritis and degenerative joint disease (osteoarthritis) and describe nursing management.
2. Describe the clinical manifestations of temporomandibular disorder (TMD).
3. State the pathophysiology of gout, fibromyalgia, bursitis, and ankylosing spondylitis.
4. Delineate the nursing care required for clients with gout, fibromyalgia, bursitis, and ankylosing spondylitis.
5. Discuss the multisystem involvement associated with systemic lupus erythematosus.
6. Identify the causes of osteomyelitis.
7. Explain the inflammatory process associated with Lyme disease.
8. Identify risk factors for development of osteoporosis.
9. Distinguish the pathophysiology of osteomalacia and Paget's disease.
10. Differentiate between bunions and hammer toe.
11. Discuss characteristics of benign and malignant bone tumors.

SECTION I: ASSESSING YOUR UNDERSTANDING

Activity A *Fill in the blanks by choosing the correct word from the options given in parentheses.*

1. A positive C-reactive protein (CRP) test, low red blood cell count and hemoglobin levels in later stages, and positive RF are laboratory findings that support the diagnosis of _____. *(Rheumatoid arthritis, Osteoarthritis, Osteomyelitis)*

2. _____ is the most common form of arthritis. It also is known as the "wear and tear" disease and typically affects the weight-bearing joints. It is characterized by a slow and steady progression of destructive changes in weight-bearing joints and those that are repeatedly used for work. *(Rheumatoid arthritis, Osteoarthritis, Temporomandibular disorder)*

3. _____ is a painful metabolic disorder involving an inflammatory reaction in the joints. It usually affects the feet (especially the great toe), hands, elbows, ankles, and knees. *(Fibromyalgia, Gout, Ankylosing spondylitis)*

4. _____ is a chronic syndrome of pain, fatigue, and sleep disturbances. The pain is widespread, affecting muscles, ligaments, and tendons. *(Fibromyalgia, Gout, Ankylosing spondylitis)*

5. The most common symptoms of _____ are low back pain and stiffness. As the disease progresses, the spine and hips become more immobile, thus restricting movement. The lumbar curve of the spine may flatten. The neck can be permanently flexed and the client appears to be in a perpetual stooped position. *(Fibromyalgia, Gout, Ankylosing spondylitis)*

6. Approximately 60% to 70% of people with
_____ have positive anti-dsDNA.
(Systemic lupus erythematosus, Osteomyelitis, Lyme disease)

7. _____ is an infection of the bone. Limited blood supply, inflammation of and pressure on the tissue, and formation of new bone around devitalized bone tissue make this condition difficult and challenging to treat. *(Systemic lupus erythematosus, Osteomyelitis, Lyme disease)*

8. _____ is a chronic bone disorder characterized by abnormal bone remodeling. It affects adults older than 60 years of age. The most common areas of involvement are the long bones, spine, pelvis, and skull. *(Osteomyelitis, Osteomalacia, Paget's disease)*

Activity B *Mark each statement as either "T" (True) or "F" (False). Correct any false statements.*

1. T F Arthritis includes more than 100 different types of recognized inflammatory disorders, making this collective group the most common orthopedic problem.

2. T F Arthroplasty is a procedure to remove the lining of the joint. This procedure is performed when the lining is inflamed and adding to the pain the client is experiencing.

3. T F Bouchard's nodes are bony enlargements of the distal interphalangeal joints associated with osteoarthritis.

4. T F Some clients with osteoarthritis may have a slightly elevated ESR.

5. T F There is no specific treatment for Lyme disease. Medical management aims at producing a remission and preventing or treating acute exacerbations of the disorder. High doses of corticosteroids are used initially.

6. T F *Escherichia coli* causes 70% to 80% of bone infections (osteomyelitis).

7. T F Lyme disease results in progressive symptoms, beginning with a characteristic rash and eventually involving the cardiac, neurologic, and musculoskeletal systems.

8. T F Small-framed, thin African American women are at greatest risk for osteoporosis.

9. T F A bunion is a flexion deformity of the proximal interphalangeal (PIP) joint and may involve several toes.

Activity C *Write the correct term for each description given below.*

1. The synovial fluid usually appears cloudy, milky, or dark yellow, and contains many inflammatory cells, including leukocytes and complement (a group of proteins in blood that affect the inflammatory process and influence antigen–antibody reactions).

_____

2. These products act as a lubricant, substituting for hyaluronic acid, the substance that provides joint fluid viscosity. Pain relief appears to last 6 to 13 months. Side effects include swelling, redness, or heat at the injection site. Clients allergic to eggs should not receive these injections. _____

3. An attack is characterized by a sudden onset of acute pain and tenderness in one joint.

_____

4. Pregabalin (Lyrica) is the first drug approved by the Food and Drug Administration to treat this disorder. It is used to reduce pain and fatigue and improve sleep quality.

_____

5. Painful movement of a joint, such as the elbow or shoulder, is the most common symptom. A distinct lump may be felt. If there is a rupture, tissue in the area may become edematous, warm, and tender.

_____

6. A chronic connective tissue disorder of the spine and surrounding cartilaginous joints, such as the sacroiliac joints and soft tissues around the vertebrae. _____

7. Known as "the great imitator" because the clinical signs resemble many other conditions.

_____

8. This type of bone tumor usually results from misplaced or overgrown clusters of normal bone or cartilage cells that cause the structure to enlarge and impair local function. They grow slowly and do not metastasize. Their growth can weaken the bone structure by compressing or displacing the normal tissue.

_____

Activity D *Match the conditions given in Column A with their characteristics in Column B.*

Column A

_____ **1.** Gout

_____ **2.** Fibromyalgia

_____ **3.** Bursitis

_____ **4.** Ankylosing spondylitis

Column B

a. It is believed that repeated nerve stimulation results in abnormal levels of neurotransmitters that signal pain. The pain receptors in the brain develop a memory of the pain and are more sensitive to the signals. There are tender and painful points that can be identified on clients with this condition that other people without this condition do not have.

b. Usually begins in early adulthood and is more common in men than in women. Its etiology is unknown, although some theorize that an altered immune response occurs when T-cell lymphocytes mistake human cells for similar-appearing bacterial antigens. There also is a strong familial tendency for some affected individuals. The disorder tends to be inherited and affects more men than women. It may occur secondary to other diseases marked by decreased renal excretion of uric acid. It also has been identified among clients who have received organ transplants and the antirejection drug cyclosporine.

c. Trauma is the most common cause. Other causes include overuse, stress, infection, and secondary effects of gout and RA. Typical of any inflammation, pain and swelling occur with compromised function.

Activity E *Compare and contrast rheumatoid arthritis and osteoarthritis (degenerative joint disease) using the following criteria.*

Criteria	Rheumatoid Arthritis (RA)	Osteoarthritis (Degenerative Joint Disease)
Etiology		
Pathophysiology		
Signs and Symptoms		
Medical Management		

Activity F *Briefly answer the following questions.*

1. Describe the following proximal finger deformities associated with rheumatoid arthritis: Swan neck deformity, Boutonnière deformity, and Ulnar deviation.

_____

_____

_____

2. Temporomandibular disorder (TMD) is a cluster of symptoms localized near the jaw. Describe these symptoms.

_____

_____

_____

3. What are the two treatment approaches for gout?

_____

_____

_____

4. Describe the etiology of systemic lupus erythematosus.

_____

_____

_____

5. Describe how osteomyelitis may occur.

_____

_____

_____

6. Describe the pathophysiology of osteoporosis.

_____

_____

_____

7. Where are malignant bone tumors usually found?

_____

_____

_____

SECTION II: APPLYING YOUR KNOWLEDGE

Activity G _Give rationales for the following questions._

1. Why does the nurse advise the client to take aspirin and NSAIDs with food?

_____

_____

_____

2. Why does the nurse place a cradle over the affected joint for the client with gout?

_____

_____

_____

3. Why does aging contribute to osteoporosis?

_____

_____

_____

4. Why is bone mass structurally weaker and why do bone deformities occur with osteomalacia?

_____

_____

_____

5. Why would a client with systemic lupus erythematosus have coping issues? What assistance can the nurse provide?

_____

_____

_____

6. Why would respiratory compromise be an issue for a client with ankylosing spondylitis?

_____

_____

_____

7. Why were some COX-2 inhibitors removed from the market?

_____

_____

_____

Activity H _Answer the following questions related to caring for clients with orthopedic and connective tissue disorders._

1. What is Prosorba column therapy used for? Describe the therapy.

_____

_____

_____

2. Describe the nursing management for the client with rheumatoid arthritis.

_____

_____

_____

3. Describe the nursing management for the client with osteoarthritis.

_____

_____

_____

4. What are the signs and symptoms of systemic lupus erythematosus?

_____

_____

_____

5. Describe the medical and surgical management of osteomyelitis.

_____

_____

_____

6. What are the 3 stages of Lyme disease?

_____

_____

_____

7. How is osteoporosis medically managed?

_____

_____

_____

8. Describe the pathophysiology of Paget's disease.

_____

_____

_____

Activity I   *Think over the following questions. Discuss them with your instructor or peers.*

1. Your client does not understand the articular and extra-articular manifestations of rheumatoid arthritis. What educational information would you provide?

_____

_____

_____

2. What high priority nursing diagnoses and interventions would you identify for a client with rheumatoid arthritis?

_____

_____

_____

3. Your client has a family history of osteoarthritis. What educational information would you provide to them about the prevention of osteoarthritis?

_____

_____

_____

4. A client with systemic lupus erythematosus is distraught related to their physical appearance and limitations. How would you support them and promote coping?

_____

_____

_____

5. Your client lives in an area where deer ticks are common. What educational information would you provide to promote prevention of Lyme disease?

_____

_____

_____

SECTION III: GETTING READY FOR NCLEX

Activity J   *Choose the correct response for the following questions.*

1. Which of the following should the nurse emphasize during the teaching of a client with degenerative joint disease?

a. Sleep on a firm mattress.

b. Maintain moderate activity.

c. Avoid administering prescribed aspirin and NSAIDs with food.

d. Avoid purine-rich foods.

2. Which of the following would increase excretion of uric acid in a client with gout?

a. A high fluid intake

b. Use of salicylates

c. A high intake of purine-rich foods

d. A low intake of carbohydrates

3. Which of the following are the most common symptoms of ankylosing spondylitis?

a. Painful movement of a joint

b. Swelling and tenderness at a joint

c. Low back pain

d. Partial paralysis

4. Which of the following should a nurse instruct a client with lupus erythematosus to use before performing ROM exercises?
   a. Prescribed analgesics
   b. Cold packs
   c. Moist heat
   d. Braces or splints

5. Which of the following symptoms should the nurse observe in a client who is in the midstage of Lyme disease?
   a. Joint erosion
   b. Fever, chills, and malaise
   c. Arthritis
   d. Facial palsy and meningitis

6. In providing care for clients with osteoporosis, the nurse emphasizes the need for a nutritious, well-balanced diet that is high in which of the following?
   a. Calcium
   b. Iron
   c. Zinc
   d. Carbohydrates

7. Which of the following findings is common in clients with Paget's disease?
   a. Elevated serum alkaline phosphatase level
   b. Decreased urinary hydroxyproline excretion
   c. Elevated leukocyte count
   d. Elevated creatinine level

8. To reduce the risk of renal calculi, a complication of prolonged immobility and gout, the nurse should advise clients to drink at least ___ quarts of fluid daily.

9. A client with a disease of the bones is beginning to feel better. Which of the following critical instructions should a nurse provide this client at this stage?
   a. Advise the client to reduce the dosage of the prescribed drugs
   b. Caution the client against discontinuing the prescribed drugs
   c. Encourage the client to resume heavy activity
   d. Encourage the client to gain weight

10. A client is admitted to the floor with Systemic Lupus Erythematosus (SLE). Which of the following teaching points does the nurse stress to the client with SLE?
    a. Apply ice as instructed
    b. Avoid sunlight and ultraviolet radiation.
    c. Use assistive devices appropriately
    d. Change dressing as prescribed

Introduction to the Integumentary System

SECTION I: ASSESSING YOUR UNDERSTANDING

Activity A *Fill in the blanks by choosing the correct word from the options given in parentheses.*

1. The epidermis is constantly shed and replaced with epithelial cells from the dermis every day. The epidermis is totally replaced approximately every _____ days. *(25 to 35, 35 to 45, 45 to 55)*

2. The _____ is the layer of skin attached to muscle and bone. It is composed primarily of connective tissue and fat cells. *(Dermal layer, Subcutaneous tissue, Epidermal layer)*

3. _____ are connected to each hair follicle and secrete an oily substance called sebum, which is a lubricant that prevents drying and cracking of the skin and hair. *(Sebaceous glands, Apocrine glands, Eccrine glands)*

4. A fungal culture requires incubation at room temperature for _____ weeks. *(1 to 2 weeks, 2 to 3 weeks, 3 to 4 weeks)*

5. _____ are prescribed when allergy is a factor in causing a skin disorder. They relieve itching and shorten the duration of the allergic reaction. *(Antibiotics, Antihistamines, Antiseptics)*

6. Fingernails and toenails are layers of hard keratin that have a _____ function. *(Sensory, Protective, Chemical synthesis)*

Activity B *Mark each statement as either "T" (True) or "F" (False). Correct any false statements.*

1. T F The dermis contains an outer layer of dead skin cells, the stratum corneum, which forms a tough protective protein called keratin.

2. T F The skin, combined with body hair, serves as a means of monitoring the outside environment, as well as warning of danger. Specialized nerve endings in the skin respond to pressure, pain, heat, and cold.

3. T F Apocrine glands release water and electrolytes, such as sodium and chloride, in the form of perspiration.

4. T F Hair assessment applies only to the head.

5. T F Clubbing of the nails is a sign of iron-deficiency anemia.

6. T F Corticosteroids are used in the treatment of infestations with scabies, mites, and lice.

7. T F Local (topical) anesthetics are used to reduce bacteria on the skin.

Activity C *Write the correct term for each description given below.*

1. Consists of connective tissue and contains elastic fibers, blood vessels, sensory and motor nerves, sweat and sebaceous (oil) glands, and hair follicles (roots). _____

2. The color of the skin is determined by this pigment which is manufactured by melanocytes located in the epidermis. _____

3. It covers all parts of the body except the palms, soles, dorsum of the fingers, lips, penis, labia, and nipples. _____

4. These commonly occur on the skin over the coccyx and sacrum in the lower spine, the hips, heels, elbows, shoulder blades, ears, and back of head. _____

5. A hand-held device that can identify certain fungal infections that fluoresce under long-wave ultraviolet light. _____

6. Medications applied directly to the scalp or incorporated into shampooing products. They are used to control dandruff. _____

Activity D *Match the stages of a pressure sore in Column A with their correct descriptions in Column B.*

Column A

____ **1.** Stage I

____ **2.** Stage II

____ **3.** Stage III

____ **4.** Stage IV

Column B

a. The most traumatic and life-threatening stage. The tissue is deeply ulcerated, exposing muscle and bone. The dead tissue produces a rank odor.

Local infection, which is the rule rather than the exception, easily spreads throughout the body, causing a potentially fatal condition referred to as sepsis.

b. Characterized by redness of the skin. The reddened skin fails to resume its normal color, or blanch, when pressure is relieved.

c. A shallow crater extends to the subcutaneous tissue. These pressure sores may be accompanied by serous drainage from leaking plasma or purulent drainage (white or yellow-tinged fluid) caused by a wound infection. The area is relatively painless.

d. The area is reddened and accompanied by blistering or a shallow break in the skin, sometimes described as a skin tear. Impairment of the skin leads to microbial colonization and infection of the wound.

Activity E *Provide the description and identify the purpose of the following medical and surgical treatments based on the given criteria.*

Treatment	Description	Purpose
Surgical Excision		
Laser Therapy		
Cryosurgery		
Electrodesiccation		
Radiation Therapy		
Photochemotherapy		

Activity F *Briefly answer the following questions.*

1. Describe the functions of the integumentory system.

_____

_____

_____

2. How does the skin facilitate the synthesis of vitamin D?

_____

_____

_____

3. How does a pressure sore occur?

_____

_____

_____

4. What causes an abnormal thickening of the nails?

_____

_____

_____

5. What is the purpose of a skin biopsy?

_____

_____

_____

6. What medications are used to treat infectious disorders?

_____

_____

_____

7. Describe how keratolytics are used to treat warts, corns, and calluses.

_____

_____

_____

8. What is the purpose of a therapeutic bath?

_____

_____

_____

SECTION II: APPLYING YOUR KNOWLEDGE

Activity G *Give rationale for the following questions.*

1. Why is the skin considered protective?

_____

_____

_____

2. Why can densely saturated moist air result in heat stroke?

_____

_____

_____

3. Why is thermoregulation altered in the older adult?

_____

_____

_____

4. Why does odor occur with perspiration?

_____

_____

_____

5. Why are older adults more vulnerable to heat?

_____

_____

_____

6. Why do nails have a pink semitransparent appearance?

_____

_____

_____

7. Why would a physician order a potassium hydroxide test?

_____

_____

_____

8. Why are emollients, ointments, powders, and lotions used on the skin?

_____

_____

_____

Activity H *Answer the following questions related to the integumentory system.*

1. Heat dissipates through the skin and through respiration. Describe the four methods of how heat is lost and provide an example of each.

_____

_____

_____

2. Describe the elements of a skin assessment and identify normal findings.

_____

_____

_____

3. Identify measures that reduce conditions under which pressure sores are likely to form.

_____

_____

_____

4. Describe the elements of a nail assessment.

_____

_____

_____

5. Describe the application and purpose of a wet dressing.

_____

_____

_____

6. Describe why lifestyle changes are important to some skin disorders.

_____

_____

_____

Activity I *Think over the following questions. Discuss them with your instructor or peers.*

1. Your client has a stage II pressure sore. What nutritional information would you provide to the client?

_____

_____

_____

2. Your older client requires assistance with moving and transferring. How would you educate the staff in the movement of this client to prevent a pressure sore?

_____

_____

_____

3. Your client requires the application of a topical medication. What is the nursing care required for this medication administration?

_____

_____

_____

SECTION III: GETTING READY FOR NCLEX

Activity J *Answer the following questions.*

1. Which of the following factors stimulates the production of melanin?
   a. Exposure to a cloudy environment
   b. Exposure to ultraviolet light
   c. Exposure to air pollutants
   d. Exposure to warm temperature

2. Which of the following actions helps the nurse assess the skin temperature?
   a. Inspecting and palpating the skin
   b. Detecting moisture with the palmar surface
   c. Grasping the skin
   d. Placing the dorsum of the hand on the surface of the skin

3. Which of the following are consequences of skin impairment?
   a. Purulent leakage
   b. Itching
   c. Infection of the wound
   d. Pain

4. During the routine nail assessment of a client, the nurse notices that the angle between the nail base and the skin is greater than 160°. What does this finding indicate?
   a. Poor circulation
   b. Iron deficiency anemia
   c. Long-standing cardiopulmonary disease
   d. Fungal infection

5. A nurse is caring for a client who has been bedridden for several years. Which of the following actions should the nurse perform if the client's skin blanches with pressure relief?
   a. Massage bony areas
   b. Use a moisturizing skin cleanser
   c. Pad body areas
   d. Turn and reposition the client frequently

6. A client is admitted to the floor and has symptoms of nausea, vomiting, and diarrhea as well as immobility due to a fractured femur. Which of the following are risk factors for pressure ulcers in this client?
   a. Dehydration
   b. Hypokalemia
   c. Hypernatremia
   d. Fluid overload

7. A nurse identifies a skin lesion on a client and documents the lesion stating that the lesion is elevated, round, and filled with serum. What is the correct type of lesion that the above definition describes?
   a. Macule
   b. Papule
   c. Wheal
   d. Vesicle

8. A nurse is taking care of a client and assesses skin color to be yellow. What is the underlying cause of yellow skin color?
   a. Anemia
   b. Liver or kidney disease
   c. Low tissue oxygenation
   d. Trauma to soft tissue

9. A client is prescribed drug therapy for the treatment of lice in addition to recovering from postoperative surgery. What is the drug class treatment for this disorder?
   a. Antihistamines
   b. Antifungals
   c. Keratolytics
   d. Pediculicides

Caring for Clients with Skin, Hair, and Nail Disorders

Learning Objectives

1. Identify risks associated with tattooing and body piercing.
2. Describe general care following tattooing and body piercing.
3. Define and name two types of dermatitis.
4. Explain factors that lead to acne vulgaris.
5. Describe characteristics of rosacea.
6. Differentiate between a furuncle, furunculosis, and carbuncle.
7. Describe the appearance and cause of psoriasis.
8. Describe the process for eradicating a skin mite infection using a scabicidal medication.
9. Identify locations on the body where parasitic fungi known as dermatophytes are most likely to infect.
10. Describe the characteristics of an outbreak of shingles.
11. Discuss factors that promote skin cancer as well as measures that help prevent it.
12. Name two conditions characterized by hair loss, and the etiology for each.
13. Describe the appearance of head lice and nits and explain how to remove them.
14. Discuss factors that promote fungal infections of the nails.
15. Name techniques for preventing onychocryptosis (ingrown toenails).

SECTION I: ASSESSING YOUR UNDERSTANDING

Activity A *Fill in the blanks by choosing the correct word from the options given in parentheses.*

1. With _____ the skin response is characterized by dilation of the blood vessels, causing redness and swelling, and sometimes by vesiculation and oozing. Itching is a prominent symptom. *(Dermatitis, Psoriasis, Rosacea)*

2. _____ is a method of removing surface layers of scarred skin. It is useful in lessening scars such as the pitting from severe acne. The outermost layers of the skin are removed by sandpaper, a rotating wire brush, chemicals (chemical face peeling), or a diamond wheel. *(Scarification, Salabrasion, Dermabrasion)*

3. _____ is a chronic, noninfectious inflammatory disorder of the skin that affects both men and women. Its onset is in young and middle adulthood. Periods of emotional stress, hormonal cycles, infection, and seasonal changes appear to aggravate the condition *(Dermatitis, Psoriasis, Rosacea)*

4. _____ is a dermatologic condition associated with excessive production of secretions from the sebaceous glands. Although it is not always confined to the scalp, it is one of the primary sites. *(Alopecia, Seborrhea, Lice)*

5. _____ is a fungal dermatophyte infection of the fingernails or toenails. A fungus is a tiny, plantlike parasite that thrives in warm, dark, moist environments. Fungi can spread unchecked from one nail to another. *(Onychomycosis, Seborrhea, Onychocryptosis)*

Activity B *Mark each statement as True (T) or False (F). Correct any false statements.*

1. T F The earliest sign of rosacea is frequent, intermittent blushing across the nose, forehead, cheeks, and chin.

2. T F A carbuncle is a boil, and carbunculosis refers to having multiple boils.

3. T F Symptoms vary with skin cancer, but usually the new appearance of a growth or a change in color of the skin is the first symptom the client notices. The lesion can be smooth or rough, flat or elevated, and itchy or tender. It may bleed.

4. T F Androgenetic alopecia is believed to be an autoimmune disorder characterized by patchy areas of hair loss about the size of a coin. Antibodies attack and destroy the hair follicle.

5. T F Lice are transmitted through direct contact. They cannot survive longer than about 24 hours without blood. Sharing clothing, combs, and brushes promotes transmission.

6. T F Pediculicides are contraindicated in pregnant and nursing women, children younger than 2 years of age, and those who have health conditions such as open wounds, epilepsy, or asthma.

Activity C *Write the correct term for each description below.*

1. The insertion of a metal ring or barbell, which is a straight or curved rod, into a body part. Common locations include lips, ear cartilage, cheeks, nose, tongue, eyebrows, navel, nipples, or genital area. _____

2. Mild cases improve with gentle facial cleansing and nonprescription drying agents containing benzoyl peroxide. _____

3. Factors that contribute to vasodilation or irritation of the skin may trigger blushing; examples include consuming hot beverages, spicy food, or alcohol; exposure to sun, wind, or cold; bathing with hot water; stress, or use of skin care products. _____

4. A combination of UV light therapy and a photosensitizing psoralen drug such as methoxsalen (Oxsoralen-Ultra), also has been used for severe, disabling psoriasis that does not respond to other methods of treatment. _____

5. The medical term for an ingrown toenail. _____

6. A person trained to care for feet. _____

Activity D *Describe the pathophysiology and signs and symptoms of the skin disorders that follow.*

Disorder	Pathophysiology	Signs and Symptoms
Scabies		
Dermatophytoses		
Shingles		

Activity E *Compare and contrast the following skin disorders based on the given criteria.*

Disorder	Description	Pathophysiology
Dermatitis		
Acne vulgaris		
Rosacea		

Activity F *Briefly answer the following questions.*

1. Describe the medical management of dermatitis.

_____

_____

_____

2. Describe the medical management of a furuncle, furunculosis, or carbuncle.

_____

_____

_____

3. Describe the etiology of psoriasis.

_____

_____

_____

4. Describe the medical management of scabies.

_____

_____

_____

5. Describe the appearance and treatment for lice.

_____

_____

_____

SECTION II: APPLYING YOUR KNOWLEDGE

Activity G *Give rationale for the following questions.*

1. Why does the American Association of Blood Banks reject potential blood donors who have received a tattoo within 1 year?

_____

_____

_____

2. Why is furunculosis associated with diabetes?

_____

_____

_____

3. Why should pediculicides not be used on pets?

_____

_____

_____

4. Why does the nurse instruct the client or family not to shampoo or rinse with a conditioner before applying a pediculicide?

_____

_____

_____

5. Why are sutures not required for the surgical treatment of onychocryptosis?

_____

_____

_____

Activity H *Answer the following questions related to caring for clients with skin, hair, and nail disorders.*

1. What are the risks associated with body tattooing?

_____

_____

_____

2. What are the risks associated with body piercing?

_____

_____

_____

3. What treatment options are available for clients with severe acne vulgaris?

_____

_____

_____

4. Describe the nursing management of a client with a furuncle, furunculosis, or carbuncle.

_____

_____

_____

5. Describe the pathophysiology and signs and symptoms of psoriasis.

_____

_____

_____

6. What factors predispose to malignant changes in the skin?

_____

_____

_____

Activity I *Think over the following questions. Discuss them with your instructor or peers.*

1. A neighbor has received a tattoo and asks you how to care for the affected area of the skin. What educational information would you provide?

_____

_____

_____

2. A co-worker is considering a body piercing but is unfamiliar with the risks and care following a piercing. What educational information would you provide?

_____

_____

_____

3. You volunteer to provide educational information about skin cancer prevention at a health promotion fair. What information will you provide?

_____

_____

_____

4. A friend calls and states their child has been sent home from school due to head lice. The friend asks you what to do. How would you advise them on the treatment and procedure for removing lice?

_____

_____

_____

SECTION III: GETTING READY FOR NCLEX

Activity J *Answer the following questions:*

1. What instruction should the nurse give to an elderly client to reduce the itching that results from dry skin?
   a. Take hot baths daily.
   b. Apply moisturizer to the skin.
   c. Take an antipruritic to control the itching.
   d. Wear minimal clothing to expose the skin to the air.

2. Several skin disorders involve an infecting agent. Which of the following is the cause of dermatophytoses?
   a. Itch mite.
   b. Parasitic fungi.
   c. Reactivated virus.
   d. Pediculosis.

3. A client has come to the ambulatory care center for the surgical treatment of a persistent ingrown toenail on her right foot. The nurse provides the review of the procedure to the client. Which of the following statements indicates the correct information?
   a. The client should fast overnight as the operation will be performed under general anesthesia.
   b. There won't be much bleeding as the physician will tie up the open vessels.
   c. The client will be able to drive to work directly from the center.
   d. The procedure does not require sutures.

4. What are the right practices for self-care to be followed by a client with onychomycosis of the foot?
   a. Antifungal medications should be taken daily for 5 to 10 days.
   b. Change footwear from leather shoes to tennis shoes.
   c. Avoid walking barefoot.
   d. Keep the feet moist.

5. An elderly client with diabetes mellitus is taught how to care for the carbuncle on her foot and to prevent the spread of infection. What is the most important action to prevent the spread of infection?

   a. Cold wet soaks.

   b. Proper disposal of the soiled material.

   c. Wash hands before and after applying a topical medication.

   d. The use of an antiseptic solution to clean the wound.

6. A client is using acne preparations containing benzoyl peroxide. What instruction should the nurse give to the client to prevent fabric discoloration?

   a. A thorough washing of the hands

   b. A thorough bath after the medication

   c. Wear disposable clothes

   d. Wear disposable plastic gloves

7. A client with psoriasis is feeling distressed as the condition has no known cure. Which of the following actions from the nurse can help the client accept the condition?

   a. Encourage the client to join a psoriasis support group.

   b. Recommend dermabrasion.

   c. Apply anthralin.

   d. Recommend a skin graft.

8. A client is being discharged from the hospital and states that they are planning to get a body piercing in the navel within the next month. The client asks the nurse if she knows the healing time associated with such a procedure. The nurse investigates the answer and answers the client's question by stating which of the following?

   a. "It should take up to 8 weeks for healing at the site of the navel."

   b. "It should take up to 4 months for healing at the site of the navel."

   c. "It should take up to 9 months for healing at the site of the navel."

   d. "It should take up to 2 weeks for healing at the site of the navel."

9. A nurse is providing information to clients in a dermatologist's office about prevention of skin cancer. Which of the following is the most important prevention measure when teaching a client who frequents a swimming pool?

   a. Wear a hat with a wide brim and cover the back of the neck.

   b. Use a sunscreen with an SPF of at least 15 and reapply every 2 hours.

   c. Use a lip balm with sunscreen and apply frequently.

   d. Stay in the shade when outdoors and only swim after 2:00 p.m.

Caring for Clients with Burns

SECTION I: ASSESSING YOUR UNDERSTANDING

Activity A *Fill in the blanks by choosing the correct word from the options given in parentheses.*

1. A burn is a _____ injury to the skin and underlying tissues. Heat, chemicals, or electricity cause burn injuries. *(Superficial, Traumatic, Deep)*

2. _____ is a quick assessment technique to estimate how much of the client's skin surface is involved. *(Comparing the client's foot with the size of the burn wound, Comparing the client's palm with the size of the burn wound, Rule of tens)*

3. _____ is the removal of necrotic tissue. *(Autograft, Debridement, Allograft)*

4. A disadvantage of surgical debridement is _____. *(Infection, Bleeding, Pain)*

5. Skin grafting is necessary for _____ burns because the skin layers responsible for regeneration have been destroyed. *(Superficial and superficial partial-thickness, Superficial partial-thickness and deep partial-thickness, Deep partial-thickness and full-thickness)*

6. _____ or homograft is human skin obtained from a cadaver. *(An autograft, An allograft, A heterograft)*

7. _____ is a bioengineered covering which promotes wound healing by interacting directly with body tissues. It can be applied all over the burn wound as soon as the skin is cleaned and debrided instead of having to wait until enough skin is available for grafting purposes. *(Skin substitutes, Cultured skins, Autografts)*

Activity B *Mark each statement as either T (True) or F (False). Correct any false statements.*

1. T F The risk for acquiring a burn injury is highest among children and adults older than 60 years of age. The most common causes of thermal burns in older adults are scalding and home fires; secondary causes include smoking, alcohol ingestion, or flammable substances that ignite materials.

2. T F Cardiac dysrhythmias and central nervous system complications are common among victims of thermal burns.

3. T F   The zone of injury is determined by assessing the color, characteristics of the skin, and sensation in the area of the burn injury.

4. T F   The palm is approximately 1% of a person's total body surface area (TBSA).

5. T F   The open method is the current preferred method of wound management.

6. T F   An autograft is obtained from animals, principally pigs.

7. T F   A slit graft is used when the area available as a donor site is limited, as in clients with extensive burns. The skin is removed from the donor site and passed through an instrument that slits it; thus, a smaller piece of skin is stretched to cover a larger area.

Activity C *Write the correct term for each description given below.*

1. Generally the drug of choice to manage severe pain for a burn victim. _____.

2. If the eschar constricts the area and impairs circulation, an incision into the eschar is done to relieve pressure on the affected area.

   _____

3. The regrowth of skin. _____

4. Only skin transplanted from one identical twin to another or this type of graft can become a permanent part of the client's own skin. _____

5. The epidermis and a thin layer of dermis are harvested from the client's skin. This type of autograft is usually obtained from the buttocks or thighs. _____

6. This type of autograft includes epidermis, dermis, and some subcutaneous tissue. It is used when the burned area is fairly small or involves the hands, face, or neck._____

7. A wound-closure product that is developed by growing the client's own skin cells in a laboratory culture medium. From a piece of postage stamp–sized skin, it is possible to grow sufficient skin to cover nearly the entire body in 3 weeks. _____

Activity D *Match the zones of burn injury in Column A with their correct descriptions in Column B.*

Column A

____ 1. Zone of coagulation

____ 2. Zone of stasis

____ 3. Zone of hyperemia

Column B

a. The area of least injury, where the epidermis and dermis are only minimally damaged.

b. The area of intermediate burn injury. It is here that blood vessels are damaged, but the tissue has the potential to survive.

c. The area at the center of the injury, where the injury is most severe and usually deepest.

Activity E *Differentiate between the various depths of burn injury based on the given criteria.*

Burn Injury	Depth and Characteristics
Superficial Burn	
Superficial Partial-Thickness Burn	
Deep Partial Thickness Burn	
Full-Thickness Burn	

Activity F *Briefly answer the following questions.*

1. Describe the difference between the pathophysiological changes in a thermal, chemical, and electrical burn.

   _____

   _____

   _____

2. What neuroendocrine changes occur with serious burns?

   _____

   _____

   _____

3. What factors increase the mortality rate from burn injuries?

_____

_____

_____

4. Name three potential complications of burns that can be life threatening.

_____

_____

_____

5. What are the goals of fluid resuscitation?

_____

_____

_____

6. What three microorganisms most commonly cause infection in burned tissue?

_____

_____

_____

7. Name the three major antimicrobial agents used for treatment with burn victims.

_____

_____

_____

SECTION II: APPLYING YOUR KNOWLEDGE

Activity G *Give rationale for the following questions.*

1. Why are burns caused by electricity characteristically the most severe?

_____

_____

_____

2. Why can burns result in serious complications for the older adult?

_____

_____

_____

3. Why may the estimate of burn depth be revised in the first 24 to 72 hours?

_____

_____

_____

4. Why is impaired ventilation associated with a burn involving the upper airway?

_____

_____

_____

5. Why do healthcare providers wear powder-free sterile gloves when caring for a burn victim?

_____

_____

_____

6. Why is the body hair around the perimeter of the burn shaved?

_____

_____

_____

7. Why is skin grafting performed?

_____

_____

_____

Activity H *Answer the following questions that relate to caring for clients with burns.*

1. Describe the pathophysiology of a burn.

_____

_____

_____

2. Describe the initial first aid for a burn victim.

_____

_____

_____

3. Describe the acute care for a burn victim.

_____

_____

_____

4. Describe the closed method of wound management.

_____

_____

_____

5. What are the disadvantages of harvesting the client's own tissue for a graft?

_____

_____

_____

6. Describe the care for a client following a skin graft.

_____

_____

_____

Activity I *Think over the following questions. Discuss them with your instructor or peers.*

1. Your client with full thickness burns is upset because everyone entering the room is in sterile attire. The client feels detached from people. How would you explain the importance of sterile attire to the client?

_____

_____

_____

2. Your client needs nutritional support via a nasogastic tube. However, the client is refusing to have the tube inserted. How would you explain the importance of nutritional support to the client?

_____

_____

_____

3. A burn victim is brought in to the emergency department. How would you assess the client to determine if there are signs of heat or smoke inhalation injury?

_____

_____

_____

4. Your client has carbon monoxide poisoning and is going for hyperbaric oxygen treatment. How would you explain this treatment to the client?

_____

_____

_____

SECTION III: GETTING READY FOR NCLEX

Activity J *Answer the following questions:*

1. Which of the following are goals of fluid resuscitation?

   a. Intravascular volume is restored.

   b. Weight is gained rapidly.

   c. Bleeding is reduced.

   d. Breathing is normalized.

2. A client with a superficial partial-thickness burn should be informed that the wound should heal within ___ days.

3. Which of the following dietary recommendations regarding protein and calorie intake should a nurse suggest to a client recovering from a burn injury?

   a. Protein needs should equal the normal Recommended Dietary Allowance; calorie needs may be 4000 to 5000/day.

   b. Protein needs should be half the normal Recommended Dietary Allowance; calorie needs may be 2000 to 3000/day.

   c. Protein needs increase two to four times above the normal Recommended Dietary Allowance; calorie needs may be 4000 to 5000/day.

   d. Protein needs increase two to four times above the normal Recommended Dietary Allowance; calorie needs may be 2000 to 3000/day.

4. Which of the following is a disadvantage of using cultured skin?

   a. The pigmentation does not perfectly match the original skin color.

   b. Growing cultured skin is time-consuming.

   c. There is an increased risk of infection.

   d. There is an increased risk of rejection of the cultured skin.

5. Which of the following instructions, meant to minimize the risk of scarring, should a nurse give a client with burns who has undergone skin grafting?

a. Wear thick clothes.

b. Apply sunscreen with a high SPF when outdoors.

c. Avoid use of topical gels.

d. Avoid cold water baths.

6. Which of the following interventions is effective in minimizing the risk of morbidity and mortality after fluid resuscitation has been provided to a client with extensive burns?

a. Providing the client with antibiotics and analgesics.

b. Addressing the client's depression.

c. Grafting of skin.

d. Providing aggressive nutritional support.

7. A client is admitted to the burn unit following a fire in the storage room at work. The nurse notes which of the following on the client's assessment that would indicate heat or smoke inhalation injury?

a. Fever, malaise, and singed eyebrows

b. Hoarseness, fever, and singed eyebrows

c. Malaise, shortness of breath, and fever

d. Sore throat, hoarseness, shortness of breath

8. A client has experienced a fourth degree burn. What depth of skin and tissue involvement is present with a fourth degree burn?

a. Epidermis, dermis, subcutaneous tissue

b. Deeper layer of the dermis with damage to sweat and sebaceous glands

c. Epidermis, dermis, subcutaneous tissue, fat, fascia, muscle, and bone

d. Epidermis and dermis, hair follicles intact

9. A nurse is caring for a client with an allograft. Which of the following describes the source of the allograft?

a. Client's own skin transplanted from one part of the body to another.

b. Obtained from animals, principally pigs

c. Skin substitute made from bioengineered materials

d. Human skin obtained from a cadaver

10. The nurse is caring for a client following debridement. The nurse is most concerned with which complication?

a. Bleeding

b. Pain control

c. Loss of fluids

d. Infection

CHAPTER 67

Interaction of Body and Mind

Learning Objectives

1. Discuss new areas of neuroscience being studied to learn more about mind–body connections and their effect on health.
2. Name chemical substances transmitted between neurons, giving examples of each.
3. Explain why mental illnesses are now considered psychobiologic disorders.
4. Name biologic and psychologic components that contribute to disorders affecting the body and mind.
5. List examples of techniques used to assess clients with psychobiologic disorders.
6. Describe treatment and nursing care for psychobiologic disorders.
7. Distinguish between stress, eustress, and distress.
8. Describe the general adaptation syndrome, naming its three stages.
9. Explain the purpose of coping mechanisms and the outcomes that may result from their use.
10. List the defining features of hardiness.
11. Discuss techniques that the nurse can suggest for helping clients cope with stressors.
12. Discuss the rationale for a mind–immune system connection.
13. Discuss four explanations for the development of psychosomatic disorders.
14. Describe treatment and nursing care for psychosomatic disorders.
15. Explain the placebo effect.

SECTION I: ASSESSING YOUR UNDERSTANDING

Activity A *Fill in the blanks by choosing the correct word from the options given in parentheses.*

1. _____ are conditions in which evidence supports a connection between abnormalities in the brain and altered cognition, perception, emotion, behavior, and socialization. *(Psychological disorders, Psychosocial disorders, Psychobiologic disorders)*

2. _____ aims at correcting the underlying biochemical abnormality. *(Drug therapy, Psychotherapy, Cognitive therapy)*

3. According to Selye's theory (1956), _____ is a physiologic response to biologic stressors such as surgical trauma or infection, psychological stressors such as worry and fear, or sociologic stressors, including a new job or increased family responsibilities. *(Fear, Stress, Emotion)*

4. _____ are the unconscious tactics humans use to protect the self from feeling inadequate or threatened. *(Physiological responses, Coping mechanisms, General adaptation syndrome)*

5. Psychosomatic disorders are also known as _____ related disorders. *(Stress, Mood, Anxiety)*

6. The effect of chronically suppressing _____ and the neurochemical changes that accompany it, however, may be the triggering mechanism for a dysfunctional immune response. *(Anger, Dependence, Ambivalence)*

Activity B *Mark each statement as either "T" (True) or "F" (False). Correct any false statements.*

1. T F There are distinctive brain activity patterns for seizure disorders, schizophrenia, depression, dementia, anxiety disorders, and attention deficit/hyperactivity disorder.

2. T F A definitive diagnosis for many psychobiologic disorders usually is achieved by ruling out other diseases that manifest similar symptoms.

3. T F The goals of psychotherapy, cognitive therapy, and behavior modification are to uncover repressed thoughts and emotions and identify healthier coping mechanisms.

4. T F Excessive, ill-timed, or unrelieved stress is called eustress.

5. T F The biopsychosocial effects of stress and mental state should be considered in the evaluation and treatment of all illnesses.

6. T F Psychoneuroimmunology is the study of how fluctuations in pituitary, adrenal, thyroid, and reproductive hormones alter cognition, perception, behavior, and mood.

Activity C *Write the correct term for each description given below.*

1. It is the basis for sensory perception, voluntary movement, personality, intelligence, language, thoughts, judgment, emotions, memory, creativity, and motivation.

_____

2. A technique that compares a client's brain activity patterns (from an EEG or other electronic image) with a computerized database of electrophysiologic abnormalities.

3. Implicated in the development or exacerbation of autoimmune diseases, anorexia nervosa, obsessive–compulsive disorder, panic attacks, thyroid conditions, heart disease, functional and inflammatory disorders of the gastrointestinal tract, chronic pain conditions, and diabetes. _____

4. A nonspecific physiologic response to a stressor. _____

5. Characteristics include: a commitment to something meaningful versus a sense of alienation; a sense of having control over sources of stress versus a feeling of helplessness; and the perception of life events as a challenge rather than a threat. _____

6. The healing or improvement that takes place simply because the individual believes a treatment method will be effective.

_____

Activity D *Match the theorist(s) in Column A with the proposed psychological factors that may influence psychological equilibrium in Column B.*

Column A

____ **1.** Sigmund Freud

____ **2.** Erik Erikson and Harry Stack Sullivan

____ **3.** B. F. Skinner

Column B

a. Proposed the theory that adaptive and maladaptive behaviors are learned and repeated because of rewarding reinforcement.

b. Proposed that mental health or illness is a consequence of social relationships and interpersonal interactions.

c. Proposed that disordered behavior is the result of intrapersonal (within oneself) conflicts that arise during particular stages of development that occur between infancy and adolescence.

Activity E *Identify some of the functions of the following neurotransmitters.*

Neurotransmitter	Functions
Serotonin	
Dopamine	
Norepinephrine	
Acetylcholine	
Gamma-aminobutyric acid	
Glutamate	

Activity F *Briefly answer the following questions.*

1. Describe the two structures in the brain that play the greatest role in connecting the mind with physiologic functions.

_____

_____

_____

2. Identify 3 types of neuropeptides.

_____

_____

_____

3. What suggests that brain, endocrine system, and immune system communicate with each other?

_____

_____

_____

4. What are the elements of an extensive mental status examination that elicit information about a person's cognitive and mental state?

_____

_____

_____

5. Describe the advantages and disadvantages of coping mechanisms.

_____

_____

_____

6. How can stress affect the immune system?

_____

_____

_____

SECTION II: APPLYING YOUR KNOWLEDGE

Activity G *Give rationale for the following questions.*

1. Why might an older adult be more vulnerable to stressors?

_____

_____

2. Why are clients with psychosomatic illnesses given anti-inflammatory and corticosteroid drugs?

_____

_____

3. Why might an excessive expression of hostility be related to increased incidents of heart disease?

_____

_____

4. Why is it important to conduct tests before assuming that a disorder is stress induced?

_____

_____

5. Why do clients taking placebos experience improvement?

_____

_____

_____

Activity H *Answer the following questions related to caring for clients with psychobiologic disorders.*

1. Describe the relationship between receptors and neurotransmitters.

   _____

   _____

   _____

2. Describe the physiologic stress response.

   _____

   _____

   _____

3. How can a nurse foster effective coping skills?

   _____

   _____

   _____

Activity I *Think over the following questions. Discuss them with your instructor or peers.*

1. A client with irritable bowel syndrome asks you how their symptoms are related to stress. How would you explain this relationship to them?

   _____

   _____

   _____

2. A client is diagnosed with a mood disorder and does not understand how neurotransmitters play a part in their diagnosis. What would you tell them?

   _____

   _____

   _____

3. Describe how you feel the effects of psychobiology, intrapersonal conflicts, learned behavior, and social relationships/interpersonal interactions play a role in mental illness.

   _____

   _____

   _____

SECTION III: GETTING READY FOR NCLEX

Activity J *Answer the following questions.*

1. Which of the following nutritional instructions should a nurse give to stress-prone clients?
   a. Eat at regular intervals
   b. Eat only when hungry and not eat otherwise
   c. Eat only one meal a day
   d. Avoid consumption of oily food

2. Which of the following is an important nursing intervention when caring for a client with psychobiologic illness?
   a. Provide individual and group counseling
   b. Provide books on psychobiologic illness
   c. Provide entertainment regularly
   d. Provide family counseling

3. Which of the following is a maladaptive coping mechanism for a client with stress?
   a. Anger
   b. Hardiness
   c. Alcohol
   d. Self mutilation

4. Which of the following is the mechanism of the placebo effect?
   a. Individual believes a treatment method will be effective.
   b. Individual believes that the treatment is spiritual in nature.
   c. Individual believes the physician and his or her capabilities.
   d. Individual believes that the treatment method is without pain.

5. Which of the following are the implications of stress?
   a. Valvular conditions
   b. Inflammatory GI disorders
   c. Fluid imbalance
   d. Electrolyte imbalance

6. Which of the following neurotransmitters influences movement, memory, thoughts, and judgment?
   a. Norepinephrine
   b. Dopamine
   c. Epinephrine
   d. Serotonin

7. Which of the following is a type of stress that helps individuals to pursue goals, learn to solve problems, or manage life's predictable and unpredictable crises?
   a. Energy stress
   b. Active stress
   c. Eustress
   d. Distress

8. A nurse is assisting a client with a psychobiologic disorder and remembers a theorist who discussed adaptive and maladaptive behaviors and suggested that they are learned and repeated because of rewarding reinforcement. Who is this theorist?
   a. B.F. Skinner
   b. Harry Stack Sullivan
   c. Erik Erikson
   d. Sigmund Freud

9. A nurse is attending an in-service on common symptoms of mental disorders. Which of the following is one of the symptoms of mental disorders?
   a. Anger
   b. Sleep deprivation
   c. Speech abnormalities
   d. Anxiety

10. A nurse is assisting in the administration of a psychological test. Which of the following is the test that is performed when a client is asked to quickly provide a response to words, such as "mother ..., work ...," etc. and responses are analyzed for psychological significance?
    a. Minnesota Multiphasic Personality Inventory
    b. Word Association Test
    c. Rorschach Test
    d. Beck Depression Inventory

68

Caring for Clients with Anxiety Disorders

Learning Objectives

1. Differentiate anxiety from fear.
2. Name four levels of anxiety, explaining the differences among the various levels.
3. Give six areas of nursing management that apply to the care of anxious clients.
4. Name examples of anxiety disorders.
5. List categories of drugs used to treat anxiety disorders.
6. Name and discuss two types of psychotherapy used to treat anxiety disorders.
7. List six nursing interventions that are helpful for reducing anxiety.
8. Discuss areas of teaching for clients with anxiety disorders.

SECTION I: ASSESSING YOUR UNDERSTANDING

Activity A *Fill in the blanks by choosing the correct word from the options given in parentheses.*

1. _____ is a vague uneasy feeling, the cause of which is not readily identifiable. It is evoked when a person anticipates nonspecific danger. *(Anxiety, Fear, Apprehension)*

2. _____ is manifested by the performance of an anxiety-relieving ritual to terminate a disturbing, persistent thought. *(A phobic disorder, A post-traumatic stress disorder, An obsessive–compulsive disorder)*

3. _____ are drugs that relieve the symptoms of anxiety. These medications include benzodiazepines and nonbenzodiazepines. *(Anxiolytics, Beta-adrenergic blockers Central-acting sympatholytics)*

4. _____ are prescribed more often to control primary hypertension; however, they potentially have beneficial effects in anxious people with elevated blood pressure. *(Anxiolytics, Central-acting sympatholytics, Antidepressants)*

5. _____ involves talking with a psychiatrist, psychologist, or mental health counselor. Some clients respond better when therapy sessions are conducted one on one; others, such as those with post-traumatic stress disorder, respond better to group interactions. *(Psychotherapy, Cognitive therapy, Behavioral therapy)*

Activity B *Mark each statement as either "T" (True) or "F" (False). Correct any false statements.*

1. T F Panic disorder is characterized by chronic worrying on a daily basis for 6 or more months. Often, the worrying is out of proportion with reality. In addition to worrying, at least six other signs and symptoms of anxiety accompany the client's distress.

2. **T F** Most people with phobic disorders are aware of how illogical the phobia is and how unrealistic their disabling response has become.

3. **T F** Although anxiety causes behavioral, cognitive, and emotional effects, most clients seek treatment for physical signs and symptoms.

4. **T F** Findings from positron emission tomography (PET) and computed tomography (CT) scans performed on clients with anxiety disorders are essentially normal.

5. **T F** Behavioral therapy attempts to extinguish undesirable responses by teaching other adaptive techniques.

Activity C *Write the correct term for each description given below.*

1. A feeling of terror in response to someone or something specific that a person perceives as dangerous or threatening. _____

2. A group of psychobiologic illnesses that result from activation of the autonomic nervous system, chiefly the sympathetic division. They tend to be chronic and sometimes appear without any logical explanation. _____

3. A condition that involves a delayed anxiety response 3 or more months after an emotionally traumatic experience. _____

4. Following an emotionally traumatic event, the affected person avoids dealing with the tragedy and detaches himself or herself from others using this technique. _____

5. Antidepressants prescribed for obsessive–compulsive disorder and post-traumatic stress disorder which sustain levels of serotonin. _____

6. A type of psychotherapy in which the therapist helps clients alter their irrational thinking, correct their faulty belief systems, and replace negative self-statements with positive ones. This therapy is based on the theory that it is not events per se that provoke anxiety but rather the person's interpretation of events. By reshaping a person's viewpoint, the disorder can be minimized or eliminated. _____

Activity D *Match the level of anxiety in column A with the associated behavioral manifestations listed in column B.*

Column A

____ **1.** Mild

____ **2.** Moderate

____ **3.** Severe

____ **4.** Panic

Column B

a. The client is more easily distracted, concentration is slightly impaired but attention can be redirected. Learning takes more effort, perception narrows, problem-solving becomes difficult, and the client is irritable and feels inadequate.

b. The client exaggerates details, perception is distorted, and learning is disabled. Thoughts are fragmented. The client cannot control emotions and feels helpless.

c. Attention is heightened and sensory perception is expanded. The focus is on the stimuli and reality is intact. Information processing is accurate, the client feels in control.

d. The attention span decreases; the person cannot concentrate or remain focused and perception is reduced. The ability to learn is impaired and information processing is inaccurate or incomplete. The client is aware of extreme discomfort and effort is needed to control emotions. The client feels incompetent.

Activity E *Compare the purpose of the following nursing interventions based on the given criteria.*

Nursing Intervention	Purpose
Building Trust	
Restoring Comfort	
Modifying Communication	
Adjusting Teaching	
Helping Problem-Solve	
Ensuring Safety	

Activity F *Briefly answer the following questions.*

1. Describe the changes that occur as anxiety escalates.

   _____

   _____

   _____

2. What are the manifestations of a phobic disorder?

   _____

   _____

   _____

3. What situations may trigger a flashback for a client with post-traumatic stress disorder?

   _____

   _____

   _____

4. Describe the medical management of clients with anxiety disorders.

   _____

   _____

   _____

5. Describe the process of desensitization.

   _____

   _____

   _____

SECTION II: APPLYING YOUR KNOWLEDGE

Activity G *Give rationale for the following questions.*

1. Why do some clients with post-traumatic stress disorder abuse substances?

   _____

   _____

   _____

2. Why is long-term treatment with benzodiazepines not recommended?

   _____

   _____

   _____

3. Why would nonbenzodiazepines be preferred to benzodiazepines?

   _____

   _____

   _____

4. Why is it important to decrease external stimuli for the client with an anxiety disorder?

   _____

   _____

   _____

5. Why is the client with an anxiety disorder advised to avoid caffeine, nicotine, or stimulating drugs such as nonprescription diet pills and cold and allergy medications?

   _____

   _____

Activity H *Answer the following questions related to caring for clients with anxiety disorders.*

1. What are the manifestations of panic disorder?

   _____

   _____

   _____

2. What are the manifestations of an obsessive-compulsive disorder?

_____

_____

_____

3. Describe the purpose and side effects of beta-adrenergic blocking agents.

_____

_____

_____

4. What assessment data will the nurse gather when caring for the client with an anxiety disorder?

_____

_____

_____

5. What interventions can the nurse use to decrease the client's anxiety?

_____

_____

_____

Activity I _Think over the following questions. Discuss them with your instructor or peers._

1. What physical manifestations would cue you that your client is experiencing an escalating level of anxiety?

_____

_____

_____

2. Your client's chart reveals that a T3, T4, blood chemistry panel, and drug screen were performed prior to admission. Why would these laboratory tests be performed?

_____

_____

_____

3. What high priority nursing diagnoses and interventions would you identify for a client diagnosed with an anxiety disorder?

_____

_____

_____

4. What educational information related to nutrition would you provide to your client with an anxiety disorder?

_____

_____

_____

SECTION III: GETTING READY FOR NCLEX

Activity J _Answer the following questions._

1. Before administering a benzodiazepine to a client with anxiety, which of the following should the nurse assess?

   a. Sleep problems

   b. Memory impairment

   c. Cognitive disorder

   d. Behavior changes

2. What should the nurse teach a client who is recommended antianxiety drugs?

   a. Use the drug on a long-term basis

   b. Avoid lifting heavy weights

   c. Use caution when driving

   d. Be aware that the drug causes excessive sleeplessness

3. Why should the nurse assess current weight status and recent weight fluctuations in a client with anxiety?

   a. Weight fluctuations indicate impaired kidney function in clients with anxiety

   b. All clients with anxiety lose weight rapidly

   c. Antianxiety drugs increase appetite

   d. Some clients may react to stress by overeating

4. After implementing nursing interventions for a client with anxiety, which of the following expected outcomes does the nurse evaluate?

   a. The client avoids all kinds of anxiety-provoking stimuli

   b. The client has no need for written instructions for follow-up care

   c. The client accurately repeats information about the drug therapy

   d. There are no consequences if anxiolytic drug is discontinued suddenly

5. When assessing a client with an anxiety disorder, which of the following does the nurse observe for evidence of various levels of anxiety?

    a. Absence of crying

    b. Talking excessively

    c. Being motionless

    d. Not complaining

6. For a client with anxiety disorder, numerous stimuli escalate anxiety. Which of the following nursing interventions can help the client avoid dealing simultaneously with multiple stimuli?

    a. Reducing activity

    b. Touching the client as often as possible

    c. Increasing bright lights

    d. Taking a position as close to the client as possible

7. A client with a panic disorder experiences a fear of having panic attacks in a public place. What is the correct term for this condition?

    a. Social phobia

    b. Acrophobia

    c. Nyctophobia

    d. Agoraphobia

8. A nurse is assisting a client with a disorder in which flashbacks are a symptom. What is the disorder called?

    a. Post-traumatic stress disorder

    b. Phobic disorder

    c. Anxiety disorder

    d. Obsessive-compulsive disorder

9. A client is prescribed an anxiolytic drug for obsessive-compulsive disorder. Which of the following drugs fits within this category?

    a. Lopressor

    b. Tenormin

    c. Inderal

    d. Xanax

10. A client is being treated for a disorder and attends psychotherapy in which the therapist helps clients alter their irrational thinking, correct their faulty belief systems, and replace negative self-statements with positive ones. This therapy is based on the theory that it is not events per se that provoke anxiety but rather the person's interpretation of events. Which type of therapy does this describe?

    a. Desensitization therapy

    b. Behavioral therapy

    c. Cognitive therapy

    d. Psychobiologic therapy

CHAPTER 69

Caring for Clients with Mood Disorders

Learning Objectives

1. Discuss common signs and symptoms of mood disorders.
2. Name three neurotransmitters that, when imbalanced, affect mood.
3. Identify the types of drugs that are used to treat depression and nursing considerations related to their administration.
4. Discuss the causes, manifestations, and management of serotonin syndrome.
5. Identify the reasons electroconvulsive therapy is used in the management of depression.
6. Name three interventions that are alternatives to electroconvulsive therapy for recurrent depression.
7. Give three criteria that indicate a high risk for suicide.
8. Discuss nursing measures that are useful in preventing suicide.
9. Discuss the nursing management of clients with depression.
10. Describe seasonal affective disorder, its treatment, and nursing management.
11. Explain bipolar disorder and describe its treatment and nursing management.

SECTION I: ASSESSING YOUR UNDERSTANDING

Activity A *Fill in the blanks by choosing the correct word from the options given in parentheses.*

1. Brain function, and consequently mood, depends on the dynamic interplay of neurotransmitters. Moods are most likely generated by the _____ system, which is the center for emotions. *(Limbic, Ventricle, Reticular activating)*

2. _____ block the reuptake of serotonin and norepinephrine. *(MAOIs, TCAs, Atypical antidepressants)*

3. The lag time before the client experiences a therapeutic effect is approximately _____ weeks after beginning MAOI therapy. *(1 to 2, 3 to 6, 6 to 8)*

4. _____ uses the application of an electric stimulus to one or both temporal regions of the head to produce a brief, generalized seizure. Although the exact mechanism of action is unknown, the belief is this type of therapy achieves its effect by either increasing circulating levels of monoamine neurotransmitters or by improving transmission to the receptor site. *(Electroconvulsive therapy, Vagus nerve stimulation, Deep brain stimulation)*

5. Treatment for seasonal affective disorder may include _____ *(Electroconvulsive therapy, Phototherapy, Vagus nerve stimulation)*

6. _____, a chemical element, usually is the initial drug of choice for bipolar disorder. It controls both depressive as well as manic symptoms in clients. *(SNRIs, Atypical antidepressants, Lithium)*

7. _____ may be prescribed for a brief period for clients with bipolar disorder to induce sedation and control hallucinations and delusions. *(Atypical antidepressants, Lithium, Antipsychotics)*

8. Providers must stress the importance of maintaining an adequate ingestion of _____ to all clients who rely on lithium to control their disorder. *(Potassium, Salt, Calcium)*

Activity B *Mark each statement as either "T" (True) or "F" (False). Correct any false statements.*

1. T F The term "mood" refers to the verbal and nonverbal behavior that communicates feelings.

2. T F Depression may be a comorbid (coexisting) condition among people with anxiety disorders and substance abuse.

3. T F Hallucinations are fixed false beliefs that often are persecutory or guilt-ridden in nature.

4. T F Transient depression is a normal reaction to loss, such as the death of a loved one; disappointment, such as being fired from a job; or overwhelming events, such as being heavily in debt.

5. T F Psychotherapy often is more productive after clients who are depressed respond to antidepressant drug therapy.

6. T F The vagus nerve stimulation device consists of an electrode that is tunneled beneath the skin at the neck. One end of the electrode is attached to the vagus nerve, a cranial nerve that exits the brainstem, travels through the neck, and moves down to supply the chest and abdomen. The other end of the electrode is connected to a pulse generator implanted in the chest, similar to a cardiac pacemaker. The pulse generator sends intermittent electrical impulses directed toward the brain via the vagus nerve.

7. T F Lithium has a narrow range of safety between a therapeutic serum level (0.8–1.2 mEq) and toxic levels (1.5 mEq) and requires periodic laboratory tests to monitor serum blood levels.

Activity C *Write the correct term for each description below.*

1. A potentially life-threatening condition that results from elevated levels of serotonin in the blood secondary to drug therapy.

_____

2. Symptoms include an elevated blood pressure, headache, often an occipital headache, nausea, vomiting, sweating, palpitations, visual changes, neck stiffness, sensitivity to light, and tachycardia. _____

3. Clinical evidence has shown that children and adolescents experience increased risk of suicidal thoughts and behavior with the use of these drugs. The U.S. Food and Drug Administration issued a "black box" prescription drug-warning label advising the close monitoring of children and adolescents for worsening depression, thoughts or attempts of suicide, or significant changes in behavior, such as social withdrawal. _____

4. This type of multiple reuptake inhibitor provides rapid relief of symptoms with fewer sexual side effects compared with SSRIs.

_____

5. It is believed that sending continuous electrical signals via this device can alter brain circuitry and relieve depression. Treatment involves implanting an electrode in the brain through a small opening in the skull. The distal end of the electrode is passed under the skin of the head, neck, and shoulder, eventually connecting to a neurostimulator implanted under the skin near the clavicle, chest, or abdomen. _____

6. A mood disorder that has its onset during darker winter months and spontaneously disappears in the spring. This mood disorder is more prevalent among people living in states north of 40 to 50 degrees of latitude.

_____

Activity D *Psychotherapy is a treatment for major depression. Match the types of psychotherapy given in Column A with their corresponding benefits given in Column B.*

Column A

____ 1. Psychodynamic psychotherapy

____ 2. Interpersonal psychotherapy

____ 3. Supportive psychotherapy

____ 4. Cognitive therapy

____ 5. Behavioral therapy

Column B

a. Facilitated by a bond that develops between the therapist and client. The empathy and trust help clients gain an understanding of their condition and the courage and support to overcome it.

b. Helps clients replace negative, and often

illogical, ways of thinking with more positive outlooks.

c. Endeavors to change unhealthy ways of behaving. Clients are rewarded verbally or in some other way when they alter their behavior positively. The praise and recognition encourage the client to continually repeat the healthy behavior. Gradually, the resulting changes increase self-esteem and promote further improvement.

d. Clients discuss their early life experiences to raise repressed feelings to a conscious level. Clients often are in this type of therapy for months to years. It can be tedious and expensive, but traumatic events buried deep in the unconscious may require extensive therapy.

e. Helps clients learn about their disorder and treatment techniques, improve or develop new social skills, obtain positive reinforcement for progress, and gain encouragement to persevere.

Activity E *Describe the following moods and mood disorders.*

Mood or Mood Disorder	Description
Euthymia	
Dysthymia	
Cyclothymia	
Reactive (Secondary) Depression	
Unipolar Depression (Major Depression)	
Psychotic Depression	
Bipolar Disorder (Manic-Depressive Syndrome)	
Mania	
Seasonal Affective Disorder	

Activity F *Briefly answer the following questions.*

1. Describe the relationship between mood disorders and genetics.

_____

_____

_____

2. Describe the role of a neuroendocrine imbalance on mood.

_____

_____

_____

3. What are the signs and symptoms of serotonin syndrome?

_____

_____

_____

4. How do MAOIs work?

_____

_____

_____

5. What is a leading cause of noncompliance with SSRIs?

_____

_____

_____

6. How does transcranial magnetic stimulation work?

_____

_____

_____

7. Describe the etiology and pathophysiology of bipolar disorder.

_____

_____

_____

8. How are anticonvulsants used in the treatment of bipolar disorder?

_____

_____

_____

SECTION II: APPLYING YOUR KNOWLEDGE

Activity G *Give rationale for the following questions.*

1. Why should alternative reasons for clinical findings be considered when a tentative diagnosis of depression is thought to be the cause for alterations in mood?

_____

_____

_____

2. Why might older adults be reluctant to admit depressive feelings?

_____

_____

_____

3. Why is closer observation of the depressed client essential once antidepressant therapy is initiated?

_____

_____

_____

4. Why are the MAOIs tranylcypromine (Parnate) and phenelzine (Nardil) the least prescribed category of antidepressants?

_____

_____

_____

5. Why are SSRIs currently the most prescribed group of drugs used to treat depression?

_____

_____

_____

6. Why is it essential that clients taking antidepressants consult with their physician before taking herbal remedies or dietary supplements?

_____

_____

_____

7. Why is a history of substance abuse considered to be a risk factor for bipolar disorder?

_____

_____

_____

8. Why are client who take carbamazepine (Tegretol) at risk for infection?

_____

_____

_____

Activity H *Answer the following questions related to caring for clients with mood disorders.*

1. Describe the hypothesis of neurotransmitter dysregulation.

_____

_____

_____

2. What are the disadvantages of TCAs?

_____

_____

_____

3. Describe the differences in action of the following multiple reuptake inhibitors: SSRIs, SNRIs, and atypical antidepressants.

_____

_____

_____

4. Describe assessment data for the suicidal client.

_____

_____

_____

_____

5. Differentiate between the various types of bipolar disorder.

_____

_____

_____

6. Describe the signs and symptoms of bipolar disorder.

_____

_____

_____

Activity I *Think over the following questions. Discuss them with your instructor or peers.*

1. Antidepressant therapy has been initiated for your client diagnosed with major depression. You are concerned about the risk for suicide. What behavioral clues will you watch for to identify an increased risk for suicide?

_____

_____

_____

2. Your client is currently in a manic phase of a bipolar disorder. What high priority nursing diagnoses and interventions will you implement to keep the client safe and healthy?

_____

_____

_____

3. The family members of a client diagnosed with bipolar disorder are feeling the strain of dealing with the disorder. What interventions and educational information can you provide to support the family members?

_____

_____

_____

4. A friend tells you they have been experiencing depression since their divorce 3 months ago. The friend is having difficulty adjusting to the changes in the family dynamics. What educational information would you provide?

_____

_____

_____

SECTION III: GETTING READY FOR NCLEX

Activity J *Answer the following questions.*

1. Which of the following factors place a client at risk for serotonin syndrome?
   a. Coprescription of antidepressants from different classes such as MAOIs and SSRIs
   b. Abnormal levels of cortisol in the body
   c. Adequate time between weaning from one antidepressant drug to initiating another antidepressant
   d. Premenstrual syndrome

2. In which clients is electroconvulsive therapy (ECT) usually contraindicated?
   a. Clients with cardiac or neurovascular diseases
   b. Clients who have not responded to drug therapy
   c. Clients who are intolerant of the side effects of antidepressant medications
   d. Clients who are extremely suicidal

3. Bipolar disorder is managed by the administration of one or more mood-stabilizing medications such as lithium. Which of the following statements are correct for lithium?

   a. Effective for all

   b. Has a delay of 10 to 28 days in achieving therapeutic benefits

   c. Has a narrow range of safety between a therapeutic serum level and toxic levels

   d. May be therapeutic when administered in combination with any other drugs

4. Which of the following risks is more prone to clients who administer carbamazepine for the treatment of bipolar disorder?

   a. Risk for injury

   b. Risk for self-directed violence

   c. Risk for imbalanced nutrition

   d. Risk for infection

5. Which of the following signs and symptoms of lithium toxicity should a nurse monitor for when caring for a client who is prescribed lithium for the treatment of a mood disorder?

   a. Constipation

   b. Vomiting

   c. Amnesia

   d. Muscular rigidity

6. A client with bipolar disorder shows signs of aggression and is at risk for self-directed violence. Which of the following nursing interventions will help the client to demonstrate self-control and control angry outbursts?

   a. Orient client to person, place, time, and events

   b. Avoid strenuous exercises

   c. Take client to a secluded area

   d. Increase distracting stimuli

7. A client is experiencing swings in mood and exhibits sensory phenomena such as hearing voices or seeing images that do not objectively exist. What are these sensory phenomena called?

   a. Mania

   b. Delusions

   c. Seasonal affective disorder

   d. Hallucinations

8. A nurse is teaching a client who takes an MAOI inhibitor that tyramine in some foods can cause a fatal side effect. What is the side effect?

   a. Cardiac dysrrhythmias

   b. Thyroid storm

   c. Hypertensive crisis

   d. Rhabdomyolysis

9. What is the technique called that manages the tremors caused by Parkinson's disease?

   a. Deep brain stimulation

   b. Transcranial magnetic stimulation

   c. Vagus nerve stimulation

   d. Electroconvulsive therapy

10. A nurse is speaking with a client who has seasonal affective disorder. The client should be taught which of the following when discharged?

    a. Use heavy drapes rather than translucent curtains or shades.

    b. Jog after sundown and before sunup.

    c. Avoid the use of eyeglasses or contact lenses that are coated to shield ultraviolet radiation.

    d. Take brief walks outside around midnight without sunglasses.

CHAPTER 70

Caring for Clients with Eating Disorders

Learning Objectives

1. Differentiate normal eating from an eating disorder.
2. Name four types of eating disorders.
3. Describe two forms of anorexia nervosa.
4. Name the neurotransmitters, neurohormones, and other chemicals that affect the appetite and satiety center in the brain.
5. Discuss two reasons that most people with anorexia nervosa induce self-starvation.
6. Identify the tool used to evaluate a person's size in relation to norms within the adult population.
7. Give the healthy range for body mass index (BMI).
8. List four components of treatment for clients with anorexia nervosa.
9. Discuss the nurse's role in managing the care of a client with anorexia nervosa.
10. Give two examples of how people with bulimia nervosa compensate for binging.
11. Name two problems, besides nutrition, that are the nursing focus when caring for clients with bulimia nervosa.
12. Differentiate between binge-eating disorder and compulsive overeating.
13. Discuss at least three psychosocial problems that may accompany overeating syndromes.
14. Describe nursing care for a client with binge-eating disorder or compulsive overeating.

SECTION I: ASSESSING YOUR UNDERSTANDING

Activity A *Fill in the blanks by choosing the correct word from the options given in parentheses.*

1. Eating disorders are more prevalent in young women between _____ years of age. *(10 and 17, 12 and 25, 15 and 30)*

2. _____ is characterized by an obsession with thinness that is achieved through self-starvation. *(Anorexia, Bulimia, Binge eating)*

3. A healthy body mass index is between _____. *(16 and 18.5, 18.5 and 24.9, 25 and 29.9)*

4. _____ is a technique in which clients with anorexia attempt to demonstrate weight gain by consuming a large volume of water and avoiding urination before being weighed. *(Water intoxication, Water loading, Water dumping)*

5. A nursing intervention for the anorexic client is to remove the eating tray after _____ minutes without commenting on food that has not been eaten; this helps to avoid a power struggle. *(30, 45, 60)*

Activity B *Mark each statement as either "T" (True) or "F" (False). Correct any false statements.*

1. T F Normal eating occurs in response to hunger and ceases when satiety, a feeling of comfortable fullness, is attained.

2. T F People with bulimia nervosa consume an average of 600 to 900 calories per day, often less. They do get hungry but control the urge to eat because of a morbid fear of becoming fat.

3. T F In contrast to anorexia, people with bulimia are generally older at the onset of the disorder, are overweight or of normal weight, admit that their eating behavior is abnormal, and are ashamed of habitually binging and purging.

4. T F Treatment of bulimia nervosa includes drug therapy with antidepressants, individual and group psychotherapy, and behavior modification techniques. Most clients are managed on an outpatient basis.

5. T F Binge-eating disorder is characterized as eating in the absence of hunger or regardless of feeling full.

Activity C *Write the correct term for the descriptions given below.*

1. Almost universally, people with this disorder consider themselves obese despite appearing emaciated. _____

2. The body mass index in people with anorexia. _____

3. Characterized by a minimum of two episodes of secret food binges per week followed by behaviors intended to prevent weight gain. The abnormal eating pattern must have persisted for at least 6 months. _____

4. Natural chemicals with marijuana-like properties that activate the appetite center. _____

5. Acts as a major anorexic signal via the hypothalamus that limits the consumption of calories, increases energy expenditure, and promotes sustained weight loss. _____

Activity D *Match the key food groups from MyPyramid in Column A with their recommended daily allowances given in Column B.*

Column A

____ 1. Grains

____ 2. Vegetables

____ 3. Fruits

____ 4. Milk

____ 5. Meat and beans

Column B

a. 3 cups every day.

b. 6 oz. every day.

c. 2 cups every day.

d. 5 oz. every day.

e. 2 cups every day.

Activity E *Compare and contrast the physical, emotional, and behavioral manifestations of the eating disorders in Table 70-1 based on the given criteria.*

Activity F *Briefly answer the following questions.*

1. Name the four types of eating disorders.

_____

_____

_____

2. Describe the two types of anorexia.

_____

_____

_____

3. What complications can result from anorexia?

_____

_____

_____

TABLE 70-1			
Eating disorder	**Physical**	**Emotional**	**Behavioral**
Anorexia nervosa			
Bulimia nervosa			
Binge eating and compulsive overeating			

4. How is a body mass index calculated?

_____

_____

_____

5. Describe the two different types of bulimia.

_____

_____

_____

6. What complications can result from bulimia?

_____

_____

_____

SECTION II: APPLYING YOUR KNOWLEDGE

Activity G _Provide rationale for the following questions._

1. Why are family and friends often not aware an eating disorder exists?

_____

_____

_____

2. Why might as few as 1500 calories per day be prescribed initially for the treatment of anorexia?

_____

_____

_____

3. Why does the nurse work with the dietitian to provide at least 6 to 8 meals each day with a total caloric value between 1500 and 2000 calories, then gradually increase the total calories to between 2500 and 4000 calories/day for the anorexic client?

_____

_____

_____

4. Why does the nurse formulate a contract with the bulimic client to seek out the nurse or another support person when the client feels the urge to purge?

_____

_____

_____

5. Why does the nurse advise the client with an overeating disorder to follow the meal plan for three meals and three snacks each day that has been developed by a dietitian in conjunction with nutritional counseling?

_____

_____

_____

6. Why do some clients with overeating disorders consider suicide or perform self-mutilation, such as cutting and burning themselves, pulling their hair, and interfering with wound healing?

_____

_____

_____

Activity H _Answer the following questions related to caring for clients with eating disorders._

1. Discuss the etiology of anorexia.

_____

_____

_____

2. What are the assessment findings with anorexia?

_____

_____

_____

3. How is anorexia medically managed?

_____

_____

_____

4. Discuss the etiology of bulimia.

_____

_____

_____

5. What are the signs and symptoms of bulimia?

_____

_____

_____

6. What are complications of overeating syndromes?

_____

_____

_____

Activity I _Think over the following questions. Discuss them with your instructor or peers._

1. What high-priority nursing diagnoses and interventions would you identify for the anorexic client?

_____

_____

_____

2. What nursing assessments would you perform to identify complications of anorexia?

_____

_____

_____

3. What high-priority nursing diagnoses and interventions would you identify for the client with bulimia?

_____

_____

_____

4. How would you provide support to the client diagnosed with an overeating disorder?

_____

_____

_____

SECTION III: GETTING READY FOR NCLEX

Activity J _Answer the following questions._

1. A nurse is working with a client who has an eating disorder. Which of the following clients is more apt to be diagnosed with an eating disorder?

   a. Male, 65 years of age, in good health

   b. Female, 20 years of age, who feels guilty most of the time

   c. Female, 40 years of age, who just went through a divorce

   d. Male, 17 years of age, who wrestles and must lose weight before matches

2. A nurse is working with a support group for eating disorders. Which of the following eating disorders would a client be diagnosed with if they engaged in self-starvation?

   a. Binge-eating disorder

   b. Bulimarexia

   c. Bulimia nervosa

   d. Anorexia nervosa

3. Which of the following traits are clients with anorexia nervosa noted to have?

   a. Refusal to look at self

   b. High self-esteem

   c. Perfectionism

   d. Intense desire to displease others

4. Complications related to anorexia nervosa include which of the following?

   a. Premature wrinkles

   b. Vitamin excess

   c. Stress fractures in spine or hip

   d. Fluid overload

5. Why would a client who has anorexia nervosa develop lanugo?

   a. In the absence of body fat, lanugo helps maintain body temperature

   b. In the absence of body fat, lanugo helps decrease body temperature.

   c. In the absence of body fat, lanugo prevents infection.

   d. In the absence of body fat, lanugo increases the chance of infection.

6. BMI is typically _____ with anorexia nervosa.

7. A nurse weighs a client diagnosed with binge eating using random weights. What does this help to prevent?
   a. Dehydration
   b. Lying about weight
   c. Water loading
   d. Denial of weight loss

8. Complications of self-induced vomiting in a binge eating disorder include which of the following?
   a. Fluid and electrolyte disorders
   b. Damage to teeth
   c. Constipation
   d. Cardiac problems

9. Complications of overeating include which of the following?
   a. Hyperlipidemia
   b. Type I diabetes
   c. Sleep disturbances
   d. Rheumatoid arthritis

10. A BMI of _____ or above is associated with overeating syndromes.

CHAPTER 71

Caring for Clients with Chemical Dependence

Learning Objectives

1. Discuss the health and social consequences of substance abuse.
2. Name four commonly abused addictive substances and at least three other categories of abused drugs.
3. Discuss the meaning of withdrawal.
4. Explain tolerance and give two mechanisms by which it occurs.
5. List four steps in the progression toward chemical dependence.
6. List two physiologic explanations and two psychosocial factors for the development of chemical dependence.
7. Explain two ways abused drugs produce their effects.
8. Define alcoholism and list three accompanying symptoms.
9. Describe treatment and nursing management for clients with alcoholism.
10. List five potential health consequences of tobacco use.
11. Discuss the components of a successful smoking cessation program.
12. Discuss elements of recovery programs.
13. Describe signs and symptoms of cocaine and methamphetamine abuse as they relate to the manner of use.
14. Describe treatment and nursing management for clients addicted to cocaine and methamphetamine.
15. Discuss methods for managing opiate dependence.

SECTION I: ASSESSING YOUR UNDERSTANDING

Activity A *Fill in the blanks by choosing the correct word from the options given in parentheses.*

1. _____ refers to the reduction in a drug's effect that follows persistent use. *(Withdrawal, Chemical dependence, Tolerance)*

2. _____ involves stabilizing the client with a sedative drug while alcohol is metabolized from his or her system. Withdrawal symptoms are controlled until they subside. *(Cross-tolerance, Detoxification, Psychotherapy)*

3. Alcoholism may result in _____ deficiency, which can lead to dementia. *(Riboflavin, Thiamine, Niacin)*

4. _____ therapy prevents neurologic complications, known as Wernicke's encephalopathy and Korsakoff's psychosis, which affect memory and cognitive functions. *(Hydration, Sedation, Vitamin)*

5. _____ is the most heavily used addictive, mood-altering substance in the United States. *(Alcohol, Nicotine, Cocaine)*

Activity B *Mark each statement as either "T" (True) or "F" (False). Correct any false statements.*

1. T F Alcohol and drug abuse are major contributors to domestic violence and child abuse, crime, traffic and boating fatalities, assaults, and murders.

2. T F Older adults may abuse over-the-counter and prescription drugs or alcohol rather than illicit drugs.

3. T F Because of their widespread use and harmful effects, cocaine and heroin contribute most to morbidity and mortality, and thus are considered the most harmful substances.

4. T F Chemical dependence refers to the physical symptoms and craving for a drug that occur when a person abruptly stops using an abused substance.

5. T F Most people benefit from chemical detoxification unassisted.

6. T F Alcohol withdrawal without detoxification is a potentially fatal process.

Activity C *Write the correct term for each description below.*

1. The use of a drug for a purpose that is different from its intended use. _____

2. A chronic, progressive, multisystem disease characterized by an inability to control the consumption of alcohol. _____

3. Deters drinking by causing unpleasant physical reactions when alcohol is consumed or absorbed through the skin. _____

4. A body temperature of at least 100°F, a pulse rate of at least 100 beats per minute, or a diastolic blood pressure of at least 100 mm Hg. The rise in any one of these three vital signs suggests the need for sedative medication because the physiologic consequences of withdrawal may be extremely difficult to counteract once they have begun.

   _____

5. Refers to the smoke given off by the burning end of a cigarette, pipe, or cigar and the exhaled smoke from the lungs of a smoker, which is potentially injurious to others.

   _____

6. Abuse of more than one substance. _____

Activity D *Match the chemicals in Column A with their descriptions in Column B.*

Column A

____ 1. Cocaine

____ 2. Crack

____ 3. Methamphetamine

____ 4. Opiates

____ 5. Opioid

Column B

a. Causes sedation after initial euphoria.

b. A purified form of cocaine with a crystalline or rocklike appearance.

c. A term for synthetic narcotics.

d. An addicting stimulant that is made by combining over-the-counter medications containing ephedrine and pseudoephedrine with other chemicals such as ammonia, acetone, and lye.

e. A CNS stimulant obtained from the leaves of the coca plant.

Activity E *Compare and contrast the commonly abused substances based on the given criteria.*

Substance abuse	Signs and symptoms	Complications
Cocaine and methamphetamine dependence		
Opiate dependence		

Activity F *Briefly answer the following.*

1. Identify the commonly abused drugs.

   _____

   _____

   _____

2. Describe the etiology of alcoholism.

   _____

   _____

   _____

3. How does an association with dopamine help explain addictive behavior?

_____

_____

_____

4. What complications may result from alcoholism?

_____

_____

_____

5. What is the purpose of psychotherapy for alcoholism?

_____

_____

_____

6. How can Alcoholics Anonymous benefit a client with alcoholism?

_____

_____

_____

7. What are the complications of smoking?

_____

_____

_____

SECTION II: APPLYING YOUR KNOWLEDGE

Activity G *Give rationale for the following questions.*

1. Why is tobacco considered one of the most harmful substances?

_____

_____

_____

2. Why does tolerance occur?

_____

_____

_____

3. Why is initiating treatment one of the most difficult hurdles in treating chemical dependence?

_____

_____

_____

4. Why must glucose solutions be avoided until thiamine is administered with alcoholism?

_____

_____

_____

5. Why must cocaine toxicity be treated immediately?

_____

_____

_____

Activity H *Answer the following questions related to caring for chemically dependent clients.*

1. What factors contribute to the development of substance abuse?

_____

_____

_____

2. Describe the signs and symptoms of alcoholism.

_____

_____

_____

3. Describe the addictive quality of tobacco.

_____

_____

_____

4. What are the risks associated with environmental tobacco smoke?

_____

_____

_____

5. Explain the purpose and advantages of methadone maintenance therapy.

_____

_____

_____

Activity I *Think over the following questions. Discuss them with your instructor or peers.*

1. Your client is admitted for an opiate overdose. What nursing care would you provide?

_____

_____

_____

2. The parents of a young adult are hopeless about their child's recovery. What educational assistance would you provide?

_____

_____

_____

3. Your client is chemically dependent. What high-priority nursing diagnoses and interventions would you identify?

_____

_____

_____

4. A client seeks information about smoking cessation. What educational information would you provide?

_____

_____

_____

SECTION III: GETTING READY FOR NCLEX

Activity J *Answer the following questions.*

1. Which of the following complications occurs when disulfiram and alcohol are mixed?

   a. Metabolic deficiencies

   b. Aspiration pneumonia

   c. Neurologic disorders

   d. Cardiopulmonary complications

2. Which of the following is an indicator of escalating withdrawal used by a nurse when assessing a client with alcohol dependence?

   a. Rule of one hundreds

   b. Cage screening test

   c. Alcoholics anonymous

   d. Rule of nines

3. The typical weight gain in the year after smoking cessation is _____

4. Which of the following must a nurse ensure before administering prescribed naltrexone to a client with opiate dependence?

   a. Client has consumed adequate fluid

   b. Client's pulse rate is at least 100 beats per minute

   c. Client has been opiate free for at least 7 days

   d. Client's diastolic blood pressure is at least 100 mm Hg

5. Which of the following instructions should a nurse provide a client with alcohol dependence after discontinuing disulfiram?

   a. Be regular for periodic checkup

   b. Avoid dietary fat for at least 3 weeks

   c. Continue rehabilitation by joining a support group

   d. Avoid all forms of alcohol for at least 2 weeks

6. Which of the following is an effect of prolonged use of alcohol in older adults?

   a. Neurologic deficits

   b. Sleep disorders

   c. Aspiration pneumonia

   d. Periodic blackouts

7. A nurse is taking care of a client with esophageal varices as a result of alcoholism. Which of the following diets will the nurse recommend for this client when giving discharge instructions?

   a. Low-fat diet

   b. Soft diet

   c. Low-acid diet

   d. High-protein diet

8. In the CAGE questionnaire for alcoholism, what does the G stand for?

    a. Have you ever had gallstones following a drinking episode?

    b. Have you ever had gastrointestinal problems when you drink?

    c. Have you ever asked God for help with your drinking?

    d. Have you ever felt guilty about your drinking?

9. A client admits to finding alcohol in a variety of products that are used for other conditions. Which of the following products might the client admit to abusing in order to obtain alcohol?

    a. Hydrogen peroxide

    b. Mouthwash

    c. Shaving cream

    d. Deodorant

10. A client is admitted through the ER after a motor vehicle accident, and the breathalyzer shows impairment from alcohol. What is the blood alcohol percentage level when a client exhibits staggering, controls emotions poorly, and is easily angered?

    a. 0.05%

    b. 0.08%

    c. 0.3%

    d. 0.2%

CHAPTER 72

Caring for Clients with Dementia and Thought Disorders

Learning Objectives

1. Differentiate between delirium and dementia, and give an example of a condition that causes each.
2. List five etiologic factors linked to Alzheimer's disease.
3. Discuss the pathophysiologic changes associated with Alzheimer's disease.
4. Name the first symptom of Alzheimer's disease.
5. Identify two methods for diagnosing Alzheimer's disease.
6. Explain the mechanism of drug therapy in Alzheimer's disease.
7. Describe nursing management for clients with Alzheimer's disease.
8. Name three characteristics of schizophrenia.
9. Describe two psychobiologic explanations for schizophrenia.
10. Differentiate between positive and negative symptoms of schizophrenia, and give two examples of each.
11. Discuss the medical management of most people with schizophrenia.
12. Name three examples of antipsychotic drugs and their mechanisms of action.
13. Explain the term *extrapyramidal symptoms* and list four examples.
14. Describe a technique used to prevent noncompliance with drug therapy in clients with schizophrenia.
15. Describe the nursing management of clients with schizophrenia.

SECTION I: ASSESSING YOUR UNDERSTANDING

Activity A *Fill in the blanks by choosing the correct word from the options given in parentheses.*

1. _____ is a sudden, transient state of confusion. *(Delirium, Dementia, Alzheimer's disease)*

2. _____ is a progressive, deteriorating brain disorder. Two types exist: early onset (before age 60 years) and late onset (after age 60 years), with late onset being more common. *(Delirium, Alzheimer's disease, Schizophrenia)*

3. _____ is a thought disorder characterized by deterioration in mental functioning, disturbances in sensory perception, and changes in affect. *(Alzheimer's disease, Dementia, Schizophrenia)*

4. _____ produce their effects with reduced incidence of extrapyramidal symptoms. *(Traditional antipsychotics, Atypical antipsychotics, Typical antipsychotics)*

Activity B *Mark each statement as either "T" (True) or "F" (False). Correct any false statements.*

1. T F Various disorders are characterized by dementia. Alzheimer's disease is the leading example, followed by cerebrovascular disorders and Parkinson's disease.

2. T F There is no specific diagnostic test for Alzheimer's disease. The disease can only be confirmed during a postmortem examination of the brain.

3. T F Clients with schizophrenia improve with drug therapy but, unfortunately, never fully recover. The condition is lifelong and appears in young adulthood.

4. T F Positive symptoms of schizophrenia are more easily managed (with drugs) than negative symptoms.

Activity C *Write the correct term for each description given below.*

1. Conditions in which decline in memory, thinking, and reasoning is severe enough to affect the daily life of an alert person. This condition is manifested by a gradual, irreversible loss of intellectual abilities. _____

2. These drugs, used to treat Alzheimer's disease, increase acetylcholine by inhibiting cholinesterase, the enzyme that degrades it. When they are administered in the early- to middle-stages of Alzheimer's disease, some clients improve, some stay the same, some progress more slowly, and some fail to respond. _____

3. These drugs are also called major tranquilizers or neuroleptics. _____

4. This antipsychotic medication has the potentially adverse effect of dangerously depressing bone marrow function, and clients who take this drug must have a blood count done weekly or biweekly. _____

Activity D *Match the extrapyramidal side effects (EPS) given in Column A with their correct descriptions given in Column B.*

Column A

____ **1.** Akinesia

____ **2.** Akathisia

____ **3.** Dystonia

Column B

a. The client cannot sit or stand still.

b. The client appears to have symptoms of Parkinson's disease

____ **4.** Tardive dyskinesia

such as hand tremors, stooped posture, and stiff shuffling gait.

c. The client makes involuntary muscle movements, usually in the face, such as tongue thrusting, continuous chewing, grimacing, lip smacking, or blinking; irreversible once manifested.

d. Sudden severe muscle spasm occurs, usually in the neck, tongue, or eyes.

Activity E *Compare and contrast the positive and negative signs of schizophrenia.*

Positive symptoms of schizophrenia	Negative symptoms of schizophrenia

Activity F *Briefly answer the following questions.*

1. What conditions can result in delirium? How is mentation restored?

_____

_____

_____

2. What is the etiology of early onset and late onset Alzheimer's disease?

_____

_____

_____

3. What is the action of *N*-methyl-D-aspartate (NMDA) antagonists? How effective are they?

_____

_____

_____

4. How is schizophrenia medically managed?

_____

_____

_____

5. What are signs of neuroleptic malignant syndrome? What action should the nurse take if signs and symptoms are identified?

_____

_____

_____

SECTION II: APPLYING YOUR KNOWLEDGE

Activity G *Give rationale for the following questions.*

1. Why are older adults at high risk for loss of identity?

_____

_____

_____

2. Why would institutionalization be necessary for a schizophrenic client?

_____

_____

_____

3. Why are anticholinergic drugs given to clients with schizophrenia?

_____

_____

_____

4. Why are depot injections used for the non-hospitalized schizophrenic client?

_____

_____

_____

Activity H *Answer the following questions related to caring for clients with dementia and thought disorders.*

1. Describe the pathophysiology of Alzheimer's disease.

_____

_____

_____

2. What are the signs and symptoms of Alzheimer's disease?

_____

_____

_____

3. Describe the pathophysiology of schizophrenia.

_____

_____

_____

4. What are the classic symptoms of schizophrenia?

_____

_____

_____

Activity I *Think over the following questions. Discuss them with your instructor or peers.*

1. What high-priority nursing diagnoses and interventions would you identify for a client with Alzheimer's disease?

_____

_____

_____

2. What educational information would you provide to a client starting on a traditional antipsychotic medication?

_____

_____

_____

3. What high-priority nursing diagnoses and interventions would you identify for a client with schizophrenia?

_____

_____

_____

4. What educational information would you provide to family members caring for a client with dementia in the home setting?

_____

_____

_____

SECTION III: GETTING READY FOR NCLEX

Activity J *Answer the following questions.*

1. Which of the following individuals are at higher risk of acquiring Alzheimer's disease?

   a. Clients with coronary heart disease

   b. Clients with partial memory loss

   c. Clients with inherited genetic abnormalities

   d. Clients with insomnia

2. A male client visits a clinic, accompanied by his wife. The client's wife expresses her concern about the sudden memory loss faced by her husband, resulting in confusion in remembering his location or, for that matter, his own name. On further investigation, the client's wife also states that the client has just recovered from a heavy fever and has metabolic disorders. From the assessment conducted, which of the following disorders does the nurse take into consideration?

   a. Dementia

   b. Delirium

   c. Alzheimer's disease

   d. Schizophrenia

3. Which of the following is the nurse's role in caring for a client with Alzheimer's disease in an extended-care facility?

   a. Administers IV infusions

   b. Provides emotional support

   c. Assists family and meets client's physical needs

   d. Provides family teachings

4. A female client accompanied by her husband visits a clinic. The client's husband expresses his concern about his wife hallucinating and having fluent but disorganized speech. From the information gathered, which of the following disorders does the nurse take into consideration?

   a. Alzheimer's disease

   b. Dementia

   c. Schizophrenia

   d. Delirium

5. Which of the following is an appropriate nursing intervention when a client with schizophrenia expresses a delusional belief or experiences a hallucination?

   a. Leave the client alone throughout the hallucination.

   b. Inform the physician.

   c. Question the validity of client's hallucination.

   d. Stay with the client throughout the hallucination.

6. A nurse is taking care of a client with schizophrenia. What is a negative symptom of schizophrenia?

   a. Echolalia

   b. Inappropriate affect

   c. Loose associations

   d. Thought blocking

7. A client is diagnosed in stage 3 on the Global Deterioration Scale. What characteristics are associated with stage 3?

   a. Assistance of others needed

   b. Getting lost in an unfamiliar location

   c. Strong denial of impairment

   d. Memory of past sketchy

8. A client is experiencing an extrapyramidal symptom where the client cannot sit or stand still. What is this extrapyramidal symptom called?

   a. Dystonia

   b. Akathisia

   c. Tardive dyskinesia

   d. Akinesia

9. In the case of which of the following drugs used for treating schizophrenia does a nurse have to monitor an older client for dehydration and aspiration potential?

   a. Zyprexa

   b. Risperdal

   c. Haldol

   d. Prolixin

10. A client is experiencing sudden severe muscle spasms, usually in the neck, tongue, or eyes. What is this extrapyramidal symptom called?

    a. Dystonia

    b. Akathisia

    c. Tardive dyskinesia

    d. Akinesia